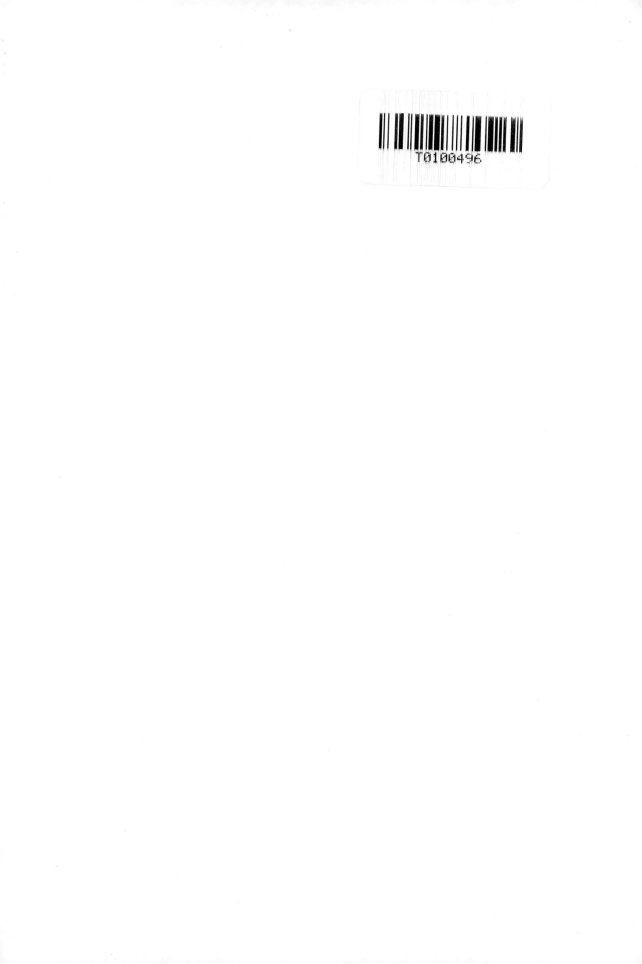

Sleep in Women

Editor

MONICA L. ANDERSEN

SLEEP MEDICINE CLINICS

www.sleep.theclinics.com

December 2023 • Volume 18 • Number 4

ELSEVIER

1600 John F. Kennedy Boulevard • Suite 1800 • Philadelphia, Pennsylvania, 19103-2899

http://www.theclinics.com

SLEEP MEDICINE CLINICS Volume 18, Number 4
December 2023, ISSN 1556-407X, ISBN-13: 978-0-443-18242-6

Editor: Joanna Gascoine
Developmental Editor: Akshay Samson

Sleep Medicine Clinics (ISSN 1556-407X) is published quarterly by Elsevier Inc., 360 Park Avenue South, New York, NY 10010-1710. Months of issue are March, June, September and December. Business and Editorial Offices: 1600 John F. Kennedy Blvd., Ste. 1800, Philadelphia, PA 19103-2899. Customer Service Office: 3251 Riverport Lane, Maryland Heights, MO 63043. Periodicals postage paid at New York, NY and additional mailing offices. Subscription prices are $243.00 per year (US individuals), $100.00 (US and Canadian students), $612.00 (US institutions), $283.00 (Canadian individuals), $278.00 (international individuals) $135.00 (International students), $692.00 (Canadian and International institutions). Foreign air speed delivery is included in all *Clinics* subscription prices. All prices are subject to change without notice. **POSTMASTER:** Send change of address to *Sleep Medicine Clinics*, Elsevier Health Sciences Division, Subscription Customer Service, 3251 Riverport Lane, Maryland Heights, MO 63043. Customer Service: **Tel: 1-800-654-2452 (U.S. and Canada); 314-447-8871 (outside U.S. and Canada). Fax: 314-447-8029. E-mail: journalscustomerservice-usa@elsevier.com (for print support); journalsonline-support-usa@elsevier.com (for online support).**

Reprints. For copies of 100 or more of articles in this publication, please contact the Commercial Reprints Department, Elsevier Inc., 360 Park Avenue South, New York, NY 10010-1710. Tel.: 212-633-3874; Fax: 212-633-3820; E-mail: reprints@elsevier.com.

Sleep Medicine Clinics is covered in *MEDLINE/PubMed (Index Medicus)*.

SLEEP MEDICINE CLINICS

FORTHCOMING ISSUES

March 2024
The Parasomnias
Alon Y. Avidan, *Editor*

June 2024
Overlap of Respiratory Problems with Sleep Disordered Breathing
Krishna Sundar, *Editor*

September 2024
Multi-perspective Management of Sleep Disorders
Brendon Yee and Amanda Piper, *Editors*

RECENT ISSUES

September 2023
Advances in Technology for the Sleep Field
Steven Holfinger, *Editor*

June 2023
Pediatric Sleep Clinics
Haviva Veler, *Editor*

March 2023
Adjunct Interventions to Cognitive Behavioral Therapy for Insomnia
Joshua Hyong-Jin Cho, *Editor*

SERIES OF RELATED INTEREST
Neurologic Clinics
https://www.neurologic.theclinics.com/

Contributors

CONSULTING EDITORS

TEOFILO LEE-CHIONG Jr, MD
Professor of Medicine, National Jewish Health, Professor of Medicine, University of Colorado, Denver, Colorado, USA; Chief Medical Liaison, Philips Respironics, Murrysville, Pennsylvania, USA

DIEGO GARCIA-BORREGUERO, MD, PhD
International Medical Director Instituto del Sueño, Calle Padre Damián, Madrid, Spain

ANA C. KRIEGER, MD, MPH, FCCP, FAASM
Chief, Division of Sleep Neurology, Medical Director, Weill Cornell Center for Sleep Medicine, Professor of Clinical Medicine, Professor of Medicine in Neurology and Genetic Medicine, Weill Cornell Medical College, Cornell University, New York, New York, USA

EDITOR

MONICA L. ANDERSEN, PhD
Departamento de Psicobiologia, Universidade Federal de São Paulo (UNIFESP/EPM), Brazil Sleep Instituto, São Paulo, Brazil Conselho Nacional de Desenvolvimento Científico e Tecnológico (CNPq) Fellowship

AUTHORS

WAHIDA AKBERZIE, MD
Department of Primary Care Medicine, Physician, Primary Care Service, Martinsburg VA Medical Center, Martinsburg, West Virginia, USA

ELISABET ALZUETA, PhD
Postdoctoral Researcher, Human Sleep Research Program, SRI International, Menlo Park, California, USA

MONICA L. ANDERSEN, PhD
Departamento de Psicobiologia, Universidade Federal de São Paulo (UNIFESP/EPM), Brazil Sleep Instituto, São Paulo, Brazil Conselho Nacional de Desenvolvimento Científico e Tecnológico (CNPq) Fellowship

FIONA C. BAKER, PhD
Human Sleep Research Program, SRI International, Menlo Park, California, USA; Honorary Professorial Research Fellow, Brain Function Research Group, School of Physiology, University of the Witwatersrand, Johannesburg, South Africa

LUCIANA BENEDETTO, PhD
Assistant Researcher, Departamento de Fisiología, Facultad de Medicina, Universidad de la República, Montevideo, Uruguay

LAÍS F. BERRO, PhD
Assistant Professor, Department of Psychiatry and Human Behavior, University of Mississippi Medical Center, Jackson, Mississippi, USA

ANDRÉIA GOMES BEZERRA, PhD
Postdoctoral Researcher, Departamento de Psicobiologia, Universidade Federal de São Paulo, São Paulo, Brazil

JOAO SABINO CUNHA-FILHO, MD, PhD
Professor, Faculdade de Medicina, Universidade Federal do Rio Grande do Sul, Porto Alegre, Brazil

ARLIN DELGADO, MD
Physician, Department of Obstetrics and Gynecology, University of South Florida Morsani College of Medicine, Tampa, Florida, USA

LUCIANO F. DRAGER, MD, PhD
Associate Professor of Medicine, Center of Clinical and Epidemiologic Research (CPCE), Unidade de Hipertensão, Disciplina de Nefrologia, Hospital das Clínicas HCFMUSP, Unidade de Hipertensão, Instituto do Coração (InCor) do Hospital das Clínicas HCFMUSP, Faculdade de Medicina, Universidade de São Paulo, São Paulo, São Paulo, Brazil

FRIDA ENTEZAMI, MD, MSc
Managing Director, American Hospital of Paris, IVF Unit, Neuilly-Sur-Seine, France

BIANCA PEREIRA FAVILLA, MSc
Genetics Division, Departamento de Morfologia e Genética, Universidade Federal de São Paulo, São Paulo, Brazil

ANNABEL FERREIRA, PhD
Sección de Fisiología y Nutrición, Facultad de Ciencias, Universidad de la República, Montevideo, Uruguay

NAIRA LAPI FERREIRA, RN
Center of Clinical and Epidemiologic Research (CPCE), Unidade de Hipertensão, Disciplina de Nefrologia, Hospital das Clínicas HCFMUSP, Faculdade de Medicina, Universidade de São Paulo, São Paulo, São Paulo, Brazil

KELSIE M. FULL, PhD, MPH
Assistant Professor of Medicine, Division of Epidemiology, Department of Medicine, Vanderbilt University Medical Center, Nashville, Tennessee, USA

RITIKA GADODIA, MD
Resident, Department of Medicine, MedStar Washington Hospital Center, Washington, DC, USA

KAMALESH K. GULIA, PhD
Scientist 'G', Division of Sleep Research, Department of Applied Biology, Biomedical Technology Wing, Sree Chitra Tirunal Institute for Medical Sciences and Technology, Trivandrum, Kerala, India

HELENA HACHUL, MD, PhD
Associate professor, Departamento de Psicobiologia e Ginecologia, Universidade Federal de São Paulo (UNIFESP) São Paulo, Sleep Institute, Brazil

BEATRIZ HACHUL DE CAMPOS, BSc (Medicine)
Department of Psychobiology, Universidade Federal de São Paulo, São Paulo, Brazil

ISABELA A. ISHIKURA, MSc
Departamento de Psicobiologia, Universidade Federal de São Paulo (UNIFESP/EPM), São Paulo, Brazil

ZSUZSANNA I.K. JARMY-DI BELLA, MD, PhD
Affiliated Professor, Department of Gynecology, Federal University of São Paulo, São Paulo, Brazil

DAYNA A. JOHNSON, PhD, MPH, MSW, MS
Assistant Professor, Department of Epidemiology, Rollins School of Public Health, Emory University, Atlanta, Georgia, USA

LYNN KATARIA, MD
Director, Sleep Laboratory, Washington DC VA Medical Center, Clinical Associate Professor of Neurology and Rehabilitation Medicine, George Washington University School of Medicine, Washington, DC, USA

CHRISTOPHER N. KAUFMANN, PhD, MHS
Assistant Professor, Department of Health Outcomes and Biomedical Informatics, College of Medicine, University of Florida, Gainesville, Florida, USA

LUCIA C. LEMOS, PhD
Department of Health, Life Cycles and Society, School of Public Health, University of São Paulo, São Paulo, Brazil

JUDETTE M. LOUIS, MD, MPH
Professor and Chair, Department of Obstetrics and Gynecology, University of South Florida Morsani College of Medicine, Tampa, Florida, USA

LEANDRO LUCENA, MSc
Department of Psychobiology, Universidade Federal de São Paulo, São Paulo, Brazil

ATUL MALHOTRA, MD
Professor of Medicine, Division of Pulmonary, Critical Care and Sleep Medicine, School of Medicine, University of California, San Diego, La Jolla, California, USA

MARIA ISABEL MELARAGNO, PhD
Professor, Genetics Division, Departamento de Morfologia e Genética, Universidade Federal de São Paulo, São Paulo, Brazil

CLAUDIA R.C. MORENO, PhD
Professor, Department of Health, Life Cycles and Society, School of Public Health, University of São Paulo, São Paulo, Brazil

MARIANA MOYSÉS-OLIVEIRA, PhD
Researcher, Functional Neurobiology, Sleep Institute, Associação Fundo de Incentivo à Pesquisa, São Paulo, Brazil

DEEPIKA NANDAMURU, MD
Sleep Fellow, Department of Neurology, George Washington University School of Medicine, GW Medical Faculty Associates, Washington, DC, USA

BARBARA K. PARISE, PhD
Center of Clinical and Epidemiologic Research (CPCE), Unidade de Hipertensão, Disciplina de Nefrologia, Hospital das Clínicas HCFMUSP, Faculdade de Medicina, Universidade de São Paulo, São Paulo, São Paulo, Brazil

FLORENCIA PEÑA, BS
Departamento de Fisiología, Facultad de Medicina, Universidad de la República, Montevideo, Uruguay

GABRIEL NATAN PIRES, PhD
Professor, Departamento de Psicobiologia, Universidade Federal de São Paulo (UNIFESP/EPM), Sleep Institute, São Paulo, Brazil

RITA C.C.P. PISCOPO, MD
GERA Institute of Reproductive Medicine, São Paulo, Brazil

PÄIVI POLO-KANTOLA, MD, PhD
Professor, Department of Obstetrics and Gynecology, Turku University Hospital, University of Turku, Turku, Finland

MAYDA RIVAS, PhD
Departamento de Fisiología, Facultad de Medicina, Universidad de la República, Montevideo, Uruguay

LISIE P. ROMANZINI, MSc
Doctoral Student, Departamento de Psicobiologia, Universidade Federal de São Paulo (UNIFESP/EPM), São Paulo, Brazil

DANIELA S. ROSA, PhD
Department of Microbiology, Immunology and Parasitology, Federal University of São Paulo, São Paulo, Brazil

MARISE SAMAMA, MD, PhD
Department of Gynecology, Federal University of São Paulo, GERA Institute of Reproductive Medicine, São Paulo, Brazil

AMANDA SARTOR, BSc
GERA Institute of Reproductive Medicine, Department of Psychobiology, Federal University of São Paulo, São Paulo, Brazil

SAPNA ERAT SREEDHARAN, MD, DM
Professor, Department of Neurology, Comprehensive Centre for Sleep Disorders, Sree Chitra Tirunal Institute for Medical Sciences and Technology, Trivandrum, Kerala, India

ELENA TOFFOL, MD, PhD
Postdoctoral Researcher, Department of Public Health, University of Helsinki, Helsinki, Finland

PABLO TORTEROLO, PhD
Professor, Departamento de Fisiología, Facultad de Medicina, Universidad de la República, Montevideo, Uruguay

SERGIO TUFIK, MD, PhD
Sleep Institute, Associação Fundo de Incentivo à Pesquisa, Departamento de Psicobiologia, Universidade Federal de São Paulo, São Paulo, Brazil

SULEIMA P. VASCONCELOS, PhD
Professor, Public Health Graduate Program, Federal University of Acre, Campus da Universidade Federal Do Acre, Rio Branco, Brazil

Contents

Preface: Women's Sleep Health xv

Monica L. Andersen

The Relationship Between Mood and Sleep in Different Female Reproductive States 385

Päivi Polo-Kantola and Elena Toffol

Mood and sleep are tightly interrelated. Mood and sleep symptoms and disorders are more common in women than in men and often associated with reproductive events. This article reviews the current literature on the reciprocal relationships between mood and sleep across reproductive phases in women, such as menstrual cycle and related disorders, pregnancy, climacteric, and use of hormonal contraception and hormone replacement therapy. Mood and sleep symptoms seem to covary in relation to physiologic and pathologic reproductive conditions, although the relationship seems more clear for subjective than objective sleep.

The Menstrual Cycle and Sleep 399

Elisabet Alzueta and Fiona C. Baker

Aspects of sleep change across the menstrual cycle in some women. Poorer sleep quality in the premenstrual phase and menstruation is common in women with premenstrual symptoms or painful menstrual cramps. Although objective sleep continuity remains unchanged across the regular, asymptomatic menstrual cycle, activity in the sleep electroencephalogram varies, with a prominent increase in sleep spindle activity in the postovulatory luteal phase, when progesterone is present, relative to the follicular phase. Menstrual cycle phase, reproductive stage, and menstrual-related disorders should be considered when assessing women's sleep complaints.

An Update on Sleep Duration, Obesity, and Mortality Risk in Women 415

Kelsie M. Full, Dayna A. Johnson, Christopher N. Kaufmann, and Atul Malhotra

Sleep health is an essential component to overall health. Because of numerous societal, economic, and biological factors, obtaining adequate sleep poses a unique challenge to aging women. Yet, women have been traditionally understudied in sleep research. An increasing body of research supports abnormal sleep duration as a risk factor for obesity, cardiovascular disease, and mortality. This review focuses specifically on 3 areas of the discussion of insufficient sleep in women: (1) the mysterious poor health of long sleepers, (2) the potential underlying mechanisms linking abnormal sleep duration and cardiometabolic health, and (3) the need to investigate multiple levels of social determinants driving sleep disparities.

Sleep During Menopause 423

Helena Hachul, Beatriz Hachul de Campos, Leandro Lucena, and Sergio Tufik

Postmenopause is defined retrospectively after 12 consecutive months of amenorrhea. It represents the end of the reproductive period and ovarian failure. A decrease in estrogen leads to several changes in the short and long term. Among the early changes, vasomotor symptoms (hot flashes) are particularly common, occurring in about 70% of women. In addition, there are changes in mood, anxiety, depression, and insomnia. Insomnia occurs in almost 60% of postmenopausal women. Psychosocial aspects may also affect sleep. Proper diagnosis may lead to adequate treatment of sleep disturbances during menopause. Hormonal or other complementary therapies can improve sleep quality.

with the quantity and quality of sleep. Awakenings and sleep disturbances are more frequent and can lead to increased fatigue and stress to reconcile household activities and work demands. These changes in sleep can lead to physical and/or psychological health problems. Sleep hygiene and social support become fundamental for the performance of the maternal tasks, reducing risks and increasing prevention of future problems, both for women and children.

COVID-19: A Challenge to the Safety of Assisted Reproduction **489**

Marise Samama, Frida Entezami, Daniela S. Rosa, Amanda Sartor, Rita C.C.P. Piscopo, Monica L. Andersen, Joao Sabino Cunha-Filho, and Zsuzsanna I.K. Jarmy-Di-Bella

There is an increased risk of becoming pregnant through fertility treatments using assisted reproductive technology (ART) during the COVID-19 pandemic. The aim of this review is to gather comprehensive data from the existing literature on the potential risks of fertility management during the pandemic period, and outline strategies to mitigate them, with a focus on the hormonal and surgical procedures of ART. A comprehensive search of the scientific literature on COVID-19 in relation to fertility was conducted in the PubMed database using the keywords "coronavirus," "COVID-19," "SARS-CoV-2" and "pregnancy," "fertility," "urogenital system," "vertical transmission," "assisted human reproduction," "controlled ovarian stimulation," "oocyte retrieval," "in vitro fertilization," "hormones," "surgical procedures," "embryos," "oocytes," "sperm," "semen," "ovary," "testis," "ACE-2 receptor," "immunology," "cytokine storm," and "coagulation," from January 2020-July 2022. Published data on pregnancy and COVID-19, and the interaction of the urogenital system and SARS-CoV-2 is reported. The immunologic and prothrombotic profiles of patients with COVID-19, and their increased risks from controlled ovarian stimulation (COS) and ART surgeries, and how these procedures could facilitate COVID-19 and/or contribute to the severity of the disease by enhancing the cytokine storm are summarized. Strategies to prevent complications during COS that could increase the risks of the disease in pre-symptomatic patients are considered. The impact of SARS-CoV-2 on pre-symptomatic infertile patients presents a challenge to find ways to avoid the increased hormonal, immunologic, and prothrombotic risks presented by the use of COS in ART protocols during the COVID-19 outbreak. Safe ART procedures and recommendations are highlighted.

The Integration of the Maternal Care with Sleep During the Postpartum Period **499**

Luciana Benedetto, Florencia Peña, Mayda Rivas, Annabel Ferreira, and Pablo Torterolo

Our entire life occurs in a constant alternation between wakefulness and sleep. The impossibility of living without sleep implies that any behavior must adapt to the need for sleep, and maternal behavior does not escape from this determination. Additionally, maternal behavior in mammals is a highly motivated behavior, essential for the survival of **the** offspring. Thus, the mother has to adapt her physiology of sleep to the constant demands of the pups, where each species will have different strategies to merge these two physiological needs. However, all studied female mammals will experience sleep disturbances at some point of the postpartum period.

Insomnia as a Risk Factor for Substance Use Disorders in Women **511**

Laís F. Berro

Gender differences exist for both insomnia and substance use disorders. Women show a higher prevalence of insomnia and increased susceptibility to the effects of drugs than men. Importantly, a growing body of evidence suggests that insufficient sleep predicts and puts individuals at a higher risk for substance use and associated psychosocial problems. However, the role of insomnia in substance use disorders among women remains poorly understood. The present article discusses gender differences in insomnia and in substance use disorders and reviews evidence suggesting that an increased prevalence of insomnia may be a risk factor for substance use disorders in women.

X-Chromosome Dependent Differences in the Neuronal Molecular Signatures and Their Implications in Sleep Patterns **521**

Mariana Moysés-Oliveira, Bianca Pereira Favilla, Maria Isabel Melaragno, and Sergio Tufik

Biological factors and mechanisms that drive sex differences observed in sleep disturbances are understudied and poorly understood. The extent to which sex chromosome constitution impacts on sex differences in circadian patterns is still a knowledge void in the sleep medicine field. Here we focus on the neurological consequences of X-chromosome functional imbalances between males and females and how this molecular inequality might affect sex divergencies on sleep. In light of the X-chromosome inactivation mechanism in females and its implications in gene regulation, we describe sleep-related neuronal circuits and brain regions impacted by sex-biased modulations of the transcriptome and the epigenome. Benefited from recent large-scale genetic studies on the interplay between X-chromosome and brain function, we list clinically relevant genes that might play a role in sex differences in neuronal pathways. Those molecular signatures are put into the context of sleep and sleep-associated neurological phenotypes, aiming to identify biological mechanisms that link X-chromosome gene regulation to sex-biased human traits. These findings are a significant step forward in understanding how X-linked genes manifest in sleep-associated transcriptional networks and point to future research opportunities to address female-specific clinical manifestations and therapeutic responses.

Night Shift Work and Sleep Disturbances in Women: A Scoping Review **533**

Suleima P. Vasconcelos, Lucia C. Lemos, and Claudia R.C. Moreno

This scoping review aimed to synthesize evidence on sleep disturbances in female shift workers. The update Preferred Reporting Items for Systematic Reviews and Meta-Analyses extension for Scoping Reviews was used. Twelve studies were included, four of which used actigraphy to assess sleep duration, efficiency, and latency. Seven studies evaluated the quality of sleep and three verified the sleepiness of women. This review adds to the body of evidence as the findings are homogeneous and allow a robust conclusion, suggesting that night shift work may be a potential factor for adverse effects on sleep of female shift workers.

Sleep Disorders and Aging in Women **545**

Ritika Gadodia, Deepika Nandamuru, Wahida Akberzie, and Lynn Kataria

Women of advancing age can suffer from an array of sleep disorders. We review the changes in sleep architecture, the impact of hormonal changes on sleep, and the various sleep disorders in women of advancing age. A focused history in this population should include the temporal relation to menopause and comorbid conditions. Treatment options should involve patient preference and review of current medications and comorbid conditions to optimize sleep in this population.

Sleep Deficiency in Pregnancy **559**

Arlin Delgado and Judette M. Louis

Sleep is a critical aspect of one's daily life for overall health, with a recommended 7 to 9 hours in adulthood (ages 26–64). Up to a third of women do not sleep sufficiently, and pregnant women are at an increased risk for sleep deficiency. Throughout pregnancy, sleep is affected in differing ways. For example, in the first trimester, hormones affect sleep cycles, but by the third trimester, physical complaints such as increasing frequent urination and fetal movement create frequent awakenings. Associations between sleep deficiency and gestational diabetes, hypertensive disorders, depression, and some evidence regarding preterm birth exist. A woman's labor course and perception of delivery are also negatively affected by short sleep duration.

Preface
Women's Sleep Health

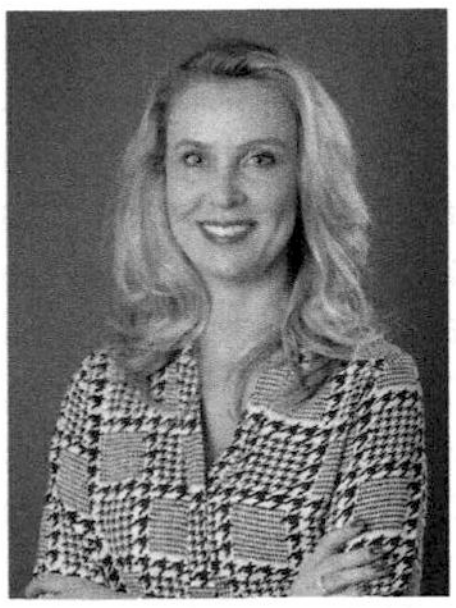

Monica L. Andersen, PhD
Editor

This special issue considers the topic of "Sleep in Women" and looks at a number of important aspects related to women's sleep health, such as how sleep changes across the lifespan in women and the influence of maternity on sleep, among other topics. It also looks at the results of some preclinical studies, which have potentially significant practical applications.

Sleep patterns tend to change with age in men and women. Women's sleep is significantly influenced by both the long-term hormonal variations that occur across a woman's life and the short-term changes that take place during the menstrual cycle. The ovarian hormones progesterone and estrogen strongly influence sleep and can modulate neurochemical transmission in many ways. The menstrual hormonal profile has been reported to affect sleep quality. A variety of other intrinsic and extrinsic factors can also play a role in the sleep pattern among women, such as pregnancy and sleep disorders.

Sleep is important for physiological well-being, and this is especially true during pregnancy given that several adverse pregnancy outcomes, such as preterm labor, gestational diabetes, preeclampsia, and postpartum depression, have been shown to be associated with poor sleep quality. Several factors can influence sleep during pregnancy, including mechanical and physiological factors. Restless legs syndrome, which is more common during pregnancy, can impact sleep negatively. In addition, sleep-disordered breathing has been associated with gestational diabetes and hypertension, while insomnia, obstructive sleep apnea, and poor sleep have been linked to preterm delivery. Assisted reproduction treatment is another issue that may well have an effect on women's sleep but has not been extensively investigated.

Sleep disorders can modify women's sleep at any stage of their lives. Studies have demonstrated that insomnia, the most prevalent sleep disorder among women, affects nearly half of all women, while obstructive sleep apnea, the second most prevalent sleep disorder, disturbs about a quarter of women. Both conditions are associated with fragmented, nonrestorative sleep and changes in circadian rhythm and have similar next-day symptoms that include excessive daytime sleepiness. Moreover, insomnia and obstructive sleep apnea in women share related comorbidities, including hormonal imbalances, mood disorders, and chronic pain.

Given the influence of ovarian hormones on sleep, the perimenopause and menopause periods are significantly associated with changes in sleep quality and sleep-wake cycles. During perimenopause, women report poor sleep, with increased insomnia, restless legs syndrome, and obstructive sleep apnea being among the main complaints. Even with the stabilization of hormone levels observed after menopause, the prevalence of sleep complaints, similar to those observed during perimenopause, increases dramatically in postmenopausal women. It is important to note that not all changes observed after menopause are necessarily associated with hormonal changes, as aging itself impacts sleep quality in

Sleep Med Clin 18 (2023) xv–xvi
https://doi.org/10.1016/j.jsmc.2023.09.001
1556-407X/23/© 2023 Published by Elsevier Inc.

women independently of the hormonal changes combined with menopause.

Several psychological factors directly or indirectly related to gender-based influences markedly affect women's sleep, including psychiatric conditions, lifestyle, sleep deprivation, and stress. In respect to psychiatric conditions, depression and anxiety are significantly connected with sleep impairment. Women with depression and anxiety present a higher prevalence of insomnia and fragmented sleep. Moreover, the relationship between psychiatric conditions and sleep disorders is bidirectional, with impaired or insufficient sleep contributing to the continuation of depression and anxiety.

It is known that gender-based influences on sleep are closely intertwined with social and cultural norms that have unequal impacts on women and men. Socioeconomic pressure, society's beauty standards, stress, and the "double shift" experienced by many working women who are also responsible for the majority of domestic tasks and childcare responsibilities are among the many societal factors that disproportionately impact women and that are directly associated with impaired or insufficient sleep among women in modern society. This is against a background of an increase in the prevalence of sleep complaints and disturbances in general over recent decades, leading to an overall reduction in sleep duration and quality in our society. This has been caused by a variety of factors, including increased work demands, in part facilitated by communication technologies blurring the division between the home and work environments, as well as by the increase in electronic and social media use, which are also known to affect sleep quality and duration. This general pressure on sleep, combined with the factors described above that affect women in particular, results in a "perfect storm" impact on women's sleep.

Many of the consequences of poor sleep are directly interconnected. Stress is associated not only with poor sleep but also with mood disorders and pain, which on their own are also influenced by and influence sleep impairment. The evidence suggests that hormone alterations related to a woman's reproductive cycle mediate pain and mood disorders in addition to being associated with poor sleep, further emphasizing how many of the components underlying sleep impairment in women can be interconnected and can, together, contribute to sleep loss. In addition to the stress response system, poor sleep affects nearly all the systems of our body, especially the cardiovascular, endocrine, and immune systems.

Women's sleep, therefore, is influenced by many factors, including the phase and hormone levels associated with a woman's reproductive cycle, lifestyle factors that can impact sleep quality directly and indirectly and comorbidities that may affect women differently from men, as well as by social and cultural factors. The complex nature of the factors than can modify women's sleep means that the effects are not the same for all individuals; however, caregiving responsibilities and the pressure of dealing with both domestic and employment responsibilities, among other factors, are known to affect women more negatively than men, resulting in impaired sleep patterns and sleep hygiene in women.

While a lot of progress has been made in respect to understanding how sex differences are associated with sleep patterns, many knowledge gaps still exist in this field, mainly because women have historically been underrepresented in scientific studies. This highlights the importance of the current movement toward including sex as a biological factor in all science, a trend that should also be encouraged in sleep science. We hope this special issue makes a contribution in this respect—let's dive in!

Monica L. Andersen, PhD
Associate Professor
Department of Psychobiology–
Universidade Federal de São Paulo (UNIFESP)
Rua Napoleão de Barros, 925
São Paulo/SP 04024-02, Brazil

E-mail address:
ml.andersen12@gmail.com

The Relationship Between Mood and Sleep in Different Female Reproductive States

Päivi Polo-Kantola, MD, PhD[a,*], Elena Toffol, MD, PhD[b]

KEYWORDS

• Mood • Sleep • Women • Menstrual cycle • Pregnancy • Menopause • Hormonal contraception • Hormone replacement therapy

KEY POINTS

- Mood and subjective sleep are tightly interrelated and tend to covary across the menstrual cycle phases. The association with objective sleep is less clear. Depressive symptoms and short sleep duration are reciprocally related to menstrual irregularity.
- Mood symptoms and sleep disturbances, especially sleep-disordered breathing, are related to polycystic ovary syndrome, the most common reproductive endocrinological disorder in the reproductive period.
- The relationship between mood and sleep in connection with the use of hormonal contraception is not well-defined.
- During pregnancy and postpartum, mood symptoms and sleep disturbances are common and they have a strong connection. In addition to this obvious bidirectional association, recent studies have emphasized that sleep disturbances during pregnancy are prodromal symptoms especially for postpartum depression.
- In climacteric, risk for mood symptoms and sleep disturbances increases. Similar to the reproductive period, also during climacteric, the relationship between mood symptoms and sleep disturbances is bidirectional.
- Menopausal hormone therapy has shown to alleviate both mood and sleep symptoms during climacteric, especially in women with vasomotor symptoms. However, depression and sleep disorders increase in menopausal transition and especially in aging, and thus, specific treatments for these disorders may be needed.

MOOD AND SLEEP: GENDER DIFFERENCE

The prevalence and phenomenology of many physiologic and pathologic conditions, including mood and sleep statuses and disorders, follow a skewed gender distribution. For example, mood disorders such as depression and anxiety are two to three times more common in women than in men.[1] Their clinical onset and manifestations also differ by gender.[2] Interestingly, these differences are more evident after puberty, tend to peak during reproductive age, and narrow later with age, approximately corresponding to the menopausal transition in women. Sleep structure and disorders follow, to a certain extent, a similar pattern. Self-reported sleep disturbances more than objective sleep alterations are more common in women[3–5] and often reported in association with menstrual cycle phases and other reproductive events.[6] Of note, sleep and

[a] Department of Obstetrics and Gynecology, Turku University Hospital, University of Turku, Turku, Finland;
[b] Department of Public Health, University of Helsinki, PO Box 20, Helsinki 00014, Finland
* Corresponding author.
E-mail address: paivi.polo@utu.fi

Sleep Med Clin 18 (2023) 385–398
https://doi.org/10.1016/j.jsmc.2023.06.002

mood are tightly interrelated. Sleep disturbances such as insomnia or short sleep duration are a prodromal as well as diagnostic symptom of depression and other mood disorders. Patients with depression and anxiety commonly suffer from sleep abnormalities (eg, decreased or increased sleep, sleep fragmentation, or altered rapid eye movement [REM] sleep) as associated and aggravating symptoms.[7–10] Reciprocally, subjects with sleep disturbances have higher risks of developing a depressive disorder.[11]

These epidemiologic and clinical observations point to a contributive role of reproductive factors, including sex hormones. Given the multiple effects that estrogens and progesterone exert on the central nervous system, their influence on mood and sleep and the consequent reciprocal relationship of mood and sleep across female reproductive stages (eg, puberty, menstrual cycle, pregnancy, and menopause, but also hormonal contraception [HC] and hormone replacement therapy) is not surprising. A study of 11 young, 21 perimenopausal, and 29 postmenopausal women detected only minor associations between depressive symptoms and subjective and objective sleep in young women, but stronger and more consistent associations in perimenopausal and postmenopausal women, suggesting that the patterns of reciprocal relationships may vary with reproductive phases.[12]

MENSTRUAL CYCLE, MOOD, AND SLEEP

Mood Across Menstrual Cycle Phases

The normal menstrual cycle, of average 28-day duration, consists of a cyclic alternation of the follicular, ovulatory, and luteal (premenstrual) phases. Psychological status tends to fluctuate across these phases, and approximately 50% to 80% of women experience physical and/or psychological symptoms, such as mood liability, irritability, depressive, and anxiety symptoms in the premenstrual period.[13] In addition, women with psychiatric, in particular mood disorders, commonly have a premenstrual symptom exacerbation or mood changes across the menstrual cycle.[14–16] However, several studies suggest that mood fluctuations across the cycle, and their premenstrual worsening, are related to the menstrual cyclicity itself, rather than to underlying depression status or history.[17] Further, Gonda and colleagues[18] studied 63 women (18–45 years) with no premenstrual dysphoric disorder (PMDD) and not using HC, via daily questionnaires for three consecutive cycles. When comparing the groups (approximately 50% each) with versus without significant premenstrual increase of physical symptoms, the group explained psychological symptom changes only to a limited extent. Similarly, a study comparing 14 PMDD and 15 healthy control women found more psychological symptoms in the luteal compared with the follicular phase in both groups, although with greater changes in PMDD women.[19]

Sleep Across Menstrual Cycle Phases

Given the cyclic secretion of gonadal hormones and their influence on body temperature and sleep-regulating centers in the central nervous system, it is plausible that sleep patterns also vary across the menstrual cycle. Ample evidence confirms this hypothesis, although with inconsistencies and differences when considering subjective or objective sleep.

Already in the 1970s, a study of six normally menstruating women found increased self-reported sleep duration, but poorer sleep quality, during the premenstrual phase.[20] The observation of poorer perceived sleep quality and more sleep disturbances during the premenstrual and early follicular phases has been rather consistent,[21] although with some exceptions.[22,23] On the contrary, when considering objective sleep, only one actigraphy-based study of 163 late-reproductive age women (median age 51.5 years) found a corresponding deteriorated sleep in the premenstrual phase.[24] More consistently, studies found that polysomnography-assessed sleep variation across the menstrual cycle is minimal or null and mostly related to REM sleep.[21,25–27]

Mood and Sleep Across Menstrual Cycle Phases

Mood and sleep in conjunction across the menstrual cycle have been less extensively investigated and mostly with respect to subjective sleep. According to the US community-based study of 900 menstruating women, more than half of the 58 participants with current clinical or subclinical depression experienced one to eight symptoms worsening in a given cycle, the most common being insomnia or hypersomnia. In detail, 15.6% of the depressed women had difficulty sleeping, and 7.3% slept too much before menses. Interestingly, the premenstrual mood symptom (especially sleep) worsening was a function of menstrual cyclicity occurring in all women, regardless of their depression status or history.[17] More recently, an Italian study of 213 university students followed via daily online questionnaires for two menstrual cycles, identified three patterns of sleep difficulty: women with a mid-cycle increase (25% of participants), with a premenstrual increase (29%), and with no changes in sleep difficulty levels across the menstrual cycle.[28] Higher overall levels of anxiety and, to a lesser extent, cognitive symptoms and depression predicted higher overall levels of sleep difficulty across the cycle. On the contrary, higher levels of mood swings were associated with lower levels of sleep difficulty. However, none of the psychological symptoms interacted with the sleep pattern group in predicting sleep difficulty levels, suggesting that their effects on sleep difficulties are quite stable across menstrual-related sleep patterns. In a previous work on the same population, the investigators described similar patterns of mood fluctuations across the cycle, with four groups: two premenstrual increase groups (altogether 61% of women), a mid-cycle increase group (13%) and a no-cycle group.[29] The identified menstrual-related affective and sleep patterns seemed to correspond, with women belonging to the mid-cycle and premenstrual affective groups having higher odds of belonging to the mid-cycle and premenstrual sleep patterns, respectively.[29] These results indicate higher interindividual variability in menstrual-related symptoms and suggest a correspondence relation between sleep and affective patterns of fluctuations across the cycle.[28] Another US study reported results of 265 young (18–25 years) healthy women with regular cycles and no contraception use, who filled in a series of online validated questionnaires on mood, sleep, emotion control, and other symptoms during the menstrual cycle. Depressive symptoms during the previous month had both direct and indirect effects on premenstrual symptoms during the most recent cycle, with mediation separately via poor sleep quality and emotional dysregulation. In specific, depressive symptoms had a direct effect on premenstrual pain, negative affect, and concentration, whereas habitual poor sleep quality mediated the associations with concentration, negative affect, and premenstrual pain.[30] To the best of our knowledge, only a recent Canadian study has specifically assessed the relationship between 6-week daily self-reported mood and both subjective and objective sleep across the menstrual cycle of 19 women (18–43 years).[22] Although self-reported sleep was not associated with gonadal hormone levels, actigraphically assessed sleep efficiency was positively, but weakly associated with 1-day lagged urinary estrogen, and negatively with progesterone levels across the overall cycle. Further, although actigraphically measured total sleep time and wake after sleep onset (WASO) were weakly associated with only 2 of 11 mood items, self-reported sleep clearly associated with mood symptoms after controlling for ovarian hormone levels, physical health, and perceived stress. In summary, these findings confirm that objective sleep correlates weakly with mood and ovarian hormones, even in women with mood disorders, whereas subjective sleep is significantly associated with mood and psychosocial measures across menstrual cycle hormonal fluctuations.[22]

Taken together, these results confirm the tight interrelation between mood and subjective (but not so clearly objective) sleep and suggest that they tend to covary during the menstrual cycle.

MENSTRUAL CHARACTERISTICS, MOOD, AND SLEEP

Mood and sleep seem to be likewise related to menstrual cycle characteristics, such as regularity and duration. Menstrual irregularity has repeatedly been related to depressed mood, anxiety, poor psychological well-being, and suicidal ideation.[31–34] Similarly, a study of over 200 fertile-aged women described associations between short sleep duration (< 6 hours) and short or (not significantly) long menstrual cycle[35] and in a sample of 5800 adolescents menstrual irregularity associated with poor sleep quality and insomnia symptoms.[36] In addition, among women with sleep complaints, those with menstrual irregularity more likely report sleep difficulties and experience more light sleep and WASO during polysomnography recordings.[6]

Accordingly, mood and sleep are reciprocally interconnected in their relation with menstrual characteristics. Among 805 Korean adolescents, those with menstrual irregularity more likely reported shorter sleep duration, and depressive mood was associated with menstrual irregularity after controlling for sleep duration.[33] In another Korean population-based study of over 4000 fertile-aged women, the proportion with severe menstrual cycle irregularity (ie, menstrual intervals longer than 3 months) was higher in women with high stress levels, depressive mood, or suicidal ideation than in those without. In addition, the proportion with severe menstrual irregularity was higher among those with short (up to 5 h/d) or long ($\geq$ 9 h/d) sleep duration compared with those who slept 6 to 8 h/d. Menstrual irregularity in general was associated with depressed mood after controlling for sleep duration, and severe menstrual irregularity was associated with both depressed mood after controlling for sleep duration and short sleep duration after controlling for psychological distress. In specific, the relationships of stress and depressed mood with menstrual irregularity were driven by the group of short sleepers.[37] Similarly, a recent US community-based study examined 579 menstruating women, who completed questionnaires on sleep quality, insomnia, fatigue, daytime sleepiness, depression, and stress. Menstrual irregularity (and, to a lesser extent, heavy menstrual bleeding) was associated with short sleep duration, worse sleep quality, and more fatigue, stress, and depression.[38]

POLYCYSTIC OVARY SYNDROME

Definition of Polycystic Ovary Syndrome

Polycystic ovary syndrome (PCOS) is the most common reproductive endocrinological disorder in the reproductive period, with the prevalence range between 4% and 21% depending on the diagnostic criteria.[39,40] The diagnosis of PCOS is defined if a woman has two of the three findings: polycystic ovaries (detected by ultrasound), irregular menstruation (oligo- or anovulation), or hyperandrogenism (biochemical or clinical, later typically hirsutism and acne).[41,42] PCOS includes endocrinologic changes of elevated androgen levels, low progesterone levels, and insulin resistance,[41,42] but PCOS is not only a hormonal disorder, it has an important comorbidity, especially with obesity, metabolic syndrome, diabetes, and cardiovascular diseases,[41–47] thus having serious long-term health consequences.

Mood in Polycystic Ovary Syndrome

PCOS may decrease quality of life; it has shown to be related to both mood symptoms and sleeping disturbances.[43] According to a meta-analysis with 30 cross-sectional studies, women with PCOS were three to six times more likely to have depressive and anxiety symptoms compared with those without PCOS.[48] In a systematic review, of the 20 to 30 years aged women with PCOS, 35% suffered from anxiety and 42% from depressive symptoms.[49] Furthermore, the incidence of both depressive and anxiety disorders has shown to be increased in PCOS patients compared with age-matched controls.[50] The mood symptoms are found across the entire fertile era.[51]

Sleep in Polycystic Ovary Syndrome

As for sleep, previous studies have shown an increase of sleep disturbances in women with PCOS compared with women of the same age, independently of obesity.[50,52,53] In a cohort of 724 women, sleep disturbances were twice as common in women with PCOS ($n = 87$) compared with those without.[53] Specifically, PCOS was associated with increasing occurrence of difficulty to fall asleep and with difficulties to maintain sleep.[53] In another cohort study with 6578 women, compared with the healthy women, women with PCOS ($n = 484$) had more difficulties to fall asleep, restless sleep, and daytime tiredness, yet the average sleep duration did not differ.[54] Further, in a study including women with infertility only, those with PCOS ($n = 739$) were more likely to have short sleep duration (<6 hours), sleep-disordered breathing (SDB), and daytime sleepiness.[55] In a study evaluating sleep architecture in 44 women, obese PCOS patients had lower sleep quality and less REM sleep compared with body mass index (BMI)-adjusted healthy women.[56] The most important sleep disorder connected to PCOS is SDB, which is even 7 to 10 folds more frequent compared with healthy women with similar BMI level.[52,57,58] In a systematic review with six studies including 252 PCOS patients, those with SDB had higher BMI, waist-hip ratio and blood pressure and worse lipid profile, glucose balance, and insulin resistance than those without SDB.[59] Nevertheless, the effect of the treatment of SDB in PCOS patients' metabolic state is unknown, and the prevalence of PCOS in SDB patients is unexplored.

Mood and Sleep in Polycystic Ovary Syndrome

Above described endocrinologic characteristics have been proposed to play a role in increased risk in both mood symptoms and sleep disturbances in PCOS.[60,61] Further, the disorder characteristics, such as hirsutism, obesity, and infertility have been suggested to associate, especially with mood symptoms in PCOS.[60,61] Some studies have also assessed the relationship between mood symptoms and sleep disturbances in PCOS patients.[53–55,62] In the two above-mentioned Australian sleep studies, the women with PCOS had more depressive symptoms than the healthy controls, but the difference in sleep remained after controlling with depressive symptoms.[53,54] In a US study, daytime sleepiness in PCOS patients was associated with depressive symptoms.[55] Further, in a Chinese study with 433 PCOS patients, mood symptoms, both anxiety and depression, which occurred frequently, were associated with sleep, especially with worse sleep quality, occurrence of sleep disturbances, and daytime dysfunction.[62] Instead, no relationship with comprehensively measured hormone levels, glucose levels, lipid profiles, insulin resistance, or ultrasound measurement were found.[62]

PREMENSTRUAL SYNDROME AND PREMENSTRUAL DYSPHORIC DISORDER

The most obvious example of the relationship between menstrual cycle, mood, and sleep is, by definition, the premenstrual syndrome (PMS) and the PMDD. The PMS is a general complex of severe recurrent physical and psychological symptoms starting 7 to 10 days before menses and ending with their onset,[63] occurring in approximately 20% or more of women. In addition, 3% to 8% of women suffer from severe physical and mood symptoms that fulfill the diagnostic criteria for PMDD.[13,64] According to the definition of PMDD,[65] sleep disturbance (insomnia or hypersomnia) is among the symptoms that may be endorsed in addition to mood symptoms (affective lability, irritability/anger, depressed mood, anxiety/tension). Other subjective sleep disturbances commonly reported by women with PMS or PMDD include frequent nighttime awakenings, fatigue, and sleepiness that typically worsen in the late premenstrual phase.

According to numerous studies, PMS women have higher depressive and sleepiness scores, poorer mood, and more fatigue in the late luteal compared with the follicular phase and compared with controls.[66,67] In addition, poorer subjective sleep quality in PMS women correlates with higher anxiety levels.[68] On the other hand, evidence regarding objective sleep impairment during the symptomatic late luteal phase in PMS and PMDD is conflicting.[69,70] For example, two studies[69,71] failed to find in PMS patients any of the sleep parameter abnormalities that are often seen in patients with affective disorders. However, although the polysomnography sleep patterns did not differ between three PMS women and six healthy controls in Chuong's study,[69] other investigators reported more Stage 2, but less Stage 3 to 4 and REM sleep, and significantly lengthened REM onset latency in PMS patients compared with controls.[25,66,71] The shorter amount of Stage 3 to 4 sleep during both the follicular and luteal phases suggests that PMS women have in general less deep sleep than healthy women, regardless of menstrual cycle phase. More recently, seven PMDD women with insomnia symptoms exclusively in the luteal phase, and five healthy controls were examined via polysomnography recordings for 8 to 11 nights during the follicular and luteal phases of one menstrual cycle.[72] PMDD women had more overall slow wave sleep (SWS) and a tendency for less Stage 2 sleep than controls. However, in both groups, Stage 2 sleep was increased in the mid-luteal compared with the early follicular phase, and REM sleep decreased in early luteal than in early follicular phase. Interestingly, PMDD women with sleep complaints had also overall decreased melatonin levels, possibly related to their increased SWS.[72]

Further evidence for the relationship between sleep and mood in PMDD comes from Parry and colleagues' study,[73] where 23 PMDD and 18 healthy control women were exposed to early-night and late-night sleep deprivation, both followed by a recovery night. Sleep quality improved during and depressive scores after recovery nights in PMDD subjects, with no significant sleep or mood score changes among controls. In addition, changes in REM sleep measures were associated with clinical improvement in responders to sleep deprivation.[74]

In general, these findings indicate different sleep architecture, though inconsistent in terms of specific parameters, between PMS/PMDD and healthy women, irrespective of the menstrual phase and without any group $\times$ menstrual phase interaction. These observations suggest that these women may have a trait-altered sleep, possibly representing an intrinsic vulnerability to cyclic hormonal fluctuations that eventually manifest with premenstrual physical and psychological symptoms.

Hormonal Contraceptives

Approximately 65% of fertile-aged women use contraception,[75] and a quarter of them choose a hormonal method.[76] The relationship between HC and mental health is quite debated.[77] Ample evidence has shown no associations between the use of contraception and an increased risk of depressive or anxiety disorders.[77–80] Preliminary results from a register-based study of over 100,000 childbearing-aged women living in Finland show that current use (in the past 6 months) of HC, in particular of estradiol- or ethinylestradiol-containing combined HC was associated with lower risk of depression compared with HC nonuse (Toffol and colleagues, Submitted).[81] However, recent observations report that women using HC (especially oral contraceptives [OC]) have higher odds of depression[82,83] and of suicidal behavior.[84,85]

The effects of HC on sleep remain similarly unclear.[6,23,86–91] According to a recent meta-analysis of 13 studies, the only significant differences out of two subjective and 12 objective sleep parameters between women using and not using HC is shorter WASO in HC users and increased total sleep time and Stage 2 sleep compared with nonusers in the follicular phase. Based on these findings, the investigators conclude that HC use does not significantly affect sleep patterns and sleep architecture.[92]

Regarding the relationship between sleep and mood in connection with HC use, a study comparing 9 naturally cycling and 10 women on OC found no differences in self-reported evening anxiety or sleep quality between the groups. However, women on OC had more Stage 2 sleep in both phases, but less SWS in the luteal phase compared with naturally cycling women.[27] Similarly, in an archival study of electroencephalogram recordings of 68 women with depression and 37 healthy controls, women using OC had less SWS percentage and REM latency than nonusers, irrespective of their depressive status. Further, healthy controls on OC had shorter sleep latency and more REM sleep than controls without OC, with no OC effect in depressed women. In general, the effects of OC on sleep were larger in healthy than in depressed women.[88] In addition, in a Dutch study of 1205 women aged 18 to 54 years,[93] OC use was associated with more severe concurrent insomnia, but not depressive symptoms or with higher prevalence of depression or dysthymia. Previous or current depression or dysthymia did not moderate the association between OC use and insomnia symptoms. However, the use of OC was associated with higher depressive symptoms and disorder prevalence in within-individual estimates, but lower in between-individual analyses.

PREGNANCY

Mood During Pregnancy

Mood symptoms, mainly depressive symptoms and anxiety, are common medical complications during pregnancy and postpartum[94] and the rates of depression peak at the beginning of postpartum.[95] Even though mental disorders during pregnancy and postpartum can contribute to other pregnancy complications[96,97] and have an effect on delivery[98] as well as have devastating effects on the maternal-newborn relationship and health of the infant[95,97,99] and possess risk to become chronic,[95] most of the cases are undiagnosed and untreated.[100]

Sleep During Pregnancy

Also sleep disturbances are frequent during pregnancy, and previous literature proposed that insomnia symptoms, both maintenance and onset insomnia, increase as pregnancy proceeds.[101,102] Several factors, both physic and mental, counteract to these changes.[102] In addition, the two important sleep disorders, SDB and restless legs syndrome (RLS), typically increase and changes in sleep architecture have also been shown.[101] Sleepiness, however, has been proposed to have a U-shape occurrence being lowest in mid-pregnancy.[102,103] Similar to mood symptoms, also sleep disturbances are associated with adverse pregnancy and delivery outcomes and worse health of the newborn.[104,105] In some women, sleep disturbances and changes in sleep architecture continue during the postnatal period[101,106] and persist.[101]

Mood and Sleep During Pregnancy

The associations between mood symptoms and sleep disturbances during pregnancy and postpartum are bidirectional: sleep disturbances can increase the severity of depressive symptoms,[107] but also mood symptoms can worsen sleep quality.[102] Furthermore, perinatal psychiatric disorders are closely related to disturbances in sleep. A systematic review with 31 studies found that women with postnatal depression, anxiety, or psychosis also suffered from concurrent insomnia.[108] A study with 124 primiparous women showed an associations between sleep and depressive and anxiety symptoms.[109] In another study with longitudinal setting, women ($n = 3645$) with a lower sleep quality and a shorter sleep duration (<8 h/d) were at a higher risk for symptoms of depression and anxiety.[110] Furthermore, another longitudinal study ($n = 1858$) showed that women with more baseline depressive and anxiety symptoms had higher levels of insomnia and sleepiness scores and those with more depressive symptoms had longer sleep latencies.[102] The association is also evident postpartum. Large cohort studies including 1398 women[107] and 4191 women[111] have shown that postpartum depressive symptoms are related to postpartum poor general sleep quality, various insomnia symptoms, lower sleep efficiency, longer sleep latency, shorter sleep duration and higher sleep loss, as well as higher daytime sleepiness, fatigue, and dysfunction after controlling with several risk factors for depressive symptoms. In addition to this obvious bidirectional association, recent studies have emphasized that sleep disturbances are prodromal symptoms for depression. In one previous study with 273 women, poor general sleep quality in early pregnancy predicted higher levels of depression in later pregnancy, but not vice versa.[112] Furthermore, according to the above-mentioned study from Pietikäinen and colleagues,[107] various sleep disturbances during pregnancy, such as poor general sleep quality, long sleep latency, short sleep, sleep loss, and daytime sleepiness were associated with postpartum depressive symptoms even when controlled with depressive symptoms during pregnancy. Another study with 2224 women from the same research group verified that long sleep latency in early pregnancy and insufficient sleep during late pregnancy predicted the risk of postpartum depression.[113]

CLIMACTERIC

Definition of Climacteric

Climacteric is a time period of a graduate depletion of ovarian follicles, resulting menopause (defined as the time of the final menstrual period). The median age of menopause is 51 years, although cessation of menstruation varies with a wide range (The Stages of Reproductive Aging Workshop + 10).[114] Although climacteric may be passed over asymptomatic, most of the women suffer from some level of climacteric symptoms. The most characteristic symptoms are vasomotor symptoms, hot flushes, and sweating, but the symptomatology includes several other symptoms, of which mood symptoms and sleep disturbances are frequent.[115,116]

Mood in Climacteric

In climacteric, risk for psychological distress, depressive symptoms, and depressive disorder increases.[117–122] Particularly, perimenopause and menopausal transition have shown to be vulnerable time, but also postmenopausal women have shown to be in risk.[122] In the Study of Women's Health Across the Nation (SWAN), women were two to four times more likely to develop major depressive disorder in the menopausal transition and early postmenopause compared with premenopause after adjusting for confounding factors.[122] The biological link between mood and climacteric has focused on the hypothesis that low levels of estrogen due to menopause are associated with mood symptoms. However, more research confirms that perimenopausal fluctuations in estrogen levels rather than the eventual drop in postmenopause are associated with impaired mood.[123,124] Moreover, women suffering from mood symptoms during other reproductive periods (eg, the premenstrual phase of the menstrual cycle or postpartum) are at greater risk for developing depressive symptoms in climacteric.[119] Important associative factors are also preclimacteric mood symptoms, somatic health problems, childhood maltreatment (physical, verbal, sexual), lack of social support and friends, recent negative life event, and other climacteric symptoms, especially vasomotor symptoms.[118–120,125]

Sleep in Climacteric

Previous literature, both cross-sectional[126–130] and longitudinal,[131–134] assures that sleep disturbances increase during climacteric. A meta-analysis including 24 cross-sectional studies showed that perimenopausal (odds ratio [OR] 1.6), postmenopausal (OR 1.7), and surgically postmenopausal (OR 2.2) women were more likely to have sleep disturbances compared with premenopausal women.[135] The sleep disturbances include insomnia symptoms, SDB, and RLS.[136] Of insomnia symptoms, the most frequent are nocturnal awakenings, but also difficulties to fall asleep and too early morning awakenings are common.[132,136] As for the effect of climacteric on sleep architecture, the previous research is not unanimous. Some studies have found no differences in sleep architecture between premenopausal and postmenopausal women[137,138] or minor deterioration in sleep architecture (elevated beta electroencephalogram [EEG] power in non-REM [NREM] and REM sleep),[139] whereas others have reported even better sleep patterns in

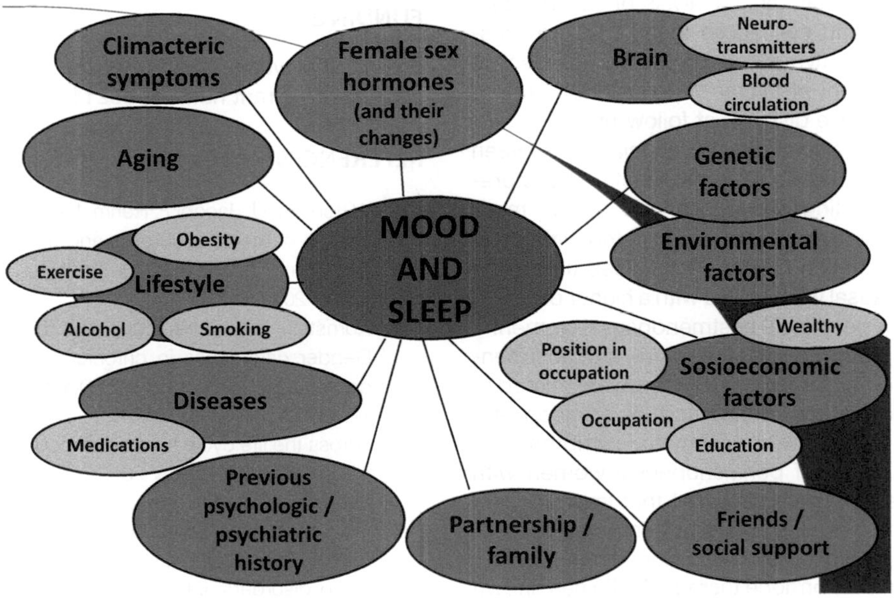

Fig. 1. Associative factors for mood and sleep.

postmenopausal women[130,140,141] (longer total sleep time and more SWS[130]; less S1 sleep and shorter SWS latency[140]; more N3 sleep[141]). Furthermore, studies evaluating the effect of menopausal transition on sleep have shown that the observed changes seem to be rather age than menopause-dependent.[142,143]

Mood and Sleep in Climacteric

Similar to the reproductive period, also during climacteric, the relationship between mood symptoms and sleep disturbances is bidirectional.[117,119,120] In addition, both symptoms are associated with several other factors, most typically with climacteric vasomotor symptoms (**Fig. 1**).[117,119,120] Thus, during climacteric, these three symptoms, mood, sleep, and vasomotor symptoms, form a triangle where one symptom worsen the other. The relationship between mood symptoms and sleep disturbances has been documented especially in the menopausal transition.[117,119,120] In two large cross-sectional cohorts of climacteric women[144,145] (over 3400 women aged 41–55 years[144] and 850 women aged 32–58 years[145]), mood symptoms and mental quality of life were the most important associative factors for sleep disturbances. In a longitudinal analysis of 309 women transitioning menopause, Avis and colleagues reported that depressive symptoms were associated with hot flashes and sleep disturbance.[146] Several other follow-up studies have ensured these associations, including a 4-year follow-up 436 women[119] and a 19-year follow-up with 1551 women.[147] Further, in a longitudinal analysis of SWAN data, Bromberger and colleagues found that the presence of subjective sleep problems at baseline was a significant predictor of persistent/recurrent major depressive disorder at follow-up.[148]

The studies evaluating the association between mood symptoms and sleep architecture have presented conflicting results. In one study, more depressive symptoms were associated with lower sleep efficiency and shorter total sleep time in 21 perimenopausal women and with a higher percentage of REM sleep in 29 postmenopausal women.[12] In another study with 343 pre-, peri-, and postmenopausal women, anxiety symptoms were related to longer sleep onset latency and lower sleep efficiency in women with vasomotor symptoms.[149] Further, a study of perimenopausal women with depressive symptoms showed that improvement in depression was predicted by improved sleep, but not by reduction of vasomotor symptoms.[150]

Menopausal hormone therapy (MHT) has shown to alleviate both mood and sleep symptoms during climacteric in randomized controlled trials.[136,151–153] The most important contributive factor is the simultaneous alleviation of vasomotor symptoms,[136,153] although an improvement of sleep quality has also been shown in asymptomatic women.[154] Nevertheless, as depression and sleep disorders increase in menopausal transition and especially in aging, specific treatments besides MHT or instead may be needed.[155]

CLINICS CARE POINTS

- Mood and sleep symptoms are tightly interrelated across female reproductive life and events. Recognizing, monitoring and treating sleep symptoms may benefit the related mood symptoms, and viceversa.
- Sleep disturbances during pregnancy may be prodromal for postpartum depression. Hence, identification and treatment of sleep symptoms during pregnancy may be of crucial importance for postpartum wellbeing.
- In spite of the potential beneficial effects of menopausal hormone therapy on mood and sleep symptoms during climacteric, depression and sleep disorders during menopause may require specific treatments.

DISCLOSURE

The authors declare that they have no conflicts of interest.

FUNDING

Elena Toffol was supported by the Finnish Cultural Foundation (grant number 00211101).

REFERENCES

1. Wittchen HU, Jacobi F, Rehm J, et al. The size and burden of mental disorders and other disorders of the brain in Europe 2010. Eur Neuropsychopharmacol 2011;21:655–79.
2. Kornstein SG, Schatzberg AF, Thase ME, et al. Gender differences in chronic major and double depression. J Affect Disord 2000;60:1–11.
3. Moline ML, Broch L, Zak R, et al. Sleep in women across the life cycle from adulthood through menopause. Sleep Med Rev 2003;7:155–77.
4. Zhang B, Wing YK. Sex differences in insomnia: a meta-analysis. Sleep 2006;29:85–93.
5. Frange C, Banzoli CV, Colombo AE, et al. Women's sleep disorders: integrative care. Sleep Sci 2017;10:174–80.

6. Hachul H, Andersen ML, Bittencourt LR, et al. Does the reproductive cycle influence sleep patterns in women with sleep complaints? Climacteric 2010; 13:594–603.
7. Ford DE, Kamerow DB. Epidemiologic study of sleep disturbances and psychiatric disorders. An opportunity for prevention? JAMA 1989;262: 1479–84.
8. Gillin JC. Are sleep disturbances risk factors for anxiety, depressive and addictive disorders? Acta Psychiatr Scand Suppl 1998;393:39–43.
9. Jehan S, Auguste E, Hussain M, et al. Sleep and premenstrual syndrome. J Sleep Med Disord 2016;3:1061.
10. Nicolau ZFM, Bezerra AG, Polesel DN, et al. Premenstrual syndrome and sleep disturbances: results from the são paulo epidemiologic sleep study. Psychiatry Res 2018;264:427–31.
11. Ford DE, Kamerow DB. Epidemiologic study of sleep disturbances and psychiatric disorders: an opportunity for prevention? JAMA 1989;262: 1479–84.
12. Toffol E, Kalleinen N, Urrila AS, et al. The relationship between mood and sleep in different female reproductive states. BMC Psychiatr 2014;14:177. Available at: http://www.biomedcentral.com/1471-244X/14/177-244X-14-177.
13. Mishell DR Jr. Premenstrual disorders: epidemiology and disease burden. Am J Manag Care 2005;11(16 Suppl):S473–9.
14. Haley CL, Sung SC, Rush AJ, et al. The clinical relevance of self-reported premenstrual worsening of depressive symptoms in the management of depressed outpatients: a STAR*D report. J Womens Health (Larchmt) 2013;22:219–29.
15. Teatero ML, Mazmanian D, Sharma V. Effects of the menstrual cycle on bipolar disorder. Bipolar Disord 2014;16:22–36.
16. Kuehner C, Nayman S. Premenstrual exacerbations of mood disorders: findings and knowledge gaps. Curr Psychiatry Rep 2021;23:78.
17. Hartlage SA, Brandenburg DL, Kravitz HM. Premenstrual exacerbation of depressive disorders in a community-based sample in the United States. Psychosom Med 2004;66:698–706.
18. Gonda X, Telek T, Juhász G, et al. Patterns of mood changes throughout the reproductive cycle in healthy women without premenstrual dysphoric disorders. Prog Neuro-Psychopharmacol Biol Psychiatry 2008;32:1782–8.
19. Reed SC, Levin FR, Evans SM. Changes in mood, cognitive performance and appetite in the late luteal and follicular phases of the menstrual cycle in women with and without PMDD (premenstrual dysphoric disorder). Horm Behav 2008;54:185–93.
20. Pátkai P, Johannson G, Post B. Mood, alertness and sympathetic-adrenal medullary activity during the menstrual cycle. Psychosom Med 1974;36: 503–12.
21. Baker FC, Lee KA. Menstrual cycle effects on sleep. Sleep Med Clin 2018;13:283–94.
22. Li DX, Romans S, De Souza MJ, et al. Actigraphic and self-reported sleep quality in women: associations with ovarian hormones and mood. Sleep Med 2015;16:1217–24.
23. Romans SE, Kreindler D, Einstein G, et al. Sleep quality and the menstrual cycle. Sleep Med 2015; 16:489–95.
24. Zheng H, Harlow SD, Kravitz HM, et al. Actigraphy-defined measures of sleep and movement across the menstrual cycle in midlife menstruating women: study of Women's Health across the Nation Sleep Study. Menopause 2015;22:66–74.
25. Lee KA, Shaver JF, Giblin EC, et al. Sleep patterns related to menstrual cycle phase and premenstrual affective symptoms. Sleep 1990;13:403–9.
26. Driver HS, Dijk DJ, Werth E, et al. Sleep and the sleep electroencephalogram across the menstrual cycle in young healthy women. J Clin Endocrinol Metab 1996;81:728–35.
27. Baker FC, Waner JI, Vieira EF, et al. Sleep and 24 hour body temperatures: a comparison in young men, naturally cycling women and women taking hormonal contraceptives. J Physiol 2001;530:565–74.
28. Van Reen E, Kiesner J. Individual differences in self-reported difficulty sleeping across the menstrual cycle. Arch Womens Ment Health 2016;19:599–608.
29. Kiesner J. One woman's low is another woman's high: paradoxical effects of the menstrual cycle. Psychoneuroendocrinology 2011;36:68–76.
30. Meers JM, Bower JL, Alfano CA. Poor sleep and emotion dysregulation mediate the association between depressive and premenstrual symptoms in young adult women. Arch Womens Ment Health 2020;23:351–9.
31. Bisaga K, Petkova E, Cheng J, et al. Menstrual functioning and psychopathology in a countywide population of high-school girls. J Am Acad Child Adolesc Psychiatry 2002;41:1197–204.
32. Toffol E, Koponen P, Luoto R, et al. Pubertal timing, menstrual irregularity, and mental health: results of a population-based study. Arch Womens Ment Health 2014;17:127–35.
33. Yu M, Han K, Nam GE. The association between mental health problems and menstrual cycle irregularity among adolescent Korean girls. J Affect Disord 2017;210:43–8.
34. Park M, Jung SJ. Association between menstrual cycle irregularity and suicidal ideation among Korean women: results from the Korea national health and nutrition examination survey (2010-2012). J Affect Disord 2021;293:279–84.
35. Lim AJ, Huang Z, Chua SE, et al. Sleep duration, exercise, shift work and polycystic ovarian

syndrome-related outcomes in a healthy population: a cross-sectional study. PLoS One 2016;11: e0167048.
36. Liu X, Chen H, Liu ZZ, et al. Early menarche and menstrual problems are associated with sleep disturbance in a large sample of Chinese adolescent girls. Sleep 2017;40(9).
37. Kim T, Nam GE, Han B, et al. Associations of mental health and sleep duration with menstrual cycle irregularity: a population-based study. Arch Womens Ment Health 2018;21:619–26.
38. Kennedy KER, Onyeonwu C, Nowakowski S, et al. Menstrual regularity and bleeding is associated with sleep duration, sleep quality and fatigue in a community sample. J Sleep Res 2022;31:e13434.
39. Lizneva D, Suturina L, Walker W, et al. Criteria, prevalence, and phenotypes of polycystic ovary syndrome. Fertil Steril 2016;106:6–15.
40. Fauser B, Tarlatzis B, Rebar R, et al. Consensus on womens health aspects of polycystic ovary syndrome (PCOS). Hum Reprod 2012;27:14–24.
41. Teede H, Misso M, Costello M, et al. Recommendations from the international evidence-based guideline for the assessment and management of polycystic ovary syndrome. Hum Reprod 2018;33: 1602–18.
42. Rotterdam ESHRE/ASRM-Sponsored PCOS Consensus Workshop Group. 2004. Revised 2003 consensus on diagnostic criteria and long-term health risks related to polycystic ovary syndrome (PCOS). Hum Reprod 2004;19:41–7.
43. Sidra S, Tariq MH, Farrukh MJ, et al. Evaluation of clinical manifestations, health risks, and quality of life among women with polycystic ovary syndrome. PLoS One 2019;14:e0223329.
44. Legro R, Kunselman A, Dunaif A. Prevalence and predictors of dyslipidemia in women with polycystic ovary syndrome. Am J Med 2001;111: 607–13.
45. Moran LJ, Misso ML, Wild RA, et al. 2010. Impaired glucose tolerance, type 2 diabetes and metabolic syndrome in polycystic ovary syndrome: a systematic review and meta-analysis. Hum Reprod Update 2010;16:347–63.
46. Ng NYH, Jiang G, Cheung LP, et al. Progression of glucose intolerance and cardiometabolic risk factors over a decade in Chinese women with polycystic ovary syndrome: a case-control study. PLoS Med 2019;16:e1002953.
47. Dokras A. Does body weight affect cardiometabolic risk in women with polycystic ovary syndrome? Fertil Steril 2019;111:56–7.
48. Cooney LG, Lee I, Sammel MD, et al. High prevalence of moderate and severe depressive and anxiety symptoms in polycystic ovary syndrome: a systematic review and meta-analysis. Hum Reprod 2017;32:1075–91.
49. Cooney L, Dokras A. Beyond fertility: polycystic ovary syndrome and long-term health. Fertil Steril 2018;110:794–809.
50. Hung JH, Hu LY, Tsai SJ, et al. Risk of psychiatric disorders following polycystic ovary syndrome: a nationwide population-based cohort study. PLoS One 2014;9:e97041.
51. Karjula S, Morin-Papunen L, Auvinen J, et al. Psychological distress is more prevalent in fertile age and premenopausal women with pcos symptoms: 15-year follow-up. J Clin Endocrinol Metab 2017; 102:1861–9.
52. Lin TY, Lin PY, Su TP, et al. Risk of developing obstructive sleep apnea among women with polycystic ovarian syndrome: a nationwide longitudinal follow-up study. Sleep Med 2017;36:165–9.
53. Moran LJ, March WA, Whitrow MJ, et al. Sleep disturbances in a community based sample of women with polycystic ovary syndrome. Hum Reprod 2015;30:466–72.
54. Mo L, Mansfield DR, Joham A, et al. Sleep disturbances in women with and without polycystic ovary syndrome in an Australian National Cohort. Clinical Endocrinol 2019;90:570–8.
55. Eisenberg E, Legro RS, Diamond MP, et al. Sleep habits of women with infertility. J Clin Endocrinol Metab 2021;106:e4414–26.
56. Hachul H, Polesel DN, Tock L, et al. Sleep disorders in polycystic ovary syndrome: influence of obesity and hyperandrogenism. Rev Assoc Med Bras 2019;65:375–83.
57. Tasali E, Van Cauter E, Hoffman L, et al. Impact of obstructive sleep apnea on insulin resistance and glucose tolerance in women with polycystic ovary syndrome. J Clin Endocrinol Metab 2008;93: 3878–84.
58. Thannickal A, Brutocao C, Alsawas M, et al. Eating, sleeping and sexual function disorders in women with polycystic ovary syndrome (PCOS): a systematic review and meta-analysis. Clinical Endocrinol 2020;92:338–49.
59. Kahal H, Kyrou I, Uthman O, et al. The association between obstructive sleep apnea and metabolic abnormalities in women with polycystic ovary syndrome: a systematic review and meta-analysis. Sleep 2018; 41. https://doi.org/10.1093/sleep/zsy085.
60. Annagür BB, Tazegül A, Uguz F, et al. Biological correlates of major depression and generalized anxiety disorder in women with polycystic ovary syndrome. J Psychosom Res 2013;74:244–7.
61. Greenwood EA, Pasch LA, Shinkai K, et al. Putative role for insulin resistance in depression risk in polycystic ovary syndrome. Fertil Steril 2015;104:707–14.
62. Yang Y, Hui Deng H, Li T, et al. The mental health of Chinese women with polycystic ovary syndrome is related to sleep disorders, not disease status. J Affect Dis 2021;282:51–7.

63. Johnson SR. The epidemiology and social impact of premenstrual symptoms. Clin Obstet Gynecol 1987;30:367–76.
64. Halbreich U, Borenstein J, Pearlstein T, et al. The prevalence, impairment, impact, and burden of premenstrual dysphoric disorder (PMS/PMDD). Psychoneuroendocrinology 2003;28(Suppl 3): 1–23.
65. Diagnostic and statistical manual of mental disorders. 5th edition. Washington, DC: American Psychiatric Association; 2013.
66. Baker FC, Kahan TL, Trinder J, et al. Sleep quality and the sleep electroencephalogram in women with severe premenstrual syndrome. Sleep 2007; 30:1283–91.
67. Baker FC, Colrain IM. Daytime sleepiness, psychomotor performance, waking EEG spectra and evoked potentials in women with severe premenstrual syndrome. J Sleep Res 2010;19:214–27.
68. Baker FC, Sassoon SA, Kahan T, et al. Perceived poor sleep quality in the absence of polysomnographic sleep disturbance in women with severe premenstrual syndrome. J Sleep Res 2012;21: 535–45.
69. Chuong CJ, Kim SR, Taskin O, et al. Sleep pattern changes in menstrual cycles of women with premenstrual syndrome: a preliminary study. Am J Obstet Gynecol 1997;177:554–8.
70. Lamarche LJ, Driver HS, Wiebe S, et al. Nocturnal sleep, daytime sleepiness, and napping among women with significant emotional/behavioral premenstrual symptoms. J Sleep Res 2007;16:262–8.
71. Parry BL, Mendelson WB, Duncan WC, et al. Longitudinal sleep EEG, temperature, and activity measurements across the menstrual cycle in patients with premenstrual depression and in age-matched controls. Psychiatry Res 1989;30:285–303.
72. Shechter A, Lespérance P, Ng Ying Kin NM, et al. Nocturnal polysomnographic sleep across the menstrual cycle in premenstrual dysphoric disorder. Sleep Med 2012;13:1071–8.
73. Parry BL, Cover H, Mostofi N, et al. Early versus late partial sleep deprivation in patients with premenstrual dysphoric disorder and normal comparison subjects. Am J Psychiatry 1995;152:404–12.
74. Parry BL, Mostofi N, LeVeau B, et al. Sleep EEG studies during early and late partial sleep deprivation in premenstrual dysphoric disorder and normal control subjects. Psychiatry Res 1999;85:127–43.
75. Daniels K, Abma JC. Current contraceptive status among women aged 15-49: United States, 2015-2017. NCHS Data Brief, 327. Hyattsville, MD: National Center for Health Statistics; 2018.
76. United Nations, Department of Economic and Social Affairs, Population Division (2019). Contraceptive Use by Method 2019: Data Booklet (ST/ESA/SER.A/435).
77. McCloskey LR, Wisner KL, Cattan MK, et al. Contraception for women with psychiatric disorders. Am J Psychiatry 2021;178:247–55.
78. Duke JM, Sibbritt DW, Young AF. Is there an association between the use of oral contraception and depressive symptoms in young Australian women? Contraception 2007;75:27–31.
79. Cheslack-Postava K, Keyes KM, Lowe SR, et al. Oral contraceptive use and psychiatric disorders in a nationally representative sample of women. Arch Womens Ment Health 2015;18:103–11.
80. Lundin C, Wikman A, Lampa E, et al. There is no association between combined oral hormonal contraceptives and depression: a Swedish register-based cohort study. BJOG 2022;129:917–25.
81. Toffol E, Partonen T, Heikinheimo O, et al. Use of systemic hormonal contraception and risk of depression. Submitted for publication.
82. Skovlund CW, Mørch LS, Kessing LV, et al. Association of hormonal contraception with depression. JAMA Psychiatr 2016;73:1154–62.
83. Anderl C, Li G, Chen FS. Oral contraceptive use in adolescence predicts lasting vulnerability to depression in adulthood. J Child Psychol Psychiatr 2020;61:148–56.
84. Skovlund CW, Mørch LS, Kessing LV, et al. Association of hormonal contraception with suicide attempts and suicides. Am J Psychiatry 2018;175:336–42.
85. Edwards A, Lönn S, Crump C, et al. Oral contraceptive use and risk of suicidal behavior among young women. Psychol Med 2022;52:1710–7.
86. Hachul H, Andersen ML, Bittencourt L, et al. A population-based survey on the influence of the menstrual cycle and the use of hormonal contraceptives on sleep patterns in São Paulo, Brazil. Int J Gynaecol Obstet 2013;120:137–40.
87. Baker FC, Mitchell D, Driver HS. Oral contraceptives alter sleep and raise body temperature in young women. Pflugers Arch 2001;442:729–37.
88. Burdick RS, Hoffmann R, Armitage R. Short note: oral contraceptives and sleep in depressed and healthy women. Sleep 2002;25:347–9.
89. Bezerra AG, Andersen ML, Pires GN, et al. Hormonal contraceptive use and subjective sleep reports in women: an online survey. J Sleep Res 2020;29:e12983.
90. Hachul H, Bisse AR, Sanchez ZM, et al. Sleep quality in women who use different contraceptive methods. Sleep Sci 2020;13:131–7.
91. Partonen T, Toffol E, Latvala A, Heikinheimo O, Haukka J. Hormonal contraception use and insomnia: A nested case-control study. Sleep Med 2023;109:192–6.
92. Bezerra AG, Andersen ML, Pires GN, et al. The effects of hormonal contraceptive use on sleep in women: a systematic review and meta-analysis. J Sleep Res 2022;e13757.

93. Morssinkhof MWL, Lamers F, Hoogendoorn AW, et al. Oral contraceptives, depressive and insomnia symptoms in adult women with and without depression. Psychoneuroendocrinology 2021;133: 105390.
94. Accortt EE, Wong MS. It is time for routine screening for perinatal mood and anxiety disorders in obstetrics and gynecology settings. Obstet Gynecol Surv 2017;72:553–68.
95. Abel KM, Hope H, Swift E, et al. Prevalence of maternal mental illness among children and adolescents in the UK between 2005 and 2017: a national retrospective cohort analysis. Lancet Public Health 2019;4(6):e291–300.
96. Grigoriadis S, Graves L, Peer M, et al. Maternal anxiety during pregnancy and the association with adverse perinatal outcomes. J Clin Psychiatry 2018. https://doi.org/10.4088/JCP.17r12011.
97. Grigoriadis S, VonderPorten EH, Mamisashvili L, et al. The impact of maternal depression during pregnancy on perinatal outcomes: a systematic review and meta-analysis. J Clin Psychiatry 2013;74: e321–41.
98. Bayrampour H, Salmon C, Vinturache A, et al. Effect of depressive and anxiety symptoms during pregnancy on risk of obstetric interventions. J Obstet Gynaecol Res 2015;41:1040–8.
99. Toffol E, Lahti-Pulkkinen M, Lahti J, et al. Maternal depressive symptoms during and after pregnancy are associated with poorer sleep quantity and quality and sleep disorders in 3.5-year-old offspring. Sleep Med 2019;56:201e210.
100. Cox EQ, Sowa NA, Meltzer-Brody SE, et al. The perinatal depression treatment cascade: baby steps toward improving outcomes. J Clin Psychiatry 2016;77:1189–200.
101. Barger MK, Caughey AB, Lee KA. Evaluating insomnia during pregnancy and postpartum. In: Attarian HP, Viola-Saltzman M, editors. Sleep disorders in women. Totowa, NJ, New York: Humana Press; 2013. p. 225–42.
102. Aukia L, Paavonen EJ, Jänkälä T, et al. Insomnia symptoms increase during pregnancy, but no increase in sleepiness - associations with symptoms of depression and anxiety. Sleep Med 2020;72: 150–6.
103. Roman-Galvez RM, Amezcua-Prieto C, Salcedo-Bellido I, et al. Factors associated with insomnia in pregnancy: a prospective Cohort Study. Eur J Obstet Gynecol Reprod Biol 2018;221:70e5.
104. Lee KA, Gay CL. Sleep in late pregnancy predicts length of labor and type of delivery. Am J Obstet Gynecol 2004;191:2041–6.
105. Lu Q, Zhang X, Wang Y, et al. Sleep disturbances during pregnancy and adverse maternal and fetal outcomes: a systematic review and meta-analysis. Sleep Med Rev 2021;58:101436.
106. Lee KA, Zaffke ME, McEnany G. Parity and sleep patterns during and after pregnancy. Obstet Gynecol 2000;95:14–8.
107. Pietikäinen JT, Polo-Kantola P, Pölkki P, et al. Sleeping problems during pregnancy-a risk factor for postnatal depressiveness. Arch Womens. Ment Health 2019;22:327–37.
108. Lawson A, Murphy KE, Sloan E, et al. The relationship between sleep and postpartum mental disorders: a systematic review. J Affect Disord 2015; 176:65–77.
109. Goyal D, Gay CL, Lee KA. Patterns of sleep disruption and depressive symptoms in new mothers. J Perinat Neonatal Nurs 2007;21:123e9.
110. Yu Y, Li M, Pu L, et al. Sleep was associated with depression and anxiety status during pregnancy: a prospective longitudinal study. Arch Womens Ment Health 2017;20:695e701.
111. Dørheim SK, Bondevik GT, Eberhard-Gran M, et al. Sleep and depression in postpartum women: a population-based study. Sleep 2009;32:847–55.
112. Skouteris H, Germano C, Wertheim EH, et al. Sleep quality and depression during pregnancy: a prospective study. J Sleep Res 2008;17:217e20.
113. Pietikäinen JT, Härkänen T, Polo-Kantola P, et al. Estimating the cumulative risk of postnatal depressive symptoms: the role of insomnia symptoms across pregnancy. Soc Psychiatry Psychiatr Epidemiol 2021;56:2251–61.
114. Harlow SD, Gass M, Hall JE, et al. Executive summary of the stages of reproductive aging workshop + 10: addressing the unfinished agenda of staging reproductive aging. J Clin Endocrinol Metab 2012;97:1159–68.
115. Avis NE, Crawford SL, Greendale G, et al. Duration of menopausal vasomotor symptoms over the menopause transition. JAMA Intern Med 2015; 175:531–9.
116. Archer DF, Sturdee DW, Baber R, et al. Menopausal hot flushes and night sweats: where are we now? Climacteric 2011;14:515–28.
117. Bromberger JT, Meyer PM, Howard M, et al. Psychologic distress and natural menopause: a multiethnic community study. Am J Public Health 2001;91:1435–42.
118. Maartens LWF, Knottnerus JA, Pop VJ. Menopausal transition and increased depressive symptomatology. A community based prospective study. Maturitas 2002;42:195–200.
119. Freeman EW, Sammel MD, Liu L, et al. Hormones and menopausal status as predictors of depression in womenin transition to menopause. Arch Gen Psychiatry 2004;61:62–70.
120. Cohen LS, Soares CN, Vitonis AF, et al. Risk for new onset of depression during the menopausal transition. The Harvard Study of Moods and Cycles Arch Gen Psychiatry 2006;63:385–90.

121. Bromberger JT, Kravitz HM, Chang Y-F, et al. Major depression during and after the menopausal transition: study of women's health across the nation (SWAN). Psychol Med 2011;41:1879–88.
122. Bromberger JT, Kravitz HM. Mood and menopause: findings from the study of Women's health across the nation (SWAN) over 10 years. Obstet Gynecol Clin North Am 2011;38:609–25.
123. Borrow AP, Cameron NM. Estrogenic mediation of serotonergic and neurotrophic systems: implications for female mood disorders. Prog Neuro-Psychopharmacol Biol Psychiatry 2014;54:13–25.
124. Soares CN. Mood disorders in midlife women: understanding the critical window and its clinical implications. Menopause 2014;21:198–206.
125. Bromberger JT, Chang Y, Colvin AB, et al. Does childhood maltreatment or current stress contribute to increased risk for major depression during the menopause transition? Psychol Med 2022;52:2570–7.
126. Cheng MH, Hsu CY, Wang SJ, et al. The relationship of self-reported sleep disturbance, mood, and menopause in a community study. Menopause 2008;15:958–62.
127. Hung HC, Lu FH, Ou HY, et al. Menopause is associated with self-reported poor sleep quality in women without vasomotor symptoms. Menopause 2014;21:834–9.
128. Kravitz HM, Ganz PA, Bromberger JT, et al. Sleep difficulty in women at midlife: a community survey of sleep and the menopausal transition. Menopause 2003;10:19–28.
129. Shin C, Lee S, Lee T, et al. Prevalence of insomnia and its relationship to menopausal status in middle-aged Korean women. Psychiatry Clin Neurosci 2005;59:395–402.
130. Young T, Rabago D, Zgierska A, et al. Objective and subjective sleep quality in premenopausal, perimenopausal, and postmenopausal women in the Wisconsin Sleep Cohort Study. Sleep 2003; 26:667–72.
131. Berecki-Gisolf J, Begum N, Dobson AJ. Symptoms reported by women in midlife: menopausal transition or aging? Menopause 2009;16:1021–9.
132. Kravitz HM, Zhao X, Bromberger JT, et al. Sleep disturbance during the menopausal transition in a multi-ethnic community sample of women. Sleep 2008;31:979–90.
133. Tom SE, Kuh D, Guralnik JM, et al. Self-reported sleep difficulty during the menopausal transition: results from a prospective cohort study. Menopause 2010;17:1128–35.
134. Woods NF, Mitchell ES. Sleep symptoms during the menopausal transition and early postmenopause: observations from the Seattle Midlife Women's Health Study. Sleep 2010;33:539–49.
135. Xu Q, Lang CP. Examining the relationship between subjective sleep disturbance and menopause: a systematic review and meta-analysis. Menopause 2014;21:1301–18.
136. Polo-Kantola P. Sleep problems in midlife and beyond. Maturitas 2011;68:224–32.
137. Freedman RR, Roehrs TA. Lack of sleep disturbance from menopausal hot flashes. Fertil Steril 2004;82:138–44.
138. Kalleinen N, Polo-Kantola P, Himanen SL, et al. Sleep and the menopause - do postmenopausal women experience worse sleep than premenopausal women? Menopause Int 2008;14:97–104.
139. Campbell IG, Bromberger JT, Buysse DJ, et al. Evaluation of the association of menopausal status with delta and beta EEG activity during sleep. Sleep 2011;34:1561–8.
140. Sharkey KM, Bearpark HM, Acebo C, et al. Effects of menopausal status on sleep in midlife women. Behav Sleep Med 2003;1:69–80.
141. Hachul H, Frange C, Bezerra AG, et al. The effect of menopause on objective sleep parameters: data from an epidemiologic study in Sao Paulo, Brazil. Maturitas 2015;80:170–8.
142. Lampio L, Polo-Kantola P, Himanen SL, et al. Sleep during menopausal transition: a 6-year follow-up. Sleep 2017;40(7). https://doi.org/10.1093/sleep/zsx090.
143. Kalleinen N, Aittokallio J, Lampio L, et al. Sleep during menopausal transition: a 10-year follow-up. Sleep 2021;44(6):zsaa283.
144. Vaari T, Engblom J, Helenius H, et al. Survey of sleep problems in 3421 women aged 41-55 years. Menopause Int 2008;14:78–82.
145. Polo-Kantola P, Laine A, Aromaa M, et al. A population-based survey of sleep disturbances in middle-aged women–associations with health, health related quality of life and health behavior. Maturitas 2014;77:255 62.
146. Avis NE, Crawford S, Stellato R, et al. Longitudinal study of hormone levels and depression among women transitioning through menopause. Climacteric 2001;4:243–9.
147. Kravitz HM, Colvin AB, Avis NE, et al. Risk of high depressive symptoms after the final menstrual period: the Study of Women's Health across the Nation (SWAN). Menopause 2022;29:805–15.
148. Bromberger JT, Kravitz HM, Youk A, et al. Patterns of depressive disorders across 13 years and their determinants among midlife women: SWAN mental health study. J Affect Disord 2016;206: 31–40.
149. Kravitz HM, Avery E, Sowers MF, et al. Relationships between menopausal and mood symptoms and EEG sleep measures in a multi-ethnic sample of middle-aged women: the SWAN Sleep Study. Sleep 2011;34:1221–32.
150. Joffe H, Petrillo LF, Koukopoulos A, et al. Increased estradiol and improved sleep, but not hot flashes,

predict enhanced mood during the menopausal transition. J Clin Endocrinol Metab 2011;96:E1044–54.
151. Schmidt PJ, Nieman L, Danaceau MA, et al. Estrogen replacement in perimenopause-related depression: a preliminary report. Am J Obstet Gynecol 2000;183:414–20.
152. Soares CN, Almeida OP, Joffe H, et al. Efficacy of estradiol for the treatment of depressive disorders in perimenopausal women: a double-blind, randomized, placebo-controlled trial. Arch. Gen Psychiatry 2001;58:529–34.
153. Cintron D, Lipford M, Larrea-Mantilla L, et al. Efficacy of menopausal hormone therapy on sleep quality: systematic review and meta-analysis. Endocrine 2017;55:702–11.
154. Polo-Kantola P, Erkkola R, Helenius H, et al. When does estrogen replacement therapy improve sleep quality? Am J Obstet Gynecol 1998;178:1002–9.
155. Fiona C, Baker FC, Lampio L, Saaresranta T, et al. Sleep and sleep disorders in the menopausal transition. Sleep Med Clin 2018;13:443–56.

The Menstrual Cycle and Sleep

Elisabet Alzueta, PhD[a], Fiona C. Baker, PhD[a,b,*]

KEYWORDS

• Sleep • Menstrual cycle • Follicular • Luteal • Reproduction

KEY POINTS

- Self-reported sleep disturbance can emerge during premenstrual and menstruation phases of the menstrual cycle, particularly in women with moderate–severe premenstrual symptoms (PMS/PMDD), irregular cycles, or painful menstrual cramps (dysmenorrhea).
- Objective measures of sleep continuity show no significant variation across the cycle in young women without menstrual-related complaints; however, perimenstrual sleep disturbances (eg, poorer sleep efficiency or more awakenings) may emerge in women in the late-reproductive years.
- There is a marked menstrual cycle-related change in sleep spindle activity in the electroencephalogram, which is increased in the luteal relative to the follicular phase, possibly due to an effect of progesterone and/or its metabolites.
- Although sleep can be affected by reproductive hormone variations, the reverse relationship is also evident such that sleep disturbance and/or altered sleep timing is associated with altered reproductive function.

INTRODUCTION

From menarche or first menstrual period, to menopause that signals the end of reproduction, women experience monthly variations in hormones that regulate reproduction. These hormones have widespread effects outside their direct reproductive functions, including influences on regulating mood, body temperature, respiration, autonomic nervous system, and sleep. This review updates an earlier review from 2018,[1] delving into the complex relationship between the menstrual cycle and sleep, focusing on perceived sleep quality, objective measures of sleep continuity and sleep architecture, as well as sleep-related physiological changes in homeostatic and circadian regulation of body temperature and heart rate, at different phases of the menstrual cycle. We discuss sleep disturbances in the context of the menstrual cycle across the reproductive years and consider relationships between sleep and infertility, use of oral contraceptives (OCs), and menstrual-associated disorders, including polycystic ovary syndrome (PCOS), premenstrual dysphoric disorder (PMDD), and dysmenorrhea.

DEFINITIONS AND MENSTRUAL CYCLE PHYSIOLOGY

Most women have menstrual cycle lengths between 21 and 30 days, with menses lasting less than 7 days.[2] The menstrual cycle is divided into a preovulatory follicular phase and postovulatory luteal phase, with onset of menstrual flow marking the beginning of a new cycle (Day 1) (**Fig. 1**).

During the follicular phase, follicle-stimulating hormone and luteinizing hormone (LH) are released from the anterior pituitary and act on the ovaries to initiate the development of several primary follicles, which produce estrogens, principally estradiol. At the end of the follicular phase, estrogen levels increase, triggering a peak in LH. Ovulation occurs 12 to 16 hours later, around day 14. Following ovulation, the corpus luteum develops, producing progesterone and estrogen, which peak 5 to 7 days after ovulation before

[a] Human Sleep Research Program, SRI International, Menlo Park, CA, USA; [b] Brain Function Research Group, School of Physiology, University of the Witwatersrand, Johannesburg, South Africa
* Corresponding author. SRI International, 333 Ravenswood Avenue, Menlo Park, CA 94025.
E-mail address: Fiona.Baker@sri.com

Sleep Med Clin 18 (2023) 399–413
https://doi.org/10.1016/j.jsmc.2023.06.003

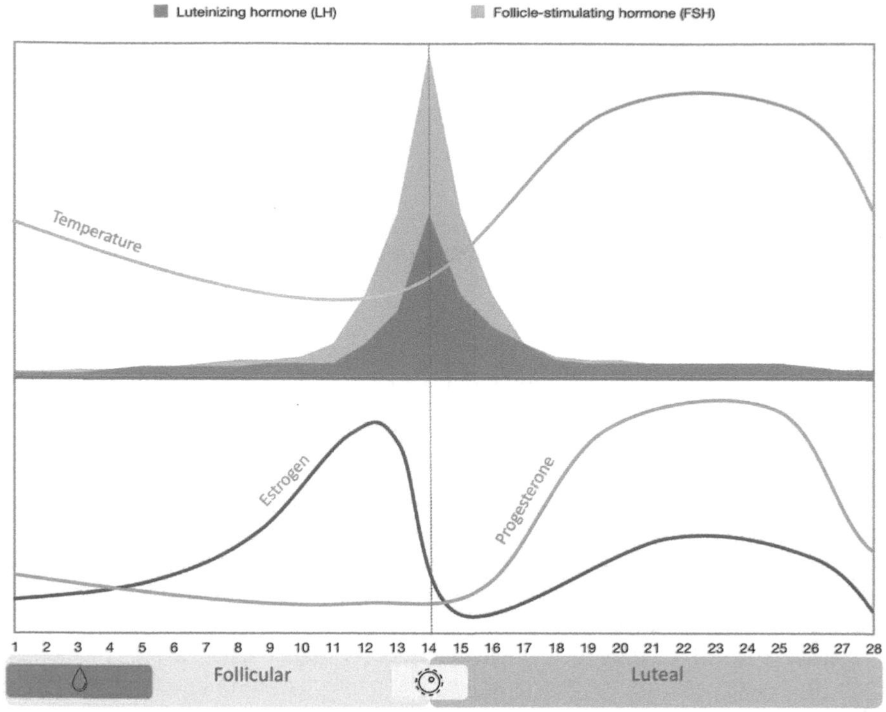

Fig. 1. Changes in hormones and temperature across a typical 28-day ovulatory menstrual cycle, where 1 represent the first day of bleeding and 14 the day of ovulation.

declining (in the absence of implantation), resulting in endometrial breakdown and menstruation.

Estrogen and progesterone receptors are widely distributed throughout the central nervous system (CNS), including the basal forebrain, hypothalamus, dorsal raphe nucleus, and locus coeruleus.[3,4] These areas are also involved in sleep regulation, and fluctuations in ovarian steroids across the menstrual cycle can modulate sleep. Indeed, studies in rodents show that sleep patterns fluctuate in concert with natural fluctuations of ovarian steroids and ovariectomy eliminates these fluctuations in sleep, with effects dependent on time of day.[5,6] Although ovarian steroids' mechanisms of action on sleep regulation are not completely clear, both sleep-promoting and wake-promoting areas of the CNS are sensitive to the effects of estrogen. Ovarian steroids can also influence circadian rhythms, including of sleep–wake activity, through direct or indirect effects on the master pacemaker—the suprachiasmatic nucleus. The mechanistic framework is therefore in place for menstrual cycle-related changes in reproductive hormones to influence sleep and circadian rhythms.

SLEEP AND MENARCHE

Women are at higher risk than men of suffering from insomnia symptoms and disorder,[7] due to many factors. Menarche is a critical time window for the emergence of a sex difference in insomnia—which persists throughout adulthood,[8] and fluctuations and transitions in gonadal hormones in women could be one factor that leads them to be vulnerable to insomnia across their reproductive life. After menarche, as menstrual cycles become established, menstrual pain becomes highly prevalent, affecting 84.1% of young women,[9] and is a leading cause of recurrent short-term school absenteeism.[10] There is limited research investigating sleep quality in the context of the menstrual cycle and menstrual-associated symptoms in adolescents; however, evidence suggests that menstrual pain is commonly associated with sleep disturbances, which could in turn negatively affect academic performance.[11] Irregular menstrual cycles are also associated with sleep disturbances (insomnia symptoms),[12] as well as daytime sleepiness.[13] However, a longer sleep duration is associated with a lower prevalence of menstrual cycle irregularity.[14] This body of research about sleep quality in the context of adolescent menstrual health has mostly relied on retrospective questionnaires and further research is needed to evaluate how menstrual cycle features and sleep correlate, what might be the directionality of this relationship, and to what extent this interaction affects academic performance and well-being during the teenager years. Effective interventions for the management of menstruation, including menstrual pain and menstrual hygiene, have been successfully applied in girls from low-income and middle-income countries,[15,16] with the aspiration of benefitting academic performance, improving school attendance and well-being. Effectiveness of such interventions for better sleep quality, which in turn could contribute to better educational outcomes, remains to be seen.

SLEEP AND CIRCADIAN RHYTHMS ACROSS THE MENSTRUAL CYCLE

Self-Reported Sleep Quality

Collectively, studies in adult women show that sleep disturbances are more commonly reported around the time of menstruation, encompassing the last few premenstrual days (late luteal phase) and first few days of menstrual bleeding (early follicular phase).[17–20] However, not all studies find a menstrual cycle effect on sleep quality[21,22] or find only small effects,[23] possibly reflecting between-individual variability in the relationship between sleep and menstrual cycle phase. Van Reen and Kiesner[24] identified 3 different patterns of variation in self-reported sleep difficulty across the menstrual cycle among their 213 participants: one group (46%) showed no relationship, a second group (25%) showed a midcycle increase in difficulty sleeping, and a third group (29%) showed a perimenstrual increase in difficulty sleeping. Psychological and vegetative symptoms (eg, anxiety, depression, headaches, cramps, and breast tenderness) significantly predicted difficulty sleeping.[24] The extent that ovarian hormones directly contribute to perceived sleep disturbance, versus other factors that vary with the menstrual cycle, remains unclear. Changes in progesterone and estrogen, rather than absolute levels, in the late-luteal phase may be a critical factor for sleep quality. Menstrual cycle characteristics are also relevant: women with irregular cycles report more sleep difficulties compared with women with regular cycles, even when controlling for age, body mass index (BMI), dysmenorrhea, and premenstrual complaints.[25] Irregular menstrual cycles and heavy bleeding were associated with poor sleep (ie, shorter sleep duration, poorer sleep quality, and fatigue) and poor mental health (stress and depression) in a racially and socioeconomically diverse community sample of women aged 22 to 60 years.[26]

Objective Sleep Measures

Sleep across the menstrual cycle has been studied objectively with research-grade actigraphy, wearable sleep technology, and polysomnography (PSG). Actigraphy and consumer wearables can be easily used to track changes in daily sleep–wake activity in a large number of participants; however, few studies have investigated menstrual cycle-related patterns in sleep using these devices. In a small study of 19 women (18–43 years), actigraphy-measured sleep efficiency (SE) was positively associated with 1-day-lagged estrogen metabolites and negatively with 1-day-lagged progesterone metabolites, although effects were weak and self-reported sleep was unassociated with hormone metabolites.[22] The Study of Women's Health Across the Nation (SWAN), which is tracking women as they transition from late-reproductive stage to postmenopause, has included actigraphy in a subsample of the group,[27] representing the largest sample of women in whom objective sleep measures are available across the menstrual cycle. In this group of 163 late-reproductive aged women (age range: 48–59 years), there was a significant decline in SE and total sleep time (TST) in the premenstrual week relative to the prior week, with greater effects associated with obesity, financial strain, smoking, and a greater apnea hypopnea index.[27] In a more recent study, the Oura ring was used to track physiological changes across the ovulatory menstrual cycle in 26 early reproductive (18–35 years old) women.[21] No significant variation across the menstrual cycle was found in sleep continuity measures, in agreement with the women's self-reported sleep quality. Importantly, this group of women had no to low premenstrual symptoms and their mood symptoms remained stable across the cycle. In a study specifically focused on collegiate female athletes (n = 45), at-home electroencephalograph (EEG) monitoring was used to examine differences in sleep on the first and second nights after menses onset compared with one night between the 7th and 10th night after menses (midfollicular phase).[28] Women had a shorter TST and a longer sleep onset latency (SOL) on the second night of menstruation (but not on the first night of menses) compared with the midfollicular phase. However, these results need to be interpreted cautiously because they refect a particular subgroup of women (ie, athletes) and authors did not control for the presence of menstrual pain, which was reported in 60% of the sample.

Laboratory-based PSG has been used in small numbers of women to compare sleep between discrete menstrual cycle phases, such as midfollicular versus midluteal phase. Major findings for PSG measures in these 2 phases are summarized in **Table 1**. A foundational study by Driver and colleagues[29] tracked changes in PSG measures of

Table 1
Summary of evidence comparing objective sleep and related physiological measures during the luteal phase relative to the follicular phase of the natural menstrual cycle

	Variable	Luteal (Relative to Follicular)
Sleep continuity		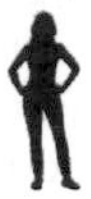 Early and late reproductive stage 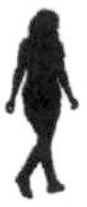
	TST	No change in young women/decreased actigraphic TST in late-reproductive women – but only when comparing the premenstrual week vs the prior week[a]
	SOL	No change
	SE	No change in young women/Decreased actigraphic SE in late-reproductive women – but only when comparing the premenstrual week vs the prior week[a]
	Wakefulness and awakenings (WASO)	Most studies show no change in young women/More PSG awakenings in late-reproductive women[b]
Sleep architecture	SWS and slow wave EEG activity	No change in young women/Decreased in late-reproductive women[a]
	REM sleep	Decrease in duration of REM sleep episodes
	Sigma EEG activity (spindle frequency range)	Increased activity associated with increased spindle density and duration
	N2 sleep	Most studies find no change
Sleep-related features	Body temperature	Increased body temperature rhythm, with reduced amplitude due to blunted nocturnal decline. No change in circadian phase
	Melatonin	No change in circadian phase or amplitude
	Heart rate	Increased (~4 bpm) - associated with decreased vagal activity
	Upper airway resistance	Lower[c]

[a] Data available from only one study.[27]
[b] Data available from only one study.[40]
[c] Data available from only one study.[122]

sleep recorded every second night across an entire menstrual cycle in 9 young women, with phases carefully characterized. They found that SOL, wakefulness after sleep onset (WASO), and SE were stable across the menstrual cycle.[30] N2 sleep was increased and rapid eye movement (REM) sleep tended to decline in the luteal phase relative to the follicular phase; however, there was no change in the amount of slow wave sleep (SWS) or slow wave activity (SWA) across the menstrual cycle,[29] indicating no change in this marker of sleep homeostasis across the menstrual cycle. Analysis of SWA by sleep cycle did reveal subtle changes, however higher SWA was found in the first non-REM sleep episode and lower activity in the second non-REM episode in the midluteal phase compared with midfollicular phase.[30]

Other studies have mostly confirmed no difference in SWS or SWA between follicular and luteal phases in young women, although inconsistencies remain (See reviews[30,31]). Others have also found variability in REM sleep with menstrual cycle phase: REM sleep had an earlier onset[32] and REM sleep episodes were shorter,[30,33] with amount of REM sleep negatively correlating with progesterone and estradiol levels in the luteal phase.[33] Using a careful ultra-rapid sleep–wake cycle procedure, Shechter and Boivin[17] also found that REM sleep was decreased (at circadian phase 0° and 30°) in the luteal phase compared with follicular phase. This reduction in REM sleep may relate to the raised body temperature in the luteal phase because heat loss mechanisms are inhibited during REM sleep.[34]

Finally, most studies support Driver and colleagues'[29] findings of no menstrual cycle variability in sleep continuity PSG measures in young women, although 2 studies found more wakefulness/awakenings in the late luteal phase[35,36] and one study found that a steeper increase in progesterone from follicular to early-mid luteal phase was associated with WASO in the luteal phase.[37] Inconsistencies in PSG findings could reflect the individual variability in effects of the menstrual cycle on sleep and reflect methodological challenges with in-laboratory studies, such as small sample sizes, differences in sampling times across the menstrual cycle (occurring at discrete intervals), as well as differences in menstrual cycle characteristics and demographic factors such as age. As for self-reported sleep, there may be clusters of women, some who may have changes in sleep continuity at transitions between the follicular and luteal phase (ie, around ovulation) and/or premenstrually or during menses, potentially in association with mood and physical symptoms. Laboratory-based PSG studies and even the few studies with wearables, actigraphy, or home-based EEG measures have had small samples or have not examined if there are different clusters of women who show variability in menstrual cycle effects on sleep.

The most dramatic and consistent menstrual cycle change in sleep is in EEG activity in the 14.25 to 15.0 Hz (sigma) band corresponding to the upper frequency range of sleep spindles, which is significantly increased in the luteal compared with the follicular phase.[29,33,38,39] This increase in spindle frequency activity is associated with an increased spindle density and duration.[40] The mechanism for luteal phase increases in spindle activity is unknown; however, it may involve modulation of Gamma-aminobutyric acid (GABA)-A receptors by progesterone metabolites.[29] Given the supposed sleep-protective function of spindles,[41] increased spindles may function to maintain sleep quality in the presence of luteal phase hormonal changes.[31] Some studies have explored the functional relevance of increased sleep spindle activity in the luteal phase, given their role in sleep-dependent memory consolidation.[42] During sleep, the brain replays and strengthens memories that were acquired during the day, a process that is essential for solidifying new memories. Spindles are thought to be involved in this process of transferring information from short-term to long-term memory storage. Studies that have investigated menstrual cycle-related modulation of sleep-dependent memory consolidation have shown poorer consolidation during menses or early follicular phase than other times of the menstrual cycle.[43,44] Genzel and colleagues[43] assessed motor and declarative performance on a memory task following a nap in men and in women at 2 time points of their cycle: early follicular (first week of the cycle) and luteal phase (third week of the cycle). Although men performed better after a nap, women only benefitted from a nap in the luteal phase of their cycle. Critically, women in the luteal phase and men experienced a significant increase in spindle activity after learning—an effect not seen in women in the early follicular phase of the menstrual cycle. Estradiol levels correlated with spindle density and frequency in women.[43] These data show that hormonal and associated changes in spindle activity across the menstrual cycle are linked with changes in declarative memory consolidation during sleep.

Circadian Rhythms

Hormonal variations across the menstrual cycle are also associated with changes in circadian rhythms. Body temperature is increased by about 0.4 C[45] due to the thermogenic action of progesterone and has a smaller amplitude due to a blunted nocturnal decline, in the luteal phase compared with follicular phase[35] (see[40] for a review). Using an ultra-short sleep–wake cycle procedure to control for light, posture, and food intake, Shechter and colleagues[47] confirmed a reduced amplitude and found no difference in phase for core temperature rhythms in the luteal phase. In freely living women, a menstrual cycle-related change in skin temperature is detectable with a wearable device: Alzueta and colleagues[21] found that distal skin temperature measured with the Oura ring increased in the postovulation luteal phase relative to menses and periovulatory phases in a group of healthy young women. There was also a smaller-magnitude periovulatory drop in skin temperature, which corresponds to the phase when estrogen surges. This study supports other studies examining changes in temperature across the cycle using wearables[48–50] and together, data suggest that the ovulatory period can be identified with skin temperature measurement, a relevant finding in the context of fertility prediction.

Melatonin plays an important role in reproduction (eg, oocyte maturation, fertilization, and embryonic development),[51] and it may have a role in the regulation of the menstrual cycle through interactions with the frequency of gonadotropin-releasing hormone pulses.[52] Studies that have examined melatonin circadian rhythms in controlled conditions (eg, forced desynchrony protocols) found that melatonin acrophase, onset, and offset did not differ between the follicular and luteal phases of the menstrual cycle of young women.[47,53,54] Two of these studies also found no menstrual-cycle differences in amplitude of the melatonin rhythm.[47,54] Although melatonin rhythm characteristics do not differ across the cycle, studies of melatonin levels in uncontrolled conditions have found variation across the cycle, which could reflect its role in reproductive function. For example, in a cross-sectional SWAN study of 20 perimenopausal (ie, still menstruating) women, Greendale and colleagues[55] analyzed overnight urinary levels of a melatonin metabolite, aMT6, and metabolites of estrogen and progesterone across the menstrual cycle. They identified a cyclic increase in aMT6 in the late-luteal phase of the menstrual cycle. A luteal increase in a metabolite of progesterone (Pregnanediol Glucuronide) predicted the aMT6 increase, suggesting that the late-luteal melatonin peak might be signaled by progesterone. In the longitudinal portion of this study, the aMT6 excretion patterns when women were no longer menstruating (ie, postmenopause) showed no organized pattern. Further, the total amount of aMT6s excretion declined by 30% in the postmenopausal collections compared with the premenopausal ones, an effect that could be due to chronological and/or reproductive aging (menopause).

SLEEP AND POLYCYSTIC OVARY SYNDROME

The most common endocrine disorder for reproductive-age women is PCOS. PCOS affects 5% to 20% of women, depending on age, type of epidemiological survey, and diagnostic criteria.[56] High testosterone levels, clinical signs of hyperandrogenism, and irregular or absent (ie, anovulation) menstrual cycles may occur, and polycystic ovaries may or may not be present. PCOS is associated with important cardiovascular and metabolic comorbidities such as obesity and insulin resistance[57,58] and psychological distress.[59] Between 50% and 60% of women with PCOS are obese[60] and are at increased risk for sleep-disordered breathing (SDB) particularly when of older age.[61] Treatments for PCOS includes hormonal treatment to lower testosterone levels.[62] OCs are effective in managing menstrual cycle irregularity, acne, and hirsutism. Metformin is indicated for weight reduction and insulin resistance as well as hirsutism.[63]

Women diagnosed with PCOS often experience sleep problems. They are significantly more likely to report difficulty falling sleep, even after adjusting for factors such as BMI and depressive symptoms.[64,65] Moreover, the prevalence of insomnia is higher in women with PCOS (10.5% scored >14 on the insomnia severity index, reflecting insomnia) compared with healthy controls.[60] Daytime sleepiness would be an expected outcome of poor sleep but findings are mixed when women with PCOS are compared with controls. Franik and colleagues[60] found no difference in the rate of daytime sleepiness. Conversely, Vgzontzas and colleagues[62] found a high prevalence of daytime sleepiness in women with PCOS (80.4%) compared with controls (27%).

PCOS has also been linked to differences in sleep architecture, with obese adolescents and adult women with PCOS experiencing a longer time to fall asleep, lower SE, and less time in REM sleep than controls. Yet, these findings may be influenced by factors such as SDB. Women with PCOS are at an increased risk of SDB during their reproductive years and are more likely to report excessive daytime sleepiness (80% vs 27% in controls).[66] It is likely that excessive weight, specifically central obesity contributes to high risk for SDB in women with PCOS.[67] Severity of SDB has been found to be connected to issues with glucose tolerance and insulin resistance in women with PCOS, indicating that SDB may play a role in the metabolic irregularities in these women (see ref[66] for a review). Beyond affecting insulin sensitivity, it is still uncertain if sleep disturbances have other effects on the development of PCOS. One study used frequent blood sampling and PSG to examine the relationship between sleep architecture and LH pulse initiation in women with PCOS.[68] In healthy women, in the mid-to-late follicular phase, LH pulses were more likely to occur after/during wake epochs and less likely to occur after/during REM epochs. However, in women with PCOS, the interaction between sleep architecture and LH pulses differed, with LH pulses more likely to occur after/during SWS and no evidence of a relationship between LH pulses and REM sleep. Authors suggest that the lack of appropriate inhibition of LH pulse initiation in REM sleep in PCOS may contribute to high-sleep LH pulse frequency, and thus ovarian hyperandrogenemia and ovulatory dysfunction.[68]

Finally, it has been proposed that dysrhythmia (abnormal or irregular rhythm of certain physiological processes) affects the function of the ovaries and is one of the underlying causes of PCOS.[69,70] As a systemic hormone modulator, melatonin may play a role in this process although it is unclear if there are abnormalities in melatonin secretion in women with PCOS.[71] Local melatonin levels in the ovary may be more relevant: Li and colleagues[72] examined levels of melatonin in the ovarian microenvironment in women receiving in vitro fertilization treatment of PCOS and non-PCOS reasons; melatonin levels in follicular fluid were lower in women with PCOS compared to other women.

SLEEP AND PREMENSTRUAL SYNDROME

Premenstrual syndrome (PMS) is characterized by emotional, behavioral, and physical symptoms that manifest almost exclusively in the late-luteal (premenstrual) phase, with resolution soon after onset of menses. Although many women experience some symptoms premenstrually, up to 18% have severe symptoms that affect daily function.[73] PMDD is a severe form of PMS evident in 3% to 8% and classified as a depressive disorder in the American Psychiatric Association's Diagnostic and Statistical Manual of Mental Disorders (DSM-5).[73] A PMDD diagnosis requires the occurrence of 5 specified symptoms, of which at least one must be a mood-related symptom experienced in the late-luteal phase, documented for at least 2 consecutive cycles. One of these symptoms is sleep disturbance (insomnia or hypersomnia). Etiology of PMDD remains unclear although symptoms are effectively managed with selective serotonin reuptake inhibitors, anxiolytics, and ovulation-suppressing agents.[74,75]

Perceived Sleep Quality and Daytime Sleepiness

Several studies have found that women with PMS report a poorer sleep quality than other women overall, based on retrospective sleep quality assessments (ie, not considering menstrual cycle phase). PMS has been associated with a 2-fold higher risk for poor sleep.[76] Similarly, in a study of female university students (67 with severe PMS/PMDD symptoms and 195 controls), the PMS/PMDD group was more likely than controls to report poor sleep quality based on a score of greater than 5 on the PSQI (80.5% vs 56.4%).[77] Sleep disturbance, daytime dysfunction, and use of sleep medications were all more prevalent in the PMS/PMDD group, although self-reported sleep duration, SOL, and SE did not significantly differ between groups. There may be both trait (across the menstrual cycle) and state (in conjunction with other symptoms) differences in women with PMS/PMDD compared with controls.[78] Trait-like symptoms may then magnify in the presence of the hormonal changes associated with the premenstrual phase. Women with severe PMS frequently report late-luteal phase sleep symptoms, including insomnia, disturbing dreams, poor sleep quality, daytime sleepiness, and fatigue.[78–80] One laboratory-based study found that women with PMS/PMDD reported more awakenings and felt less refreshed on awakening compared with controls in both the follicular and late-luteal phases, and also reported worse sleep quality in their late-luteal phase relative to their own follicular phase.[33]

A few researchers have investigated the second type of sleep disturbance (hypersomnia) listed in the DSM-5 for the diagnosis of PMDD. Mauri[81] found that PMS clinic patients reported greater daytime sleepiness in luteal and menstruation phases than other times of the menstrual cycle. Similarly, women with PMS symptoms were sleepier and less alert in late-luteal phase than in follicular phase, an effect not found in controls in another study.[82] In a survey of 269 young women, women with PMS were more likely to report daytime sleepiness and fatigue premenstrually than controls.[80] Based on objective measures, women with PMS showed psychomotor slowing, with increased lapses and slower reaction times, corresponding with their perceived greater late-luteal levels of sleepiness and fatigue compared with their follicular phase and compared with controls.[83] However, waking EEG measures of alertness and cognitive processing, as well as SOL on the maintenance of wakefulness task, did not differentiate PMS women when symptomatic, although there were some trait differences.[83]

Objective Sleep and Melatonin Function

Despite evidence of perceived poor sleep quality and greater daytime sleepiness in the late-luteal phase in women with PMS/PMDD, laboratory studies show little evidence of disturbed PSG sleep parameters specific to this phase. Most studies show no change in sleep efficiency, arousals, SOL, or sleep EEG in late-luteal phase relative to follicular phase.[31,33,78] Perception of poor sleep quality in late-luteal phase may be a component of the symptom profile of PMS in the absence of actual sleep disruption, as sleep quality correlated with anxiety in women with PMS/PMDD in late-luteal phase.[33] However, 2 studies[33,84] found increased SWS in PMS and PMDD subjects in both the follicular and luteal phase of the menstrual cycle compared with controls. Differences found in PSG measures at both phases of the menstrual cycle suggest trait differences in sleep, although the nature of these differences varies between studies.[31,78] Age may influence the severity of sleep disruption in association with symptoms; findings indicate that women aged older than 40 years with PMS report more frequent awakenings than younger women[85];

however, PSG studies have not been powered to investigate age-PMS interactions.

Shechter and colleagues have gone further to examine abnormalities in melatonin secretion in women with PMDD. They found that women with PMDD had lower nocturnal melatonin levels under controlled conditions at both menstrual phases compared with controls, suggesting a trait difference,[86] which could underlie the higher SWS found in PMDD.[84] A decreased melatonin amplitude in the symptomatic luteal phase was also evident, suggesting an additional sensitivity to the altered ovarian hormone environment (ie, state difference) in PMDD.[86] Parry and colleagues[87] also found disturbances in melatonin rhythms and timing of rhythms for cortisol and thyroid stimulating hormone, suggesting that circadian regulation disturbances may be a factor in PMDD. Melatonin therefore has been proposed as a potential treatment to modulate PMS/PMDD symptoms. In a recent study, Moderie and colleagues[88] investigated the efficacy of exogenous melatonin on sleep in 5 women with PMDD. Melatonin administration in the luteal phase during 3 consecutive cycles led to a reduction of SWS together with a reduction in PMDD symptoms. Importantly, these changes were independent from melatonin effects on circadian phase, temperature, or steroidogenesis. Moreover, light therapy in women with and without PMDD has been investigated with positive outcomes for mood.[89] Further clinical trials in larger samples are needed to establish the role of disturbed melatonin function in PMDD as well as the potential efficacy of circadian-related treatments, including light therapy, for PMDD.

SLEEP AND DYSMENORRHEA

Dysmenorrhea, defined as painful menstrual cramps of uterine origin, is either primary (menstrual pain without organic disease that typically emerges in adolescence) or secondary (associated with conditions such as endometriosis and pelvic inflammatory disease). The relationship between primary dysmenorrhea and sleep is detailed elsewhere in a prior review (Shaver and Iacovides, 2018). Briefly, evidence indicates that when severe, dysmenorrhea negatively affects sleep, daytime function, and mood,[12,90–92] and PSG studies also indicate sleep disturbances (lower SE) in association with painful menses.[93,94] Sleep and pain share a reciprocal relationship.[95] Breaking this pain–sleep cycle could be critical for long-term health of women with primary dysmenorrhea who show increased pain sensitization.[96] One study showed promising effects of a nonsteroidal anti-inflammatory drug that alleviated nocturnal pain and restored sleep quality in women with primary dysmenorrhea.[94] Moreover, exercise therapy has been shown to be effective in reducing pain severity and improving sleep quality in women with dysmenorrhea.[97]

SLEEP AND HORMONAL CONTRACEPTIVES

Combined OCs contain ethinyl estradiol and a synthetic progestin taken for 21 days, and a placebo taken for 7 days. During the 21-day period, hypothalamic pituitary ovarian axis activity is suppressed and endogenous estradiol and progesterone levels are low, similar to levels in follicular phase for nonusers.[98] Across most of the 7-day placebo period, estrogen levels remain suppressed. New formulations contain the minimum steroid doses necessary to inhibit ovulation.[99] As such, levels of estrogen and progestin in today's OCs are lower than in older formulations, which needs to be considered when comparing studies.

The few studies that have examined PSG measures in women taking OCs have not found an increased sleep disruption or poorer sleep quality; however, sleep architecture is altered. Women had about 12% more N2 sleep on a night during the 21-day period of active pill compared with a night in the 7-day placebo period.[100] They also have more N2 sleep and less N3 (SWS) than naturally cycling women in luteal phase,[100–102] and possibly a shorter REM onset latency.[102] One study also examined effects of OC use on the sleep EEG, showing that the use of a synthetic progestin (medroxyprogesterone) was associated with an increased upper spindle frequency activity and greater sleep spindle density in women,[103] similar to natural luteal phase effects. Hachul and colleagues[25] found that women using OCs had a lower apnea hypopnea index,[104] as well as shorter latency to REM sleep and fewer arousals.[25] From this study, it could be hypothesized that taking OCs might have a beneficial effect on sleep. However, as shown in a recent meta-analysis, the use of OCs seems to have minimal benefit on the main features of sleep.[105]

Other effects of OC use include increased 24-hour body temperature profiles, similar to the natural luteal phase, probably due to progestin. This increased temperature profile persists during the 7-day placebo period,[101] which contrasts with the rapid decline in temperature as progesterone levels decline before menstruation in ovulatory cycles. OCs may also influence the melatonin profile, although findings are inconsistent.[35] In one study using a modified constant routine procedure, melatonin levels did not differ between naturally cycling women and women taking OCs, although there was a trend for increased melatonin in the latter part of the night in the OC group.[54]

In summary, OCs alter aspects of sleep architecture as well as body temperature, although their impact on sleep quality seems to be minimal. Given the lower doses of hormones in current OCs, it remains to be seen if their effects on sleep architecture and temperature differ from that of prior formulations.

IMPACT OF SLEEP ON REPRODUCTIVE FUNCTION

Sleep duration, timing, and quality can influence the reproductive system, and particular sleep stages are also important for reproductive maturity: During puberty, LH is released in a pulsatile fashion during N3, playing a critical role in reproductive regulation.[106,107] In adulthood, the direction of this relationship changes in the early follicular phase, with sleep inhibiting LH secretion, which may be necessary for the recruitment of ovarian follicles.[108]

Shiftwork and Menstrual Cycle Rhythms

There are reports of associations between short sleep duration and altered menstrual cycles. Women reporting less than 6 hours sleep were more likely to report abnormal (short or long) menstrual cycle lengths.[109] There has been a larger body of work investigating the impact of shiftwork on reproductive function in women, given the typical disrupted sleep and circadian patterns in this group, as reviewed in detail elsewhere.[110] In general, observational studies have provided evidence for reproductive disturbances such as menstrual irregularity and subfertility in women shift workers.[111] For example, a 2014 meta-analysis of 4 studies involving 28,479 women suggested that shift workers experience higher rates of infertility.[112] Similarly, a meta-analysis of 4 studies involving 71,681 women suggested that shift workers experience higher rates of menstrual disruption (cycles less than 25 days or greater than 31 days) compared with nonshift workers.[112] Some evidence suggests that shift work, particularly night-shift work, may lead to fertility problems and increased risk for miscarriage; however, the effect size is uncertain.[113] Meta-analyses of the literature investigating the association between various working conditions and fetal and maternal health concluded that shiftwork poses minimal risk to the female reproductive system[114] and that there is insufficient evidence for clinicians to advise restricting shiftwork in reproductive-age women.[112] However, several professional bodies on health and safety state that shift work, particularly night shift work, may increase the risk for menstrual cycle disruption or pregnancy complications. The nature of the relationship between shiftwork and reproductive health remains unclear but it could relate to increased stress, disrupted circadian rhythms and/or sleep, which influence reproductive hormone secretion, particularly LH and follicle stimulation hormone (FSH).

Sleep During in Vitro Fertilization

In vitro fertilization (IVF) is a widely used assisted reproductive technology because it offers a solution for infertility and other reproductive issues. Emerging study has begun to examine the impact of sleep on IVF outcomes because sleep can affect various physiological processes that play a role in the success of the treatment, such as hormone regulation, immune function, and stress levels. Sleep disturbances are commonly reported throughout the IVF treatment process.[115] A pilot study of 22 women that used subjective and objective measures found that almost half of the group has short actigraphic TST (<7 hours) at baseline, and this percentage remained high across IVF treatment until postembryo transfer. Daytime sleepiness was also common in the group and increased significantly from baseline to stimulation.[116] There was a trend for a positive association of TST with oocytes retrieved in this small sample, suggesting that sleep duration may be an important factor for IVF success. Another study using actigraphy[117] showed an association between shorter sleep duration and higher rates of implantation failure. Poor sleep quality may be a risk factor for adverse IVF embryo transfer,[118] whereas good sleep quality has been associated with successful outcomes in IVF treatments, including higher rates of clinical pregnancy and live birth.[118] It should be acknowledged, however, that the association between sleep and reproductive function may be bidirectional. Disturbed sleep may interfere with fertility but the distress associated with infertility can also contribute to a poor sleep quality and shorter sleep.[119] Reschini and colleagues[120] examined sleep quality and psychological health (ie, infertility-related distress and symptoms of anxiety and depression) in women undergoing IVF treatment. Although results showed that only sleep quality was linked with IVF treatment success, they concluded the association between poor sleep quality and lower chances of pregnancy were mediated by a poorer psychological health. Further longitudinal studies of larger samples of women preparing for and undergoing IVF are required to fully understand the role of sleep in the success of IVF outcomes.

SLEEP AND LATE-REPRODUCTIVE STAGE

Women show a dramatic increase in sleep disturbance when they approach menopause (ie, during the transition to perimenopause to menopause).[121] Self-reported sleep complaints in the midlife years are more likely during the premenstrual week and during the first few days of menstruation compared with other times of the cycle. For example, the Study of Women's Health Across the Nation (SWAN), which included women in their late reproductive years and women entering the menopausal transition, reported that self-report sleep disturbance varied with cycle phase, being more likely to occur during the late luteal and early follicular phases of the menstrual cycle.[18] After controlling for cycle day and other confounders, poorer sleep quality was associated with hormonal factors, although relationships differed depending on reproductive stage: higher levels of a progesterone metabolite, pregnanediol glucuronide, in urine were related to more trouble sleeping in the perimenopausal group, and higher urine FSH levels were related to more sleeping complaints in the premenopausal group.[18]

Menstrual cycle-related changes may affect sleep more prominently with advancing age: although hormone levels were not measured, a large actigraphy study of late-reproductive aged women in SWAN, found a 5% decline in SE and a 25-minute decrease in TST in the premenstrual week relative to the prior week,[27] and a small PSG study found that women in the menopausal transition who were still cycling had more awakenings and arousals, as well as less N3 sleep in the luteal phase compared with the follicular phase[40] effects that are not observed in most studies of younger women. Although there was no change in slow-wave EEG activity, the upper frequency range of sleep spindles significantly increase in the luteal phase compared with the follicular phase.[40] Interestingly, midlife women with insomnia showed a blunted increase in sigma EEG activity in the luteal phase, possibly reflecting a weaker influence of the menstrual cycle on sleep EEG in the presence of insomnia.[40] Further investigation is necessary to examine distinct trajectories of sleep disturbance across the menstrual cycle in the context of sex hormone levels, menopausal symptoms, and age.

SUMMARY

Aspects of sleep and circadian rhythms are altered in association with the hormonal changes of the menstrual cycle, with negative effects on sleep most evident in the presence of menstrual-associated disorders. The magnitude of effect varies, particularly for self-reported sleep quality, which worsens in some, but not all, women when premenstrual symptoms emerge. For research purposes, effects of menstrual cycle phase should be kept in mind when data are collected, and ideally, phase should be documented. There are diverse menstrual cycle profiles such that intersubject variability needs to be accounted when studying sleep. When comparing aspects of sleep (eg, sleep spindles) between women and men, women of reproductive age should ideally be studied in the follicular phase before there is potential influence from the increase in progesterone. Women's lives are marked by significant hormonal fluctuations during (ie, menstrual cycle) and across (ie, puberty, menopause) their reproductive years that can affect sleep, which has consequences for their physical, mental and emotional wellbeing. Sleep is an essential behavior that needs to be prioritized in the context of women's health. Providing women with menstrual health education, necessary resources, and psychosocial support to manage the effects of hormonal changes can help them navigate potential challenges to sleep that may accompany these transformative phases.

CLINICS CARE POINTS

- Sleep is an essential behavior that needs to be prioritized for women's health.
- Women should be provided with menstrual health education, necessary resources, and psychosocial support to manage the effects of hormonal changes on sleep.

FUNDING

This study was supported by the National Institutes of Health (NIH) grant RF1AG061355 (Baker/Mednick). The content is solely the responsibility of the authors and does not necessarily represent the official views the National Institutes of Health.

DISCLOSURE

F.C. Baker has received research funding unrelated to this study from Verily Inc. and Noctrix Health, and owns stocks and is a consultant for Lisa Health. She is also a consultant for Bayer.

REFERENCES

1. Baker FC, Lee KA. Menstrual cycle effects on sleep. Sleep Med Clin 2018;13(3):283–94.

2. Wood C, Larsen L, Williams R. Menstrual characteristics of 2,343 women attending the shepherd foundation. Aust N Z J Obstet Gynaecol 1979;19(2):107–10.
3. Shughrue PJ, Lane MV, Merchenthaler I. Comparative distribution of estrogen receptor-alpha and -beta mRNA in the rat central nervous system. J Comp Neurol 1997;388(4):507–25.
4. Curran-Rauhut MA, Petersen SL. The distribution of progestin receptor mRNA in rat brainstem. Brain research Gene expression patterns 2002;1(3–4):151–7.
5. Mong JA, Baker FC, Mahoney MM, et al. Sleep, rhythms, and the endocrine brain: influence of sex and gonadal hormones. J Neurosci 2011;31(45):16107–16.
6. Mong JA, Cusmano DM. Sex differences in sleep: impact of biological sex and sex steroids. Philos Trans R Soc Lond, B, Biol Sci 2016;371(1688):20150110.
7. Zhang B, Wing YK. Sex differences in insomnia: a meta-analysis. Sleep 2006;29(1):85–93.
8. de Zambotti M, Goldstone A, Colrain IM, et al. Insomnia disorder in adolescence: diagnosis, impact, and treatment. Sleep Med Rev 2018;39:12–24.
9. Grandi G, Ferrari S, Xholli A, et al. Prevalence of menstrual pain in young women: what is dysmenorrhea? J Pain Res 2012;5:169–74.
10. Zannoni L, Giorgi M, Spagnolo E, et al. Dysmenorrhea, absenteeism from school, and symptoms suspicious for endometriosis in adolescents. J Pediatr Adolesc Gynecol 2014;27(5):258–65.
11. Ishikura IA, Hachul H, Pires GN, et al. The impact of primary dysmenorrhea on sleep and the consequences for adolescent academic performance. J Clin Sleep Med 2020;16(3):467–8.
12. Liu X, Chen H, Liu ZZ, et al. Early menarche and menstrual problems are associated with sleep disturbance in a large sample of Chinese adolescent girls. Sleep 2017;40(9):1–11.
13. Wang Z-Y, Liu Z-Z, Jia C-X, et al. Age at menarche, menstrual problems, and daytime sleepiness in Chinese adolescent girls. Sleep 2019;42(6):zsz061.
14. Nam GE, Han K, Lee G. Association between sleep duration and menstrual cycle irregularity in Korean female adolescents. Sleep Med 2017;35:62–6.
15. Kansiime C, Hytti L, Nalugya R, et al. Menstrual health intervention and school attendance in Uganda (MENISCUS-2): a pilot intervention study. BMJ Open 2020;10(2):e031182.
16. Shannon AK, Melendez-Torres GJ, Hennegan J. How do women and girls experience menstrual health interventions in low- and middle-income countries? Insights from a systematic review and qualitative metasynthesis. Cult Health Sex 2021;23(5):624–43.
17. Baker FC, Driver HS. Self-reported sleep across the menstrual cycle in young, healthy women. J Psychosom Res 2004;56(2):239–43.
18. Kravitz HM, Janssen I, Santoro N, et al. Relationship of day-to-day reproductive hormone levels to sleep in midlife women. Arch Intern Med 2005;165(20):2370–6.
19. Manber R, Baker FC, Gress JL. Sex differences in sleep and sleep disorders: a focus on women's sleep. Int J Sleep Disorders 2006;1:7–15.
20. National Sleep Foundation NSF. Sleep in America 2008 poll. 2008. Available at: http://www.sleepfoundation.org/atf/cf/%7Bf6bf2668-a1b4-4fe8-8d1a-a5d39340d9cb%7D/2008%20POLL%20SOF.PDF. Accessed 20 August 2008.
21. Alzueta E, de Zambotti M, Javitz H, et al. Tracking sleep, temperature, heart rate, and daily symptoms across the menstrual cycle with the oura ring in healthy women. Int J Womens Health 2022;14:491–503.
22. Li DX, Romans S, De Souza MJ, et al. Actigraphic and self-reported sleep quality in women: associations with ovarian hormones and mood. Sleep Med 2015;16(10):1217–24.
23. Romans SE, Kreindler D, Einstein G, et al. Sleep quality and the menstrual cycle. Sleep Med 2015;16(4):489–95.
24. Van Reen E, Kiesner J. Individual differences in self-reported difficulty sleeping across the menstrual cycle. Arch Womens Ment Health 2016;19(4):599–608.
25. Hachul H, Andersen ML, Bittencourt LR, et al. Does the reproductive cycle influence sleep patterns in women with sleep complaints? Climacteric 2010;13(6):594–603.
26. Kennedy KER, Onyeonwu C, Nowakowski S, et al. Menstrual regularity and bleeding is associated with sleep duration, sleep quality and fatigue in a community sample. J Sleep Res 2022;31(1):e13434.
27. Zheng H, Harlow SD, Kravitz HM, et al. Actigraphy-defined measures of sleep and movement across the menstrual cycle in midlife menstruating women: Study of Women's Health across the Nation Sleep Study. Menopause 2015;22(1):66–74.
28. Koikawa N, Takami Y, Kawasaki Y, et al. Changes in the objective measures of sleep between the initial nights of menses and the nights during the midfollicular phase of the menstrual cycle in collegiate female athletes. J Clin Sleep Med 2020;16(10):1745–51.
29. Driver HS, Dijk DJ, Werth E, et al. Sleep and the sleep electroencephalogram across the menstrual cycle in young healthy women. J Clin Endocrinol Metab 1996;81(2):728–35.

30. Driver HS, Werth E, Dijk D, et al. The menstrual cycle effects on sleep. Sleep medicine clinics 2008;3:1–11.
31. Shechter A, Boivin DB. Sleep, hormones, and circadian rhythms throughout the menstrual cycle in healthy women and women with premenstrual dysphoric disorder. Internet J Endocrinol 2010;2010:259345.
32. Lee KA, Shaver JF, Giblin EC, et al. Sleep patterns related to menstrual cycle phase and premenstrual affective symptoms. Sleep 1990;13(5):403–9.
33. Baker FC, Sassoon SA, Kahan T, et al. Perceived poor sleep quality in the absence of polysomnographic sleep disturbance in women with severe premenstrual syndrome. J Sleep Res 2012;21(5):535–45.
34. Sagot JC, Amoros C, Candas V, et al. Sweating responses and body temperatures during nocturnal sleep in humans. Am J Physiol 1987;252(3 Pt 2):R462–70.
35. Baker FC, Driver HS. Circadian rhythms, sleep, and the menstrual cycle. Sleep Med 2007;8(6):613–22.
36. Parry BL, Berga SL, Mostofi N, et al. Morning versus evening bright light treatment of late luteal phase dysphoric disorder. Am J Psychiatry 1989;146(9):1215–7.
37. Sharkey KM, Crawford SL, Kim S, et al. Objective sleep interruption and reproductive hormone dynamics in the menstrual cycle. Sleep Med 2014;15(6):688–93.
38. Baker FC, Kahan TL, Trinder J, et al. Sleep quality and the sleep electroencephalogram in women with severe premenstrual syndrome. Sleep 2007;30(10):1283–91.
39. Ishizuka Y, Pollak CP, Shirakawa S, et al. Sleep spindle frequency changes during the menstrual cycle. J Sleep Res 1994;3(1):26–9.
40. de Zambotti M, Willoughby AR, Sassoon SA, et al. Menstrual cycle-related variation in physiological sleep in women in the early menopausal transition. J Clin Endocrinol Metab 2015;100(8):2918–26.
41. Steriade M, McCormick DA, Sejnowski TJ. Thalamocortical oscillations in the sleeping and aroused brain. Science 1993;262(5134):679–85.
42. Mednick SC, McDevitt EA, Walsh JK, et al. The critical role of sleep spindles in hippocampal-dependent memory: a pharmacology study. J Neurosci 2013;33(10):4494–504.
43. Genzel L, Kiefer T, Renner L, et al. Sex and modulatory menstrual cycle effects on sleep related memory consolidation. Psychoneuroendocrinology 2012;37(7):987–98.
44. Sattari N, McDevitt EA, Panas D, et al. The effect of sex and menstrual phase on memory formation during a nap. Neurobiol Learn Mem 2017;145:119–28.
45. de Mouzon J, Testart J, Lefevre B, et al. Time relationships between basal body temperature and ovulation or plasma progestins. Fertil Steril 1984;41(2):254–9.
46. Baker FC, Siboza F, Fuller A. Temperature regulation in women: effects of the menstrual cycle. Temperature (Austin) 2020;7(3):226–62.
47. Shechter A, Varin F, Boivin DB. Circadian variation of sleep during the follicular and luteal phases of the menstrual cycle. Sleep 2010;33(5):647–56.
48. Grant AD, Newman M, Kriegsfeld LJ. Ultradian rhythms in heart rate variability and distal body temperature anticipate onset of the luteinizing hormone surge. Sci Rep 2020;10(1):20378.
49. Maijala A, Kinnunen H, Koskimaki H, et al. Nocturnal finger skin temperature in menstrual cycle tracking: ambulatory pilot study using a wearable Oura ring. BMC Wom Health 2019;19(1):150.
50. Shilaih M, Goodale BM, Falco L, et al. Modern fertility awareness methods: wrist wearables capture the changes in temperature associated with the menstrual cycle. Biosci Rep 2018;38(6):1–12.
51. Yong W, Ma H, Na M, et al. Roles of melatonin in the field of reproductive medicine. Biomed Pharmacother 2021;144:112001.
52. Sandyk R. The pineal gland and the menstrual cycle. Int J Neurosci 1992;63(3–4):197–204.
53. Shibui K, Uchiyama M, Okawa M, et al. Diurnal fluctuation of sleep propensity and hormonal secretion across the menstrual cycle. Biol Psychiatry 2000;48(11):1062–8.
54. Wright KP Jr, Badia P. Effects of menstrual cycle phase and oral contraceptives on alertness, cognitive performance, and circadian rhythms during sleep deprivation. Behav Brain Res 1999;103(2):185–94.
55. Greendale GA, Witt-Enderby P, Karlamangla AS, et al. Melatonin patterns and levels during the human menstrual cycle and after menopause. J Endocr Soc 2020;4(11):bvaa115.
56. National Institutes of Health N. Final Report: evidence-based methodology workshop on polycystic ovary syndrome. 2012. Available at: https://prevention.nih.gov/research-priorities/research-needs-and-gaps/pathways-prevention/evidence-based-methodology-workshop-polycystic-ovary-syndrome-pcos. Accessed December 15, 2022.
57. Diamanti-Kandarakis E, Dunaif A. Insulin resistance and the polycystic ovary syndrome revisited: an update on mechanisms and implications. Endocr Rev 2012;33(6):981–1030.
58. Torchen LC. Cardiometabolic risk in PCOS: more than a reproductive disorder. Curr Diab Rep 2017;17(12):137.
59. Cooney LG, Lee I, Sammel MD, et al. High prevalence of moderate and severe depressive and

anxiety symptoms in polycystic ovary syndrome: a systematic review and meta-analysis. Hum Reprod 2017;32(5):1075–91.
60. Franik G, Krysta K, Madej P, et al. Sleep disturbances in women with polycystic ovary syndrome. Gynecol Endocrinol 2016;32(12):1014–7.
61. Helvaci N, Karabulut E, Demir AU, et al. Polycystic ovary syndrome and the risk of obstructive sleep apnea: a meta-analysis and review of the literature. Endocr Connect 2017;6(7):437–45.
62. Vgontzas AN, Legro RS, Bixler EO, et al. Polycystic ovary syndrome is associated with obstructive sleep apnea and daytime sleepiness: role of insulin resistance. J Clin Endocrinol Metab 2001;86(2):517–20.
63. Kamboj MK, Bonny AE. Polycystic ovary syndrome in adolescence: diagnostic and therapeutic strategies. Transl Pediatr 2017;6(4):248–55.
64. Mo L, Mansfield DR, Joham A, et al. Sleep disturbances in women with and without polycystic ovary syndrome in an Australian National Cohort. Clin Endocrinol 2019;90(4):570–8.
65. Moran LJ, March WA, Whitrow MJ, et al. Sleep disturbances in a community-based sample of women with polycystic ovary syndrome. Hum Reprod 2015;30(2):466–72.
66. Tasali E, Van Cauter E, Ehrmann DA. Polycystic ovary syndrome and obstructive sleep apnea. Sleep Med Clin 2008;3:37–46.
67. Kumarendran B, Sumilo D, O'Reilly MW, et al. Increased risk of obstructive sleep apnoea in women with polycystic ovary syndrome: a population-based cohort study. Eur J Endocrinol 2019;180(4):265–72.
68. Lu C, Hutchens EG, Farhy LS, et al. Influence of sleep stage on LH pulse initiation in the normal late follicular phase and in polycystic ovary syndrome. Neuroendocrinology 2018;107(1):60–72.
69. Sellix MT. Circadian clock function in the mammalian ovary. J Biol Rhythms 2015;30(1):7–19.
70. Wang F, Xie N, Wu Y, et al. Association between circadian rhythm disruption and polycystic ovary syndrome. Fertil Steril 2021;115(3):771–81.
71. Mojaverrostami S, Asghari N, Khamisabadi M, et al. The role of melatonin in polycystic ovary syndrome: a review. Int J Reprod Biomed 2019;17(12): 865–82.
72. Li H, Liu M, Zhang C. Women with polycystic ovary syndrome (PCOS) have reduced melatonin concentrations in their follicles and have mild sleep disturbances. BMC Wom Health 2022;22(1):79.
73. Halbreich U. The etiology, biology, and evolving pathology of premenstrual syndromes. Psychoneuroendocrinology 2003;28(Suppl 3):55–99.
74. Rapkin A. A review of treatment of premenstrual syndrome and premenstrual dysphoric disorder. Psychoneuroendocrinology 2003;28(Suppl 3): 39–53.
75. Sepede G, Sarchione F, Matarazzo I, et al. Premenstrual dysphoric disorder without comorbid psychiatric conditions: a systematic review of therapeutic options. Clin Neuropharmacol 2016;39(5):241–61.
76. Conzatti M, Perez AV, Maciel RF, et al. Sleep quality and excessive daytime sleepiness in women with Premenstrual Syndrome. Gynecol Endocrinol 2021;37(10):945–9.
77. Khazaie H, Ghadami MR, Khaledi-Paveh B, et al. Sleep quality in university students with premenstrual dysphoric disorder. Shanghai Arch Psychiatry 2016;28(3):131–8.
78. Baker FC, Lamarche LJ, Iacovides S, et al. Sleep and menstrual-related disorders. Sleep Med Clin 2008;3:25–35.
79. Erbil N, Yucesoy H. Relationship between premenstrual syndrome and sleep quality among nursing and medical students. Perspect Psychiatr Care 2022;58(2):448–55.
80. Gupta R, Lahan V, Bansal S. Subjective sleep problems in young women suffering from premenstrual dysphoric disorder. N Am J Med Sci 2012;4(11): 593–5.
81. Mauri M. Sleep and the reproductive cycle: a review. Health Care Women Int 1990;11(4):409–21.
82. Lamarche LJ, Driver HS, Wiebe S, et al. Nocturnal sleep, daytime sleepiness, and napping among women with significant emotional/behavioral premenstrual symptoms. J Sleep Res 2007;16(3): 262–8.
83. Baker FC, Colrain IM. Daytime sleepiness, psychomotor performance, waking EEG spectra and evoked potentials in women with severe premenstrual syndrome. J Sleep Res 2009.
84. Shechter A, Lesperance P, Ng Ying Kin NM, et al. Nocturnal polysomnographic sleep across the menstrual cycle in premenstrual dysphoric disorder. Sleep Med 2012;13(8):1071–8.
85. Kuan AJ, Carter DM, Ott FJ. Premenstrual complaints before and after 40 years of age. Can J Psychiatry 2004;49(3):215.
86. Shechter A, Lesperance P, Ng Ying Kin NM, et al. Pilot investigation of the circadian plasma melatonin rhythm across the menstrual cycle in a small group of women with premenstrual dysphoric disorder. PLoS One 2012;7(12):e51929.
87. Parry BL, Martinez LF, Maurer EL, et al. Sleep, rhythms and women's mood. Part I. Menstrual cycle, pregnancy and postpartum. Sleep Med Rev 2006;10(2):129–44.
88. Moderie C., Boudreau P., Shechter A., et al., Effects of exogenous melatonin on sleep and circadian rhythms in women with premenstrual dysphoric disorder, *Sleep*, 44 (12), 2021, 1-11.
89. Parry BL, Berga SL, Mostofi N, et al. Plasma melatonin circadian rhythms during the menstrual cycle and after light therapy in premenstrual dysphoric

disorder and normal control subjects. J Biol Rhythms 1997;12(1):47–64.
90. (NSF) NSF. Women and sleep poll. 1998; Available at: www.sleepfoundation.org. 2006. Accessed December 15, 2022.
91. Davis S, Mirick DK. Circadian disruption, shift work and the risk of cancer: a summary of the evidence and studies in Seattle. Cancer Causes Control 2006;17(4):539–45.
92. Woosley JA, Lichstein KL. Dysmenorrhea, the menstrual cycle, and sleep. Behav Med 2014;40(1): 14–21.
93. Baker FC, Driver HS, Rogers GG, et al. High nocturnal body temperatures and disturbed sleep in women with primary dysmenorrhea. Am J Physiol 1999;277(6 Pt 1):E1013–21.
94. Iacovides S, Avidon I, Bentley A, et al. Diclofenac potassium restores objective and subjective measures of sleep quality in women with primary dysmenorrhea. Sleep 2009;32(8):1019–26.
95. Iacovides S, George K, Kamerman P, et al. Sleep fragmentation hypersensitizes healthy young women to deep and superficial experimental pain. J Pain 2017;18(7):844–54.
96. Iacovides S, Avidon I, Baker FC. What we know about primary dysmenorrhea today: a critical review. Hum Reprod Update 2015;21(6):762–78.
97. Kirmizigil B, Demiralp C. Effectiveness of functional exercises on pain and sleep quality in patients with primary dysmenorrhea: a randomized clinical trial. Arch Gynecol Obstet 2020;302(1): 153–63.
98. Gogos A, Wu YC, Williams AS, et al. The effects of ethinylestradiol and progestins ("the pill") on cognitive function in pre-menopausal women. Neurochem Res 2014;39(12):2288–300.
99. Cedars MI. Triphasic oral contraceptives: review and comparison of various regimens. Fertil Steril 2002;77(1):1–14.
100. Baker FC, Waner JI, Vieira EF, et al. Sleep and 24 hour body temperatures: a comparison in young men, naturally cycling women and women taking hormonal contraceptives. J Physiol 2001;530(Pt 3):565–74.
101. Baker FC, Mitchell D, Driver HS. Oral contraceptives alter sleep and raise body temperature in young women. Pflugers Arch 2001;442(5):729–37.
102. Shine-Burdick R, Hoffmann R, Armitage R. Short note: oral contraceptives and sleep in depressed and healthy women. Sleep 2002;25(3):347–9.
103. Plante DT, Goldstein MR. Medroxyprogesterone acetate is associated with increased sleep spindles during non-rapid eye movement sleep in women referred for polysomnography. Psychoneuroendocrinology 2013;38(12):3160–6.
104. Hachul H, Andersen ML, Bittencourt L, et al. A population-based survey on the influence of the menstrual cycle and the use of hormonal contraceptives on sleep patterns in Sao Paulo, Brazil. Int J Gynaecol Obstet 2013;120(2):137–40.
105. Bezerra AG, Andersen ML, Pires GN, et al. The effects of hormonal contraceptive use on sleep in women: A systematic review and meta-analysis. J Sleep Res 2023;32(3):e13757.
106. Boyar R, Finkelstein J, Roffwarg H, et al. Synchronization of augmented luteinizing hormone secretion with sleep during puberty. N Engl J Med 1972; 287(12):582–6.
107. Shaw ND, Butler JP, McKinney SM, et al. Insights into puberty: the relationship between sleep stages and pulsatile LH secretion. J Clin Endocrinol Metab 2012;97(11):E2055–62.
108. Hall JE, Sullivan JP, Richardson GS. Brief wake episodes modulate sleep-inhibited luteinizing hormone secretion in the early follicular phase. J Clin Endocrinol Metab 2005;90(4):2050–5.
109. Lim AJ, Huang Z, Chua SE, et al. Sleep duration, exercise, shift work and polycystic ovarian syndrome-related outcomes in a healthy population: a cross-sectional study. PLoS One 2016; 11(11):e0167048.
110. Kervezee L, Shechter A, Boivin DB. Impact of shift work on the circadian timing system and health in women. Sleep Med Clin 2018;13(3):295–306.
111. Kloss JD, Perlis ML, Zamzow JA, et al. Sleep, sleep disturbance, and fertility in women. Sleep Med Rev 2015;22:78–87.
112. Stocker LJ, Macklon NS, Cheong YC, et al. Influence of shift work on early reproductive outcomes: a systematic review and meta-analysis. Obstet Gynecol 2014;124(1):99–110.
113. Axelsson G, Rylander R, Molin I. Outcome of pregnancy in relation to irregular and inconvenient work schedules. Br J Ind Med 1989;46(6):393–8.
114. Bonzini M, Coggon D, Palmer KT. Risk of prematurity, low birthweight and pre-eclampsia in relation to working hours and physical activities: a systematic review. Occup Environ Med 2007;64(4): 228–43.
115. Lin JL, Lin YH, Chueh KH. Somatic symptoms, psychological distress and sleep disturbance among infertile women with intrauterine insemination treatment. J Clin Nurs 2014;23(11–12):1677–84.
116. Goldstein AN, Walker MP. The role of sleep in emotional brain function. Annu Rev Clin Psychol 2014;10:679–708.
117. Stocker LJ, Cagampang FR, Lu S, et al. Is sleep deficit associated with infertility and recurrent pregnancy losses? Results from a prospective cohort study. Acta Obstet Gynecol Scand 2021;100(2): 302–13.
118. Liu Z, Zheng Y, Wang B, et al. The impact of sleep on in vitro fertilization embryo transfer outcomes: a prospective study. Fertil Steril 2023;119(1):47–55.

119. Huang LH, Kuo CP, Lu YC, et al. Association of emotional distress and quality of sleep among women receiving in-vitro fertilization treatment. Taiwan J Obstet Gynecol 2019;58(1):168–72.
120. Reschini M, Buoli M, Facchin F, et al. Women's quality of sleep and in vitro fertilization success. Sci Rep 2022;12(1):17477.
121. Baker FC, de Zambotti M, Colrain IM, Bei B. Sleep problems during the menopausal transition: prevalence, impact, and management challenges. Nat Sci Sleep 2018;10:73–95.
122. Driver HS, McLean H, Kumar DV, et al. The influence of the menstrual cycle on upper airway resistance and breathing during sleep. Sleep 2005;28(4):449–56.

An Update on Sleep Duration, Obesity, and Mortality Risk in Women

Kelsie M. Full, PhD, MPH[a,*], Dayna A. Johnson, PhD, MPH, MSW, MS[b], Christopher N. Kaufmann, PhD, MHS[c], Atul Malhotra, MD[d]

KEYWORDS

• Cardiometabolic • Sleep disorders • Sleep disparities • Sex differences

KEY POINTS

- Because of the pressures of today's 24/7 society, an increasing number of adults in the United States are suffering from insufficient sleep, and unique social, occupational, and clinical factors make getting healthy sleep a challenge for women.
- Consistent evidence supports the association and potential contribution of short sleep duration to poor metabolic health, obesity risk, chronic cardiovascular conditions, and mortality.
- More research is needed to understand better the comprehensive sleep health of phenotypic short and long sleepers to understand the pathways underlying the observed associations with cardiometabolic health.
- To accomplish sleep equity across racial and ethnic minority populations, who disproportionately experience sleep disparities, there is a need to design research studies and interventions to address the multiple layers of social determinants that contribute to sleep disparities.

INTRODUCTION

Sleep is increasingly recognized as an essential factor to overall health and well-being. Diet, exercise, and sleep are often discussed as the 3 lifestyle pillars of health, with the dogma being that if one is ignored the other two will suffer. However, because of the pressures of today's 24/7 society, sleep is often viewed as a luxury. In fact, US population estimates indicate that the proportion of adults with short sleep durations has been increasing over the past 40 years.[1] Further, several recent epidemiologic studies have shown historically marginalized populations have shorter sleep duration in comparison to non-Hispanic White populations.[2] With the increase in the availability of the Internet and mobile devices, individuals can be constantly engaged throughout the 24-hour day. In addition, employment trends have led to increases in work hours, flexible or alternative work schedules, and demand for work travel, all contributing to the risk for inadequate sleep.[3–5]

Women are a group of particular interest in the context of a discussion on sleep. This focus is for several reasons: first, women have been traditionally understudied in the context of sleep research.[6] Second, women may be given disproportionate family responsibilities to balance with their own careers, including childcare, meal planning, and other household activities. As an example, women bared the unbalanced burden of household responsibilities during the COVID-19 pandemic that resulted

[a] Division of Epidemiology, Department of Medicine, Vanderbilt University Medical Center, 2525 West End Avenue, Suite 600, Nashville, TN 37203, USA; [b] Department of Epidemiology, Rollins School of Public Health, Emory University, 1518 Clifton Road, Atlanta, Georgia, 30322, USA; [c] Department of Health Outcomes and Biomedical Informatics, College of Medicine, University of Florida, 2004 Mowry Road, Gainesville, Florida, 32603, USA; [d] Division of Pulmonary, Critical Care and Sleep Medicine, School of Medicine, University of California San Diego, 9500 Gilman Drive, La Jolla, California, 92093, USA
* Corresponding author.
E-mail address: k.full@vumc.org

Sleep Med Clin 18 (2023) 415–422
https://doi.org/10.1016/j.jsmc.2023.06.015

in job loss, delays in career advancement, and employment dissatisfaction as compared with their male counterparts.[7–9] These responsibilities may be a chronic burden or stress that may result in less time available to sleep as well as directly impairing sleep duration.[10,11] Third, despite being understudied, the limited existing evidence suggests women are at increased risk of certain sleep disorders including insomnia, mood disturbance, and restless legs syndrome.[6] Although obstructive sleep apnea (OSA) is more prevalent among men,[12] the prevalence of OSA is still high in women, potentially even greater with likely missed diagnosis.[13] Research indicates that the stereotypical phenotype of OSA leads to disproportionate diagnosis of OSA in men, above and beyond the epidemiologic differences in occurrence.[13] Specific to sleep duration, as women age they report increasing difficulty with getting sufficient sleep.[14–16] In general, obtaining adequate healthy sleep poses a unique challenge to aging women.

EVIDENCE ON SLEEP DURATION, OBESITY, AND MORTALITY

The impact of abnormal sleep duration on various health outcomes has been well investigated. Highlights from the literature on the link between sleep duration, obesity, and mortality in women will be succinctly reviewed here. However, it is important to note that many studies have not focused specifically on sleep duration among women or sex differences in the associations. Several conclusions on abnormal sleep duration and obesity among women can be drawn from the existing epidemiologic literature.

Mixed Results of Observational Studies Assessing Abnormal Sleep Duration and Weight Change in Women

In a 2006 landmark study among more than 68,000 women in the Nurses' Health Study, over 16 years of follow-up Patel and colleagues reported women sleeping less than 5 hours had a 1.15 relative risk of incident obesity compared with those sleeping 7 hours or more. At the baseline examination, the nurses were asked a single question on the number of hours they slept in a typical 24-hour period. In addition, over the 16-year period, women reporting short sleep duration (<6 hours) gained more weight over time as compared with women with adequate sleep duration (7–8 hours). Of note, women who reported long sleep duration (>8 h/d) also had increased body weight over time as compared with adequate sleepers, although these findings have been controversial.[17] Although this study used only a 1-item self-report to assess usual sleep duration, the item was later validated with sleep diaries.[18] Since then, several studies have reported associations between self-reported abnormal sleep duration and obesity.[19,20] Although the evidence suggests an association, conflicting results have also been reported, particularly among women. In 2013, Appelhans and colleagues prospectively assessed sleep duration and weight change in midlife women in the Study of Women's Health Across the Nation, using 7-day actigraphy. There were no meaningful associations reported between objective short or long sleep durations with incident obesity.[21]

Data from Randomized Trials Supports Mechanisms and Causality

To investigate potential mechanisms linking sleep to weight gain, investigators have studied leptin and ghrelin: leptin is a satiety hormone made by adipocytes, whereas ghrelin stimulates appetite. In a physiologic clinical crossover study by Spiegel and colleagues, adult men underwent 2 days of sleep restriction (4 hours sleep restriction) followed by 2 days of sleep extension to investigate whether sleep duration curtailment altered appetite regulation. The investigators observed a reduction in leptin levels and an increase in ghrelin levels during sleep restriction days as compared with adequate sleep duration days. Both hormones changed in a direction to stimulate appetite.[22] These findings were among the first to provide potential mechanisms explaining why short sleep duration might stimulate appetite and thus contribute to increases in body weight over time. The findings were followed by another crossover randomized trial by Nedeltcheva and colleagues among overweight adults at midlife to investigate if sleep restriction affected the effect of diet on weight loss. The investigators observed an impairment in loss of fat-free body mass with reduced dietary intake during the period of reduced sleep duration (5.5 hours) versus adequate sleep duration (8.5 hours).[23]

Studies Have Helped to Rule Out Confounding by Genetics

Among nearly 120,000 participants in the UK Biobank, Celis-Morales and colleagues investigated the interaction of sleep duration and genetic predisposition to obesity.[24] Self-reported sleep characteristics, including short (<7 hours) and long sleep duration (>9 hours), were shown to modify the association of the genetic predisposition to obesity and anthropometric measurements including waist circumference, suggesting that abnormal sleep duration may exacerbate one's genetic risk of obesity.[24] By incorporating genetic predictors of obesity, these results partially rule out potential confounding and reverse causality and speak to how abnormal sleep duration itself may contribute to obesity.

Abnormal Sleep Duration Is Associated with Chronic Health Conditions and Mortality

A growing body of evidence supports that beyond obesity, and potentially by contributing to obesity, abnormal sleep duration increases the risk of chronic cardiovascular health conditions and increased mortality risk. Given this evidence, in 2022 the American Heart Association added sleep health to their list of the key factors that are essential to improving and maintaining cardiovascular health, as a part of "Life's Essential 8".[25] In the Massachusetts Male Aging Study, Yaggi and colleagues observed an impact of abnormal sleep duration on incident diabetes over the course of 15 years.[26] Of note, short sleepers (<6 hours) were twice as likely to develop clinical diabetes as compared with those with adequate sleep durations.[26] Long sleepers (>8 hours) were again at risk with a 3-fold increased risk of incident diabetes during follow-up.[26] Again in the Nurses' Health Study, abnormal sleep duration was linked with incident coronary artery disease in more than 71,000 women.[27] Ayas and colleagues observed an 82% increased risk of incident coronary artery disease in women reporting less than or equal to 5 hours of sleep per night as compared with those sleeping the recommended 8 hours per night.[27] The findings were followed by an important study by King and colleagues, assessing sleep duration and 5-year incident coronary artery calcification as a subclinical marker of atherosclerosis.[28] The investigators observed that short sleep duration (assessed via actigraphy) was predictive of incident coronary artery calcification; however, short sleep by self-report did not have the same predictive value regarding calcification risk.[28] Of note, the investigators did not observe an increase in calcification risk with long sleep durations as seen in prior studies. A higher cardiovascular burden has been consistently documented among racial/ethnic minorities, and numerous studies have connected abnormal sleep duration and poor sleep health with adverse cardiovascular outcomes, including resistant hypertension, among Black adults.[29–32] Lastly, several large cohort studies have reported an increased risk of cardiovascular and all-cause mortality associated with both short and long habitual sleep durations.[18,33–35]

In aggregate, the data consistently support the association and potential contribution of short sleep duration to poor metabolic health, obesity risk, chronic cardiovascular conditions, and mortality. In addition, long sleep is consistently linked with similar poor health outcomes, although the mechanism remains unclear. Despite the overwhelming collection of evidence, clarity on the underlying mechanisms and a lack of effective interventions remain missing from the literature.

AREAS FOR GREATER DISCUSSION

Given the substantial data available on the topic of sleep duration and cardiometabolic health, the authors have opted not to provide an exhaustive review of the existing literature. Instead, they have chosen to focus on 3 major areas deserving of more extensive discussion: (1) long sleep duration, (2) underlying mechanisms, and (3) racial/ethnic disparities.

Long Sleep

Although sleep deprivation has many known health effects, several large cohort studies have shown associations between long sleep duration and poor cardiometabolic health outcomes, including obesity. The observed association is consistent across different populations and different outcome measures.[26,27,32,34] Despite this evidence, there has been greater societal concern of not getting enough sleep rather than getting too much sleep. The potentially detrimental effect of long sleep is often dismissed due to study design bias, possible residual confounding, or in some cases reverse causation; however, the authors believe further investigation is imperative. Evidence supports that long sleepers have increased risk of depression and certain inflammatory disorders.[36] However, the magnitude of these associations is quite modest as compared with the documented cardiometabolic risk associated with long sleep. Given the overwhelming emphasis on increasing sleep duration at the population level, it is also critically important to better understand the mechanisms that may explain the increased risk for poor cardiometabolic health in long sleepers. A few mechanisms have been proposed that warrant further investigation. First, sleep architecture has not been adequately assessed in habitual long sleepers.[37] The possibility exists that poor sleep quality and/or undiagnosed sleep disorders may be contributing to the need for long sleep. Second, it is possible that some adults have more irregular sleep patterns that are not well captured by self-report measures, including those composed of periods of sleep deprivation followed by long periods of recovery sleep. Sleep irregularity, defined as substantial variation in sleep durations throughout the week, has recently been associated with obesity and several cardiometabolic conditions.[38–42] Third, the authors' clinical experience suggests that habitual long sleepers often have overall suboptimal health behaviors. For example, it has been observed that many individuals who sleep more than 10 hours per night experience social isolation, lack daily physical activity, have poor quality diets, and struggle with inconsistent employment. These lifestyle factors individually contribute to cardiometabolic health and may be difficult to capture with traditional measurements and cut points when measuring confounders. Finally, several medications also contribute to the propensity for long sleep duration and may not be adequately captured in epidemiologic cohorts (eg, over-the-counter hypnotics).

The Underlying Mechanisms of Abnormal Sleep Duration

Numerous studies have investigated the physiologic effects of sleep deprivation to explain the connection between short sleep duration and adverse cardiometabolic health outcomes. Clinically, patients who are short sleepers fall into 3 distinct categories: those with insomnia who have trouble falling asleep or staying asleep, those with short sleep duration due to societal pressures (eg, mothers with young children, women working multiple jobs), and those who sleep short durations and do not perceive a biological need for more sleep. Although some debate exists regarding the deleterious effects of short sleep based on why it is occurring, our view is that sleep duration per se is the predominant variable; however, further work is needed in this area. In addition to the metabolic disturbances described earlier, short sleep duration has been shown to produce sympathoexcitation, or stimulation of the sympathetic nervous system, as well as increased cortisol concentration, increased inflammatory biomarkers, and increased markers of oxidative stress.[36,43–46] In a small 22-day study by Yang and colleagues the investigators assessed microvascular and inflammatory responses during periods of sleep restriction (3 days of $\leq$4 hours). Although no significant differences were observed in macrocirculation, microcirculation, cell adhesion molecules, or markers of inflammation between the sleep-restricted group and healthy sleepers, in sex-stratified models, female participants were more likely to have increased inflammatory markers (interleukin-6) during sleep restriction period than men.[47] Calvin and colleagues investigated the effect of sleep restriction ($\leq$5 hours) compared with healthy sleep (7 hours) on endothelial function, a potential mediator in cardiovascular disease risk. Participants in the sleep restriction group experienced significant endothelial impairment as compared with healthy controls.[48] In aggregate, the data suggest major physiologic effects of short sleep duration on physical health that may over time contribute to cardiometabolic outcomes. Although the mechanisms are still being delineated, the adverse effects are likely multifactorial and include metabolic, autonomic, inflammatory, and oxidative stress mechanisms. These complex causal pathways and relationships likely explain why short sleep has been connected to multiple different organ systems and outcomes. Thus, overall mortality is likely affected by short sleep duration due to multiple underlying mechanisms; however, thoughtfully designed studies are needed to confirm and clarify these mechanisms.

RACIAL/ETHNIC DISPARITIES

Given the long-lasting disparities in sleep health and the need to address these sleep disparities, deserved attention has been given to socioeconomic and racial/ethnic differences in the context of sleep duration. Adults with low socioeconomic status may be particularly susceptible to societal and economic pressures described earlier and thus sleep duration may be compromised as a direct result.[5] It is also well documented that racial/ethnic minority groups are at a greater risk for suboptimal sleep health, including particularly abnormal sleep durations. In the racially/ethnically diverse MESA study, Chen and colleagues reported sleep durations varied significantly across racial/ethnic groups. As compared with 20% of non-Hispanic Whites, 40% of Black and African American participants and 30% of Hispanic/Latinx participants had habitual sleep durations less than 6 hours per night.[49] Evidence supports that racial/ethnic differences in sleep may be explained by socioeconomic status, racism, discrimination, neighborhood environments, and access to care,[2,50,51] but they are also in part explained by cultural differences in sleep-related beliefs. Historically, sleep has been stigmatized among Black and African American populations, contributing to the underreporting of poor sleep among Black and African American adults, and similarly, because of these stigmas around sleep, there tends to be a culture emphasis on work as opposed to sleep.[52] In a study composed of predominately older women, Grandner and colleagues found that Black older women were more likely to believe sleepiness was related to laziness and bad habits and were less likely to report motivation to make enough time for sleep or believe sleep was related to one's health than the White older women.[53] Within racial/ethnic subgroups, differences in sleep have been reported, stressing the importance of developing a better understanding of the multiple layers of social determinants that contribute to disparities in sleep health. Using NHANES data collected among 5160 US adults, Seicean and colleagues observed that Mexico-born US immigrants were less likely to report short habitual sleep durations than Mexican-Americans born in the United States, highlighting differences that exist within the US Hispanic Latino community.[54] The investigators hypothesized the differences between the US and foreign born Hispanic Latinos may in part be related to differences in cultural beliefs and values toward sleep health.[54] Within the US Hispanic Latino community there are unique barriers to obtaining adequate sleep including the stress and lifestyle changes caused by acculturation.[55] In the HCHS/SOL study including 16,415 US Hispanic Latinos, large differences were reported in both OSA prevalence (13.7% for moderate-to-severe sleep disturbed breathing) and diagnosis (1.3%), as well as OSA risk across subgroups of Hispanic backgrounds. These results suggest the proportion of undiagnosed sleep disorders may be even greater in some racial/ethnic population subgroups and may explain a larger burden of disease in these groups, including obesity.[56]

In summary, there is a need to address the multilevel social determinants of health that contribute to sleep disparities.[50,52,57] At the individual level, an opportunity exists through advocacy and educational efforts to improve health literacy, knowledge, and perceptions regarding the importance of adequate sleep to overall health and well-being. There is a need to develop culturally tailor sleep interventions. For example, racially tailoring interventions has shown participants to be more engaged and more likely to complete the intervention,[58] and increases in OSA self-efficacy have been observed.[59] In addition to individual-level targets, contextual factors are also of importance. The literature supports that the neighborhood environment explains a large portion of documented sleep disparities.[60] Thus, designing interventions and targeting policy to address adverse environments could potentially improve sleep duration at the community level.[50] Data from a natural experiment illustrated that living closer to a neighborhood investment was associated with better sleep outcomes,[61] thus investing in neighborhoods could potentially have a positive effect on sleep health. Based on the evidence, targeting the multilevel determinants of sleep disparities is a promising avenue for accomplishing sleep equity.

FUTURE DIRECTIONS

Despite considerable progress in our understanding of how sleep duration and sleep health more generally are associated with cardiometabolic health, substantial unresolved questions remain.

For clinicians:

- Given the high prevalence and major impact of poor sleep and sleep disorders, should universal screening be implemented in clinics or in the community setting?
- With the major expansion in the use of wearable consumer products, should data from these devices be used to guide clinical decision-making?
- Based on the interdependence of diet, exercise, and sleep, a question often posed by patients is: "Should I get up early and sleep less to go to the gym?" The answer likely depends on total sleep time and individual characteristics; however, a greater understanding of the interdependence of these health behaviors is needed.
- Are women more susceptible biologically to the effects of poor sleep and sleep disturbances or are observed differences more related to societal factors?

For researchers:

1. How can we achieve more comprehensive evaluations of sleep health beyond self-reported sleep duration? Polysomnography and other limited channel sleep tests can be cumbersome, particularly when one considers trying to collect these data in large studies.
2. Given the uncertainty regarding underlying mechanisms, a need for further longitudinal studies with repeated assessments and the impact of interventions needs to be undertaken. Actionable targets could be identified to help to mitigate the adverse health effects associated with inadequate sleep.
3. Given the paucity of data from underrepresented minorities, further longitudinal data enriched for various subgroups are essential to evaluate and understand better within group and between group differences. Beyond just describing differences between groups, interventions focused on social and environmental determinants of health are needed to help achieve sleep health equity.

For policy makers:

1. Increasing public education regarding the importance of sleep to overall health could be achieved through educational curriculum,

mass media, social media, and via strong advocates.
2. Given the disproportionate burden of family responsibilities that are often placed on women, there may be a need for further discussion regarding policies related to maternal leave, flexibility around childcare, and pay equity.
3. Given the ever-increasing numbers of shift workers in today's 24/7 society, optimizing schedules considering their impact on sleep and overall health needs to be considered further. Policies could be developed to optimize lighting, scheduling, and to prioritize safety (eg, avoiding drowsy driving or occupational accidents).

CLINICS CARE POINTS

- With the consistent data linking poor sleep to adverse cardiometabolic conditions and the documented high prevalence of poor sleep and sleep disorders, clinicians should consider briefly screening patients for sleep disorders.
- Clinicians should be aware that as women age, they are specifically at a greater risk for insufficient sleep and certain sleep disorders (eg, insomnia).
- More research is needed to understand better if women are more susceptible biologically to the adverse effects of poor sleep and sleep disturbances or if observed differences are due to societal factors.

DISCLOSURE

Dr Malhotra is funded by the NIH. He reports income related to medical education from Livanova, Eli Lilly, Zoll and Jazz. Additionally, ResMed provided a philanthropic donation to UCSD. All other authors have nothing to disclose.

FUNDING

Dr Full receives funding from the Eunice Kennedy Shriver National Institute of Child and Human Development award for the Building Interdisciplinary Research Careers in Women's Health career development program (K12HD043483). Dr Johnson receives funding from the National Institutes of Health, National Institute for Heart Lung and Blood (Grant #R01HL157954). Dr Kaufmann receives funding from the National Institute on Aging (Grant #'s: K01AG061239, R01AG079391, P30AG028740), and Sleep Research Society Foundation (Grant #: 23-FRA-001). Dr Malhotra receives funding from the National Institutes of Health.

REFERENCES

1. Bin YS, Marshall NS, Glozier N. Secular trends in adult sleep duration: a systematic review. Sleep Med Rev 2012;16(3):223–30.
2. Johnson DA, Jackson CL, Williams N, et al. Are sleep patterns influenced by race/ethnicity – a marker of relative advantage or disadvantage? Evidence to date. Nat Sci Sleep 2019;11:79–95.
3. Kuhn P, Lozano F. The expanding workweek? Understanding trends in long work hours among US men, 1979–2006. J Labor Econ 2008;26(2):311–43.
4. McMenamin TM. A time to work: recent trends in shift work and flexible schedules. Monthly Lab Rev 2007;130:3.
5. Grandner MA. Sleep, health, and society. Sleep Medicine Clinics 2017;12(1):1–22.
6. Mallampalli MP, Carter CL. Exploring sex and gender differences in sleep health: a society for women's health research report. J Wom Health 2014;23(7):553–62.
7. Power K. The COVID-19 pandemic has increased the care burden of women and families. Sustain Sci Pract Pol 2020;16(1):67–73.
8. Yildirim TM, Eslen-Ziya H. The differential impact of COVID-19 on the work conditions of women and men academics during the lockdown. Gend Work Organ 2021;28(Suppl 1):243–9.
9. Minello A. The pandemic and the female academic. Nature 2020. https://doi.org/10.1038/d41586-020-01135-9.
10. Johnson DA, Knutson K, Colangelo LA, et al. Associations of chronic burden, sleep characteristics, and metabolic syndrome in the coronary artery risk development in young adults study. Psychosom Med 2022;84(6):711–8.
11. Johnson DA, Lisabeth L, Lewis TT, et al. The contribution of psychosocial stressors to sleep among african Americans in the jackson Heart study. Sleep 2016;39(7):1411–9.
12. Young T, Palta M, Dempsey J, et al. Burden of sleep apnea: rationale, design, and major findings of the Wisconsin sleep cohort study. Wis Med J 2009;108(5):246–9.
13. Carden K, Malhotra A. The debate about gender differences in obstructive sleep apnea. Sleep Med 2003;4(6):485–7.
14. Edwards BA, O'Driscoll DM, Ali A, et al. Aging and sleep: physiology and pathophysiology. Semin Respir Crit Care Med 2010;31(5):618–33.
15. Foley DJ, Monjan AA, Brown SL, et al. Sleep complaints among elderly persons: an epidemiologic study of three communities. Sleep 1995;18(6):425–32.

16. Kocevska D, Lysen TS, Dotinga A, et al. Sleep characteristics across the lifespan in 1.1 million people from The Netherlands, United Kingdom and United States: a systematic review and meta-analysis. Nat Human Behav 2021;5(1):113–22.
17. Patel SR, Malhotra A, White DP, et al. Association between reduced sleep and weight gain in women. Am J Epidemiol 2006;164(10):947–54.
18. Patel SR, Ayas NT, Malhotra MR, et al. A prospective study of sleep duration and mortality risk in women. Sleep 2004;27(3):440–4.
19. Cappuccio FP, Taggart FM, Kandala NB, et al. Meta-analysis of short sleep duration and obesity in children and adults. Sleep 2008;31(5):619–26.
20. Bacaro V, Ballesio A, Cerolini S, et al. Sleep duration and obesity in adulthood: an updated systematic review and meta-analysis. Obes Res Clin Pract 2020; 14(4):301–9.
21. Appelhans BM, Janssen I, Cursio JF, et al. Sleep duration and weight change in midlife women: the SWAN sleep study. Obesity 2013;21(1):77–84.
22. Spiegel K, Tasali E, Penev P, et al. Brief communication: sleep curtailment in healthy young men is associated with decreased leptin levels, elevated ghrelin levels, and increased hunger and appetite. Ann Intern Med 2004;141(11):846–50.
23. Nedeltcheva AV, Kilkus JM, Imperial J, et al. Insufficient sleep undermines dietary efforts to reduce adiposity. Ann Intern Med 2010;153(7):435–41.
24. Celis-Morales C, Lyall DM, Guo Y, et al. Sleep characteristics modify the association of genetic predisposition with obesity and anthropometric measurements in 119,679 UK Biobank participants. Am J Clin Nutr 2017;105(4):980–90.
25. Lloyd-Jones DM, Allen NB, Anderson CAM, et al. Life's essential 8: updating and enhancing the American Heart association's construct of cardiovascular health: a presidential advisory from the American Heart association. Circulation 2022;146(5). https://doi.org/10.1161/cir.0000000000001078.
26. Yaggi HK, Araujo AB, McKinlay JB. Sleep duration as a risk factor for the development of type 2 diabetes. Diabetes Care 2006;29(3):657–61.
27. Ayas NT, White DP, Manson JE, et al. A prospective study of sleep duration and coronary Heart disease in women. Arch Intern Med 2003;163(2):205.
28. King CR, Knutson KL, Rathouz PJ, et al. Short sleep duration and incident coronary artery calcification. JAMA 2008;300(24):2859–66.
29. Yano Y, Gao Y, Johnson DA, et al. Sleep characteristics and measures of glucose metabolism in blacks: the jackson Heart study. J Am Heart Assoc 2020; 9(9). https://doi.org/10.1161/jaha.119.013209.
30. Butler MJ, Spruill TM, Johnson DA, et al. Suboptimal sleep and incident cardiovascular disease among African Americans in the Jackson Heart Study (JHS). Sleep Med 2020;76:89–97.
31. Johnson DA, Thomas SJ, Abdalla M, et al. Association between sleep apnea and blood pressure control among blacks. Circulation 2019;139(10): 1275–84.
32. Full KM, Malhotra A, Gallo LC, et al. Accelerometer-measured sleep duration and clinical cardiovascular risk factor scores in older women. J Gerontol: Series A 2020;75(9):1771–8.
33. Wallace ML, Buysse DJ, Redline S, et al. Multidimensional sleep and mortality in older adults: a machine-learning comparison with other risk factors. J Gerontol A Biol Sci Med Sci 2019;74(12):1903–9.
34. Silva AAD, Mello RGBD, Schaan CW, et al. Sleep duration and mortality in the elderly: a systematic review with meta-analysis. BMJ Open 2016;6(2): e008119.
35. Wang C, Bangdiwala SI, Rangarajan S, et al. Association of estimated sleep duration and naps with mortality and cardiovascular events: a study of 116 632 people from 21 countries. Eur Heart J 2019; 40(20):1620–9.
36. Patel SR, Malhotra A, Gottlieb DJ, et al. Correlates of long sleep duration. Sleep 2006;29(7):881–9.
37. Van Dongen HP, Maislin G, Mullington JM, et al. The cumulative cost of additional wakefulness: dose-response effects on neurobehavioral functions and sleep physiology from chronic sleep restriction and total sleep deprivation. Sleep 2003; 26(2):117–26.
38. Zuraikat FM, Makarem N, Redline S, et al. Sleep regularity and cardiometabolic heath: is variability in sleep patterns a risk factor for excess adiposity and glycemic dysregulation? Curr Diab Rep 2020; 20(8):38.
39. Huang T, Mariani S, Redline S. Sleep irregularity and risk of cardiovascular events: the multi-ethnic study of atherosclerosis. J Am Coll Cardiol 2020;75(9): 991–9.
40. Huang T, Redline S. Cross-sectional and prospective associations of actigraphy-assessed sleep regularity with metabolic abnormalities: the multi-ethnic study of atherosclerosis. Diabetes Care 2019;42(8): 1422–9.
41. Carnethon MR, De Chavez PJ, Zee PC, et al. Disparities in sleep characteristics by race/ethnicity in a population-based sample: chicago Area Sleep Study. Sleep Med 2016;18:50–5.
42. Full KM, Huang T, Shah NA, et al. Sleep Irregularity and Subclinical Markers of Cardiovascular Disease: The Multi-Ethnic Study of Atherosclerosis. J Am Heart Assoc 2023 Feb 21;12(4):e027361. https://doi.org/10.1161/JAHA.122.027361. PMID: 36789869; PMCID: PMC10111477.
43. Kanagasabai T, Ardern CI. Contribution of inflammation, oxidative stress, and antioxidants to the relationship between sleep duration and cardiometabolic health. Sleep 2015;38(12):1905–12.

44. Carter JR, Fonkoue IT, Greenlund IM, et al. Sympathetic neural responsiveness to sleep deprivation in older adults: sex differences. Am J Physiol Heart Circ Physiol 2019;317(2):H315–h322.
45. Cullen T, Thomas G, Wadley AJ. Sleep deprivation: cytokine and neuroendocrine effects on perception of effort. Med Sci Sports Exerc 2020; 52(4):909–18.
46. Mullington JM, Haack M, Toth M, et al. Cardiovascular, inflammatory, and metabolic consequences of sleep deprivation. Prog Cardiovasc Dis 2009;51(4): 294–302.
47. Yang H, Baltzis D, Bhatt V, et al. Macro- and microvascular reactivity during repetitive exposure to shortened sleep: sex differences. Sleep 2021; 44(5). https://doi.org/10.1093/sleep/zsaa257.
48. Calvin AD, Covassin N, Kremers WK, et al. Experimental sleep restriction causes endothelial dysfunction in healthy humans. J Am Heart Assoc 2014;3(6): e001143.
49. Chen X, Wang R, Zee P, et al. Racial/ethnic differences in sleep disturbances: the multi-ethnic study of atherosclerosis (MESA). Sleep 2015. https://doi.org/10.5665/sleep.4732.
50. Billings ME, Cohen RT, Baldwin CM, et al. Disparities in sleep health and potential intervention models. Chest 2021;159(3):1232–40.
51. Jackson CL. Determinants of racial/ethnic disparities in disordered sleep and obesity. Sleep Health 2017;3(5):401–15.
52. Johnson DA, Reiss B, Cheng P, et al. Understanding the role of structural racism in sleep disparities: a call to action and methodological considerations. Sleep 2022;45(10). https://doi.org/10.1093/sleep/zsac200.
53. Grandner MA, Patel NP, Jean-Louis G, et al. Sleep-related behaviors and beliefs associated with race/ethnicity in women. Journal of the National Medical Association 2013;105(1):4–16.
54. Seicean S, Neuhauser D, Strohl K, et al. An exploration of differences in sleep characteristics between Mexico-born US immigrants and other Americans to address the Hispanic Paradox. Sleep 2011; 34(8):1021–31.
55. Loredo JS, Soler X, Bardwell W, et al. Sleep health in U.S. Hispanic population. Sleep 2010;33(7):962–7.
56. Redline S, Sotres-Alvarez D, Loredo J, et al. Sleep-disordered breathing in hispanic/latino individuals of diverse backgrounds. The hispanic community health study/study of Latinos. Am J Respir Crit Care Med 2014;189(3):335–44.
57. Hale L, Hale B. Treat the source not the symptoms: why thinking about sleep informs the social determinants of health. Health Educ Res 2010;25(3): 395–400.
58. Zhou ES, Ritterband LM, Bethea TN, et al. Effect of culturally tailored, internet-delivered cognitive behavioral therapy for insomnia in Black women: a randomized clinical trial. JAMA Psychiatr 2022; 79(6):538–49.
59. Jean-Louis G, Robbins R, Williams NJ, et al. Tailored Approach to Sleep Health Education (TASHE): a randomized controlled trial of a web-based application. J Clin Sleep Med 2020;16(8):1331–41.
60. Billings ME, Hale L, Johnson DA. Physical and social environment relationship with sleep health and disorders. Chest. May 2020;157(5):1304–12.
61. Dubowitz T, Haas A, Ghosh-Dastidar B, et al. Does investing in low-income urban neighborhoods improve sleep? Sleep 2021;44(6). https://doi.org/10.1093/sleep/zsaa292.

Sleep During Menopause

Helena Hachul, MD, PhD[a,b,*], Beatriz Hachul de Campos, BSc (Medicine)[a], Leandro Lucena, MSc[a], Sergio Tufik, MD, PhD[a]

KEYWORDS

• Sleep • Insomnia • Menopause • Postmenopause • Premenopause • Hot flashes
• Hormonal therapy • Obstructive sleep apnea

KEY POINTS

- As women are living longer, nearly one-third of their lives will be spent in the climacteric period.
- Apart from symptoms due to hypoestrogenism, psychological status (anxiety and/or depression), social status (partner, children, grandchildren, friends, family) and environment (neighbors, work, leisure) may affect the symptoms of menopause, especially sleep.
- There are several possible interventions that can be used to treat sleep disorders in women during menopause: behavioral, hormonal, and nonhormonal ones (sedatives, antidepressants, hypnotics).
- Given the diversity of factors that can influence sleep in women during menopause, the use of an integrative approach seems to be the most promising approach.

INTRODUCTION

Menopause Definition

Life expectancy in women has been steadily increasing for decades. In 1940, life expectancy in women was around 44 years, but women now live for about 77 years, and this is expected to reach 90 years by 2030.[1] This means that women will live one-third of their lives in the climacteric period, which includes both the menopausal transition and the postmenopause. The interval around the menopause onset is the menopause transition. The first 8 years after menopause is the early postmenopause, and after that, it is called the late postmenopause.[2]

Factors that influence the age of menopause are.

- Family and hereditary factors: if a mother reached the menopause at 50 years, it likely that her daughter will experience menopause at a similar age.
- Nutritional status: obese women tend to reach menopause later than thinner women. This is because of the production of estrogen in adipose tissue.
- Smoking and alcohol consumption anticipate the menopause onset.
- Parity may affect menopause, but this is still a subject of debate.
- Extensive pelvic surgery, such as oophorectomy, anticipates menopause.[3]

  Menopause age onset varies in each country, a meta-analysis identified the overall average age as 48.8 years, ranging from 46 to 52 years, considering data from six continents.[4]

Menopause Physiology

Menopause is directly related to the depletion of ovarian follicles over the course of a woman's life. In the fetal period, women have 5 to 7 million follicles, at birth they have 1 to 2 million, at puberty 300,000 to 400,000 and by about 45 years of age they have only about 10,000 remaining follicles.[5]

The physiopathology of the menopause transition is a consequence of this follicular atresia and leads to a decrease in estrogen and hypoestrogenism, which is responsible for the early and the late manifestations.[6] Such alterations can contribute to the appearance of vasomotor

[a] Department of Psychobiology, Universidade Federal de Sao Paulo, Sao Paulo, Brazil; [b] Department of Ginecology, Universidade Federal de Sao Paulo, Sao Paulo, Brazil
* Corresponding author. Rua Napoleao de Barros 925, 04024-002 - Vila Clementino, Sao Paulo, Sao Paulo, Brazil.
E-mail address: helenahahul@gmail.com

Sleep Med Clin 18 (2023) 423–433
https://doi.org/10.1016/j.jsmc.2023.06.004
1556-407X/23/

symptoms, the worsening of sleep quality and mood alterations which can culminate in a decreased quality of life.[7]

Clinical Manifestations

The early manifestations, hot flashes and sweating, can impair sleep; increase levels of depression, anxiety, and irritability; promote memory loss and decrease libido. These vasomotor symptoms are due to hypoestrogenism and are the most frequent complaints and the main cause for women seeking treatment.[8] Hot flashes tend to occur most frequently in late perimenopause and in the early postmenopause stage[8,9] and are typically associated with a sudden feeling of heat and sweating lasting for between 3 and 10 minutes.[10] They may happen many times during both the day and the night, which frequently leads to sleep fragmentation.

A study by Baker and colleagues compared sleep patterns in a population of women in menopausal transition with and without insomnia. The insomnia group not only presented a reduction in total sleep time but also an increase in the number of hot flashes that were related to awakening.[11] Clinically, it is important to consider the frequency and intensity of vasomotor symptoms. Although they tend to reduce with the passage of time, in some cases a moderate to severe complaint may persist for more than 5 to 10 years after menopause.[8,12] Furthermore, hot flashes and night sweats have a relationship with decreased quality of sleep,[13] and their severity may impact insomnia symptoms.[14] According to polysomnography (PSG) records, hot flashes tend to occur in the first 4 hours of sleep,[15] mostly close to wake periods, or in the N1 sleep stage.[16] These events are associated with an increase in wake after sleep onset (WASO),[15,17] and sensitization to their occurrence predisposes women to lighter sleep.[16]

A study by Lampio and colleagues[18] assessed typical patients in premenopause using PSG and carried out follow-up 6 years later during perimenopause. The results of the study showed an increase in sleep fragmentation and WASO and a decrease in total sleep time and sleep efficiency. A longitudinal study evaluated sleep patterns in women before, during, and after menopause and identified an increase in difficulty falling asleep and the number of awakenings and earlier waking up during and after the menopausal transition.[19] Moreover, postmenopause women have been shown to present more sleep disorders than premenopausal and perimenopausal women.[20] The main causes for sleep disorders and insomnia in postmenopause is the presence of hot flashes, hormonal changes, mood swings, and nocturia resulting in difficulty going back to sleep after waking to go to the bathroom.[21–25]

Insomnia is more frequent in women and increases with aging. A study has shown that 25% of women aged between 50 and 64 report sleep problems, and 15% of them present severe sleep disturbances that impact their quality of life.[25] Insomnia disorder is defined by the American Psychiatric Association as interference in sleep maintenance and/or onset that occurs at a frequency of at least three times a week in the previous 3 months and has an impact on daily life.[26] Even in those who do not meet the criteria to be diagnosed with the disorder, insomnia symptoms are associated with a reduced quality of life.[27] More than 50% of women complain about insomnia after menopause and in women who had insomnia before the onset of menopause, it can become worse.[28,29] Moreover, some women who complain about insomnia may also have other sleep disturbances, such as obstructive sleep apnea (OSA). It was observed a 4% increases in the apnea–hypopnea index (AHI) each year after menopause.[30] Nearly 71% of women after menopause have an AHI higher than 5 hours and in one study, 50% of women complaining of insomnia also presented OSA.[31,32] OSA is a chronic condition that affects the capacity to breathe properly while sleeping, with recurrent events of upper airway obstruction.[33] OSA is associated with an increase in the risk of cardiovascular disorders, stroke, hypertension, arrhythmia, and excessive daytime sleepiness.[34,35] Although men have a higher incidence of OSA, with aging, changes in body fat distribution and hormonal alterations tend to lead to an increase in the number of obstructive events per hour in postmenopausal women.[27,31,33]

Another complaint that is very common after menopause is an increase in depression levels. In addition to the physical and hormonal changes common during menopause transition and postmenopause, increased depression may come together with sleep disorders, including difficulty falling asleep and previous major depression can return in postmenopause.[36,37] Social and cultural aspects have a role in this outcome, given that women at this age are typically exposed to a wide range of experiences that may impact heir mental health, such as retirement from work, empty nest syndrome (the grief that parents can feel after their children have grown up and left home), and caring for older family members (a responsibility that often falls unevenly on women) that can impact mental health through stress, and loss of sleep, among other factors.[38–40] Increased levels of depression and anxiety have been reported to be more frequent in the late postmenopause compared with early and premenopausal women.[41]

The relationships between anxiety, depression, hot flashes, and sleep quality were studied in 467 women aged 40 to 60 years with menopausal problems. Total sleep quality scores were positively correlated with hot flashes, sweating, and anxiety and depression symptoms. Anxiety and depression performed a mediating function between hot flashes/sweating and sleep quality, the indirect effect of anxiety symptoms accounting for 17.86% and depression symptoms for 5.36% on sleep quality. The investigators concluded that hot flashes, sweating, anxiety, and depression in peri/postmenopausal women are risk factors that can affect sleep quality.[42] In agreement with these findings, a longitudinal study evaluating 458 middle-aged Chinese women found that the prevalence of sleep disturbances was significantly increased during and after menopause, and levels of anxiety and depression were positively associated with difficulty falling asleep. Moreover, the participants who experienced insomnia in premenopause had a higher risk of moderate to severe insomnia in the menopausal transition and postmenopause.[43]

Several epidemiologic studies have been undertaken to investigate how aging impacts women's sleep patterns. A longitudinal study evaluated 873 women (40 to 60 years old) distributed into reproductive (n = 408) or postmenopause (n = 465) groups, according to data at baseline. The participants were examined annually and followed-up over a 5-year period. The analyses revealed an increase in sleep disturbances in the two years before and after the menopausal transition.[44] Moreover, the Study of Women's Health Across the Nation carried out in the United States evaluated age-related changes in sleep, using actigraphy data, across 12 years in midlife women while they going through menopause.[45] The sleep of the women was monitored on two occasions: 3 years apart and then in a third assessment 12 years after the first. The results of this longitudinal study suggested that sleep may not worsen, in general, in midlife women.[45] A Canadian longitudinal study assessed the effect of menopause on sleep in a sample of 6179 women. The study found that menopause was associated with increased sleep-onset insomnia and that postmenopausal women were more likely to screen positive for OSA; however, menopausal status was not associated with difficulties in sleep maintenance, somnolence, or restless leg syndrome than premenopausal women.[46] Finally, a Brazilian group studied the effect of menopause on objective sleep parameters (PSG) using data from a representative sample of the population of Sao Paulo, the biggest city in Brazil. Compared with premenopausal women, postmenopausal women presented higher N3 sleep stage and AHIs, even after adjusting for age and body mass index (BMI). The conclusion was that the menopause per se can promote objective alterations in sleep architecture.[47]

In late postmenopause, the common manifestations related to hypoestrogenism are dry skin, dyslipidemia, osteopenia and osteoporosis, urogenital atrophy, and nocturia.[48] Moreover, alterations in fat distribution can occur after menopause and continue until late postmenopause. There is an increase in waist circumference with hypoestrogenism.[49] Also, during the early to late postmenopause, with the increase in weight and waist circumference, these factors can increase the risk of developing OSA. In relation to waist circumference, an increase of 1 cm leads to a more than 5% increased risk of apnea.[50] The association of obesity and sleep disorders in postmenopause is clear. Increased BMI leads to a decrease in deep sleep and sleep efficiency and an increase in OSA.[41] Compared with nonobese women, obese women have been shown to present higher AHIs in postmenopause. Higher BMI was also associated with an increase in rapid eye movement (REM) sleep latency.[41] In addition, it has been suggested that there is a relationship between obesity and self-reported sleep—with more hours spent sleeping being associated with lower obesity.[51]

So far, we have reviewed several social, environmental, and physical variables that can influence the sleep patterns of postmenopausal women. In addition to these factors, pain is another important symptom that should be considered, given that it can increase the number of nocturnal awakenings. Many studies have shown that there is a high prevalence of musculoskeletal pain in women around the world. In North and South America, the prevalence of pain in women can reach almost 75%. In Europe, it can reach 63%, in Asia 71%, and in Oceania 50%.[52–56] In a study by Mathias and colleagues[57] using PSG, adults with chronic pain present reduced sleep efficiency and an increase in sleep onset latency and the number of awakenings. Specifically in women, chronic pain is also related with a reduction in sleep duration and an increase in the arousal index.[58] Pain has been studied in women with and without insomnia. Women with insomnia presented higher pain scores when compared with controls, and insomnia and pain in women have been shown to have an impact on relationships.[59] In addition, postmenopausal women with chronic pain and insomnia presented higher pain intensity and impaired sleep patterns.[60]

Patient Assessment

The best way to assist a woman in postmenopause is to look at the patient carefully and as a whole considering her multiple aspects. It is essential to perform a comprehensive anamnesis, and a detailed medical and gynecological examination. The Blatt-Kupperman index is a questionnaire that can be used by the clinician to measure menopausal symptoms, grading them from mild to severe.[61] A score higher than 18 suggest that the woman may benefit from hormonal therapy (HT), as long as the patient does not present any contraindications.

Regarding sleep, a coherent diagnosis is necessary to conduct the case properly. For instance, OSA is highly prevalent in postmenopausal women and can often bring complaints such as insomnia. Benzodiazepines are one pharmacologic option to treat insomnia, but in women with OSA, this treatment can make the OSA worse. Therefore, ideally PSG should be used to clarify the diagnosis, and the STOP-Bang questionnaire can help with anamnesis.[62] Restless leg syndrome is also a possible differential diagnosis, and comorbidities such as anxiety, depression and pain, among others should be considered. If necessary, a psychiatric evaluation may be helpful.

Treatment

Although menopause and postmenopause represent a challenging transition in a woman's life, there are good hormonal and nonhormonal treatment options that can help to sustain an individual's health and quality of life. First of all, adopting a healthy lifestyle that includes healthy nutrition, exercise, and social support is very important. In **Fig. 1**, we present multiple aspects related to impoverishment in sleep pattern during menopause transition and postmenopause. In respect of sleep, studies have shown that there is an association between low levels of physical activities, smoking, and certain occupations and reduced sleep quality in postmenopausal women.[63] Moreover, obesity and sedentarism seem to enhance levels of anxiety, depression, insomnia, and menopause symptoms, in middle-age women, whereas active lifestyles, social participation physical activity, and healthy eating promote metabolic balance and sleep quality and have been related to a positive improvement in women's well-being.[19,63–66]

Hormonal Therapy and Sleep

The risks and benefits of HT must be assessed before deciding whether a patient should undergo the treatment. HT is associated with an increased risk of cancer and cardiovascular disease, but is one of the most effective treatments in respect of vasomotor symptoms, urogenital tropism, and bone mass.[2,67] It is important to emphasize that there is an optimal window for the introduction of HT which, according to The North American Menopause Society, is in women aged 60 or younger, or who are within 10 years of menopause onset. After this window, the risks are higher than the benefits.[68] For example, the use of oral estradiol therapy was associated with less progression of subclinical atherosclerosis than placebo when therapy was initiated within 6 years of menopause onset, but not when it was initiated 10 or more years after menopause.[69]

Some studies have demonstrated that estrogen can decrease sleep latency and increase total sleep time, whereas others have shown that progesterone is a ventilatory stimulant and a hypnotic.[70–72] A meta-analysis revealed that HT leads to better sleep quality in women with hot flashes, but does not seem to promote better sleep in the population without hot flashes.[73] It is also important to mention that there has been no indication that HT can be used to treat OSA, with a mandibular advancement device (MAD) remaining the treatment for mild to moderate OSA, and continuous positive airway pressure (CPAP) for more severe cases.[74–76]

Nonhormonal Therapy

When HT is not recommended, other options can be chosen. Behavioral changes, phytotherapeutics, and other pharmacologic interventions may be useful.

The main tool for treating insomnia is cognitive behavioral therapy for insomnia (CBT-I).[77] A review on the possible treatments for insomnia in postmenopause concluded that CBT was superior to all other treatments.[78] CBT-I is the gold standard intervention for insomnia and uses sleep restriction, stimulus control, and relaxation techniques. Also, physical exercise can be used together with CBT to get better sleep. Sleep hygiene education has also shown positive results. A meta-analysis comparing both interventions (CBT-I and sleep hygiene) found that CBT-I showed better results in respect of improving sleep patterns, but sleep hygiene was associated with an enhanced sleep routine.[79] Moreover, menopausal women with sleep complaints should avoid negative sleep behaviors, such as taking naps and drinking coffee near to bedtime.[80]

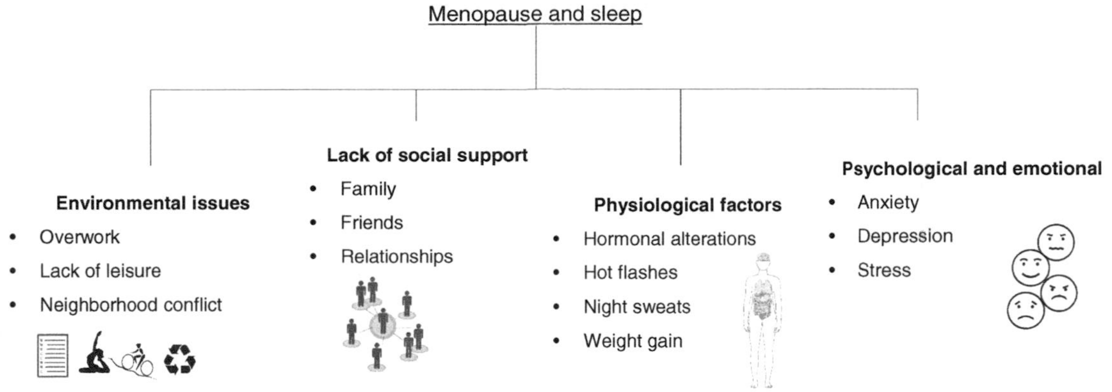

Fig. 1. Multiple aspects related to impairments in sleep pattern during the menopause transition and postmenopause.

Pharmacologic options include hypnotics, antidepressants, melatonin agonists, and the use of herbal medicine. Benzodiazepines are widely used in the treatment of chronic or acute insomnia. Treatment of associated anxiety and depression can be conducted with the following medications: tricyclic antidepressants, selective serotonin-reuptake inhibitors(SRIs), melatonin, duloxetine, fluoxetine, imipramine, nortriptyline or amitriptyline, and other drugs such as eszopiclone, escitalopram, gabapentin, quetiapine, citalopram, and mirtazapine, followed by long-acting melatonin and ramelteon.[78,81,82]

Venlafaxine is a pharmacologic option to treat vasomotor symptoms in addition to having a modest effect in respect of improved sleep quality.[83,84] Both venlafaxine and desvenlafaxine can be effective treatments in cases of depression, associated or not with insomnia. In some cases, the use of hypnotics can improve sleep duration. The Menopause Strategies: Finding Lasting Answers for Symptoms and Health clinical trials network was founded to find new ways to alleviate the most common, bothersome menopausal symptoms by designing and conducting multiple concurrent clinical intervention studies.[85] Trials were conducted in various locations in the United States, with the primary outcomes focused on vasomotor symptoms, sleep quality, insomnia, and vaginal symptoms. It was found that escitalopram, an SRI antidepressant, decreased hot flashes by nearly 50%, as compared with a 30% decrease with the use of placebo, whereas low-dose oral estradiol was effective in reducing the frequency of hot flashes compared with a placebo. Venlafaxine, another antidepressant, was found to be able to reduce the number of vasomotor symptoms. These findings corroborate the association between anxiety, depression, and sleep complaints in the postmenopause period.

A study comparing HT, isoflavone, and placebo in the treatment of menopause symptoms reported that HT achieved a 77% of improvement, isoflavone a 60% improvement, and a placebo a 30% improvement.[86] Moreover, isoflavones were shown to be able to decrease insomnia in postmenopause in a comparison with a control group.[87] Valerian root (*Valeriana officinalis* L) is an example of a potential herbal treatment and has been shown to have a positive effect in the treatment of sleep disorders, with only minimal side effects.[88] Furthermore, a study indicated that the decrease in WASO and mild anxiolytic effect were the factors that most contributed to the subjective perception of sleep in patients with benzodiazepines withdrawn, in use Valerian.[89] In postmenopausal women, a positive effect on sleep quality was also observed following valerian treatment.[90]

Complementary and Integrative Medicine (CIM) encompasses a set of traditional and alternative health-oriented techniques that work in conjunction with conventional medicine. Such practices are based on scientific evidence and, in contrast with some forms of medicine, direct the treatment with a holistic view of the individual/patient.[91,92] Among the practices that make up the CIM are meditation, yoga, massage, aromatherapy, and others,[93] which can bring a range of benefits to patients, such as reductions in the level of anxiety[94] and depression,[95] better pain management,[96] and improvements in quality of life[94] and sleep.[97–100] Moreover, due to their integrative and complementary nature, CIM can help in the drug treatment offered by a doctor; for example, the nutritional guidance provided by a nutritionist, or the psychotherapy provided by a psychologist, can complement the traditional treatment and produce more effective outcomes. Furthermore, CIM is more likely to be taken up by women, which has been shown in a range of studies in Germany,[101] Brazil,[102] England,[93] Australia,[103] and the United States.[91] During the menopausal transition and postmenopause, women use these practices alongside conventional medicine to help reduce levels of anxiety, depression, vasomotor symptoms, and sleep disorders.[104] A cohort study which followed women of different ethnicities in the menopausal transition reported that up to 80% of them used some type of CIM during this period.[105]

In respect of the disturbed sleep patterns frequently observed in postmenopausal women, studies have reported an improvement in sleep quality using therapeutic massage on patients with a diagnosis of insomnia.[99] Another intervention found positive results using foot massage in postmenopausal women to increase average daily sleep duration (hours) and reduce levels of fatigue and anxiety.[106] Regarding yoga practices, a study distributed the participants into three groups: yoga intervention, passive stretching, and a control, found that the yoga intervention had the best outcomes in postmenopausal women with insomnia.[98] Corroborating this finding, another study reported an improvement in sleep quality in perimenopausal and postmenopausal women, but not in premenopausal ones, who underwent a yoga intervention, after controlling for social support, depression, anxiety, stress, and menopausal symptoms.[107] Despites the good results found with the application of yoga on the quality of sleep, there is still a lack of evidence on its effects on vasomotor symptoms. A review found that no benefits were detected in respect of vasomotor symptoms following yoga or exercise programs when compared with usual activity.[85] In the same review, CBT-I was shown to reduce self-reported insomnia symptoms and improve overall sleep quality compared with a control receiving only menopause education.[85] In another study, both yoga and wellness education presented similar findings, reducing hot flashes by about 60% following a 10-week intervention.[108] A meta-analysis on sleep and exercise in middle-aged women revealed that moderate to intense exercise was associated with better sleep quality.[109] Another mind-body intervention, mindfulness meditation, has shown good results in improving sleep quality. A meta-analysis indicated that mindfulness practice demonstrated moderate strength evidence of a significant enhancement in sleep quality in postmenopausal women, whereas another study found that postmenopausal women with insomnia diagnosis also presented improved sleep patterns after a mindfulness intervention.[97,110]

Aromatherapy is also a part of CIM and has been used to treat insomnia and sleep disorders. Although a great diversity of methods was applied in the studies, a meta-analysis reported that aromatherapy was effective in improving these outcomes.[111] Lavender essential oil is one the most studied substances in this area.[112] The effect of lavender oil on sleep in postmenopausal women was studied in a double-blind clinical trial with 35 postmenopausal women with insomnia diagnosis. To measure the effect of the intervention, the participants underwent PSG and completed validated questionnaires. There was no significant difference between groups over time; however, the intervention group presented better sleep quality at the end of intervention and improvements in the level of depression and menopausal symptoms. According to the PSG recordings, the group who inhaled lavender essential oil had a significant improvement in sleep efficiency over time and an average decrease in WASO of 42.2 minutes compared with the control group.[100] Acupuncture has also exhibited some good results in the treatment of climacteric women. In a randomized, controlled study in postmenopausal women with insomnia, the participants who underwent acupuncture presented a higher percentage of N3 sleep stage than the sham group in the PSG findings.[113] Moreover, a meta-analysis indicated that acupuncture seems to have a positive effect on sleep in postmenopausal women.[114] Despites these positive finding regarding the use of CIM to treat sleep disorders during menopausal transition and postmenopause, it is still necessary to evaluate these outcomes in larger samples and to assess in more detail the benefits of using CIM with other treatment approaches.

SUMMARY

An integrative approach is the best way to treat sleep problems in patients during menopause, as several different aspects need to be considered. In this respect, the use of a combination of traditional and complementary therapies may be optimum in helping women deal with their symptoms during this period. Lifestyle changes including healthy nutrition and exercises are useful. CBT-I remains the gold standard intervention to treat insomnia in menopausal transition and postmenopause and HT to treat hot flashes. Pharmacologic options may be useful, especially in cases with comorbidities such as anxiety and depression disorders. OSA, if present, may be treated with MADs or CPAP. Both hot menopausal symptoms and sleep problems have to be addressed in conjunction and women should be treated as a whole, taking into account mind, body and soul, to achieve the greatest improvements in respect of their sleep-related quality of life.[115]

SUMMARY CONFLICT OF INTEREST STATEMENTS

Neither of the authors have any conflict of interest to disclose. The authors confirm that we have read the Journal's position on issues involved in ethical publication and affirm that this report is consistent with those guidelines.

CLINICS CARE POINTS

- Insomnia is highly prevalent in women during menopause and is underdiagnosed.
- Women in postmenopause can suffer from obstructive sleep apnea and may complaint of insomnia.
- Sleep complaints may be due to psychosocial influence, not only decreased hormones.

DISCLOSURE

The authors have no conflict of interest to declare.

FINANCIAL SUPPORT

This research was supported by the Associação Fundo de Incentivo à Pesquisa, Brazil (AFIP), the Coordenação de Aperfeiçoamento de Pessoal de Nível Superior, Brazil (CAPES)–Finance Code 001, and the Conselho Nacional de Desenvolvimento Científico e Tecnológico, Brazil (CNPq). H. Hachul, L. Lucena, and S. Tufik are recipients of CNPq fellowships. The funding agencies had no role in the design, preparation, review, or approval of this study.

REFERENCES

1. Kontis V, Bennett JE, Mathers CD, et al. Future life expectancy in 35 industrialised countries: projections with a Bayesian model ensemble. Lancet 2017;389(10076):1323–35.
2. Harlow SD, Elliott MR, Bondarenko I, et al. Monthly variation of hot flashes, night sweats, and trouble sleeping: effect of season and proximity to the final menstrual period (FMP) in the SWAN Menstrual Calendar substudy. Menopause 2020;27(1):5–13.
3. Sammel MD, Freeman EW, Liu Z, et al. Factors that influence entry into stages of the menopausal transition. Menopause 2009;16(6):1218–27.
4. Schoenaker DAJM, Jackson CA, Rowlands Jv, et al. Socioeconomic position, lifestyle factors and age at natural menopause: a systematic review and meta-analyses of studies across six continents. Int J Epidemiol 2014;43(5):1542.
5. Hansen KR, Knowlton NS, Thyer AC, et al. A new model of reproductive aging: the decline in ovarian non-growing follicle number from birth to menopause. Humanit Rep 2008;23(3):699–708.
6. Hachul H, Bittencourt LRA, Soares JM, et al. Sleep in post-menopausal women: differences between early and late post-menopause. Eur J Obstet Gynecol Reprod Biol 2009;145(1):81–4.
7. Baker FC, de Zambotti M, Colrain IM, et al. Sleep problems during the menopausal transition: prevalence, impact, and management challenges. Nat Sci Sleep 2018;10:73–95.
8. Freeman EW, Sammel MD, Sanders RJ. Risk of long-term hot flashes after natural menopause. Menopause 2014;21(9):924–32.
9. Gold EB, Colvin A, Avis N, et al. Longitudinal analysis of the association between vasomotor symptoms and race/ethnicity across the menopausal transition: study of women's health across the nation. Am J Public Health 2006;96(7):1226–35.
10. Kronenberg F. Menopausal hot flashes: a review of physiology and biosociocultural perspective on methods of assessment. J Nutr 2010;140(7):1380S–5S.
11. Baker FC, Willoughby AR, Sassoon SA, et al. Insomnia in women approaching menopause: beyond perception. Psychoneuroendocrinology 2015;60:96–104.
12. Avis NE, Crawford SL, Green R. Vasomotor symptoms across the menopause transition. Obstet Gynecol Clin North Am 2018;45(4):629–40.
13. Kim MJ, Yim G, Park HY. Vasomotor and physical menopausal symptoms are associated with sleep quality. PLoS One 2018;13(2):e0192934. Hachul H.
14. Ensrud KE, Stone KL, Blackwell TL, et al. Frequency and severity of hot flashes and sleep disturbance in postmenopausal women with hot flashes. Menopause 2009;16(2):286–92.
15. Freedman RR, Roehrs TA. Effects of REM sleep and ambient temperature on hot flash-induced sleep disturbance. Menopause 2006;13(4):576–83.
16. Bianchi MT, Kim S, Galvan T, et al. Nocturnal hot flashes: relationship to objective awakenings and sleep stage transitions. J Clin Sleep Med 2016;12(07):1003–9.
17. El Khoudary SR, Greendale G, Crawford SL, et al. The menopause transition and women's health at midlife. Menopause 2019;26(10):1213–27. Publish Ah.
18. Lampio L, Polo-Kantola P, Himanen SL, et al. Sleep during menopausal transition: a 6-year follow-up. Sleep 2017;40(7).

19. Kravitz HM, Janssen I, Bromberger JT, et al. Sleep trajectories before and after the final menstrual period in the study of women's health across the nation (SWAN). Curr Sleep Med Rep 2017;3(3): 235–50.
20. Nik Hazlina NH, Norhayati MN, Shaiful Bahari I, et al. Prevalence of psychosomatic and genitourinary syndrome among menopausal women: a systematic review and meta-analysis. Front Med 2022; 9. https://doi.org/10.3389/fmed.2022.848202.
21. Arakane M, Castillo C, Rosero MF, et al. Factors relating to insomnia during the menopausal transition as evaluated by the insomnia severity index. Maturitas 2011;69(2):157–61.
22. Joffe H, Massler A, Sharkey K. Evaluation and management of sleep disturbance during the menopause transition. Semin Reprod Med 2010;28(05): 404–21.
23. Salo P, Sivertsen B, Oksanen T, et al. Insomnia symptoms as a predictor of incident treatment for depression: prospective cohort study of 40,791 men and women. Sleep Med 2012;13(3):278–84.
24. Pavlova M, Sheikh L. Sleep in women. Semin Neurol 2011;31(04):397–403.
25. Polo-Kantola P. Sleep problems in midlife and beyond. Maturitas 2011;68(3):224–32.
26. American Psychiatric Association. Diagnostic and statistical manual of mental disorders. DSM-5. 5th edn. Washington, D.C: American Psychiatric Publishing; 2013. https://doi.org/10.1176/appi.books.9780890425596.744053.
27. Lucena L, Polesel DN, Poyares D, et al. The association of insomnia and quality of life: sao paulo epidemiologic sleep study (EPISONO). Sleep Health 2020;6(5):629–35.
28. von Mühlen DG, Kritz-Silverstein D, Barrett-Connor E. A community-based study of menopause symptoms and estrogen replacement in older women. Maturitas 1995;22(2):71–8.
29. Kuh DL, Wadsworth M, Hardy R. Women's health in midlife: the influence of the menopause, social factors and health in earlier life. BJOG 1997;104(8): 923–33.
30. Mirer AG, Young T, Palta M, et al. Sleep-disordered breathing and the menopausal transition among participants in the Sleep in Midlife Women Study. Menopause 2017;24(2):157–62.
31. Heinzer R, Marti-Soler H, Marques-Vidal P, et al. Impact of sex and menopausal status on the prevalence, clinical presentation, and comorbidities of sleep-disordered breathing. Sleep Med 2018;51: 29–36.
32. Hachul de Campos H, Brandão LC, D'Almeida V, et al. Sleep disturbances, oxidative stress and cardiovascular risk parameters in postmenopausal women complaining of insomnia. Climacteric 2006;9(4):312–9.
33. Perger E, Mattaliano P, Lombardi C. Menopause and sleep apnea. Maturitas 2019;124:35–8.
34. Javaheri S, Barbe F, Campos-Rodriguez F, et al. Sleep apnea. J Am Coll Cardiol 2017;69(7):841–58.
35. Lal C, Weaver TE, Bae CJ, et al. Excessive daytime sleepiness in obstructive sleep apnea. mechanisms and clinical management. Ann Am Thorac Soc 2021;18(5):757–68.
36. Terauchi M, Hiramitsu S, Akiyoshi M, et al. Associations between anxiety, depression and insomnia in peri- and post-menopausal women. Maturitas 2012;72(1):61–5.
37. Bromberger JT, Kravitz HM, Chang YF, et al. Major depression during and after the menopausal transition: study of women's health across the nation (SWAN). Psychol Med 2011;41(9):1879–88.
38. Maganhin CC, Carbonel AAF, Hatty JH, et al. Efeitos da melatonina no sistema genital feminino: breve revisão. Rev Assoc Med Bras 2008;54(3): 267–71.
39. Llaneza P, García-Portilla MP, Llaneza-Suárez D, et al. Depressive disorders and the menopause transition. Maturitas 2012;71(2):120–30.
40. Sandilyan MB, Dening T. Mental health around and after the menopause. Menopause Int 2011;17(4): 142–7.
41. Naufel MF, Frange C, Andersen ML, et al. Association between obesity and sleep disorders in postmenopausal women. Menopause 2018;25(2): 139–44.
42. Zhou Q, Wang B, Hua Q, et al. Investigation of the relationship between hot flashes, sweating and sleep quality in perimenopausal and postmenopausal women: the mediating effect of anxiety and depression. BMC Womens Health 2021; 21(1):293.
43. Luo M, Li J, Tang R, et al. Insomnia symptoms in relation to menopause among middle-aged Chinese women: findings from a longitudinal cohort study. Maturitas 2020;141:1–8.
44. Ballot O, Ivers H, Ji X, et al. Sleep disturbances during the menopausal transition: the role of sleep reactivity and arousal predisposition. Behav Sleep Med 2022;20(4):500–12.
45. Matthews KA, Kravitz HM, Lee L, et al. Does midlife aging impact women's sleep duration, continuity, and timing?: a longitudinal analysis from the Study of Women's Health across the Nation. Sleep 2020; 43(4). https://doi.org/10.1093/sleep/zsz259.
46. Zolfaghari S, Yao C, Thompson C, et al. Effects of menopause on sleep quality and sleep disorders: Canadian Longitudinal Study on Aging. Menopause 2020;27(3):295–304.
47. Hachul H, Frange C, Bezerra AG, et al. The effect of menopause on objective sleep parameters: data from an epidemiologic study in São Paulo. Brazil. Maturitas 2015;80(2):170–8.

48. Sorpreso ICE, Vieira LHL, Haidar MA, et al. Multidisciplinary approach during menopausal transition and postmenopause in Brazilian women. Clin Exp Obstet Gynecol 2010;37(4):283–6.
49. Liedtke S, Schmidt ME, Vrieling A, et al. Postmenopausal sex hormones in relation to body fat distribution. Obesity 2012;20(5):1088–95.
50. Polesel DN, Hirotsu C, Nozoe KT, et al. Waist circumference and postmenopause stages as the main associated factors for sleep apnea in women. Menopause 2015;22(8):835–44.
51. Van Cauter, E., Knutson, K., Leproult, R., & Spiegel K. The impact of sleep deprivation on hormones and metabolism. Published 2005. Available at: https://www.medscape.org/viewarticle/502825. Accessed November 11, 2022.
52. Dugan SA, Powell LH, Kravitz HM, et al. Musculoskeletal pain and menopausal status. Clin J Pain 2006;22(4):325–31.
53. da Silva AR, dAndretta Tanaka AC. Factors associated with menopausal symptom severity in middle-aged Brazilian women from the Brazilian Western Amazon. Maturitas 2013;76(1):64–9.
54. Farioli A, Mattioli S, Quaglieri A, et al. Musculoskeletal pain in Europe: the role of personal, occupational, and social risk factors. Scand J Work Environ Health 2014;40(1):36–46.
55. Lu C bo, fei Liu P, Zhou Y sheng, et al. Musculoskeletal pain during the menopausal transition: a systematic review and meta-analysis. Neural Plast 2020;2020:1–10. https://doi.org/10.1155/2020/8842110. Hu L.
56. Brown WJ, Mishra GD, Dobson A. Changes in physical symptoms during the menopause transition. Int J Behav Med 2002;9(1):53–67.
57. Mathias JL, Cant ML, Burke ALJ. Sleep disturbances and sleep disorders in adults living with chronic pain: a meta-analysis. Sleep Med 2018; 52:198–210.
58. Lavigne GJ, Nashed A, Manzini C, et al. Does sleep differ among patients with common musculoskeletal pain disorders? Curr Rheumatol Rep 2011; 13(6):535–42.
59. Frange C, Naufel MF, Andersen ML, et al. Impact of insomnia on pain in postmenopausal women. Climacteric 2017;20(3):262–7.
60. Frange C, Hachul H, Hirotsu C, et al. Temporal analysis of chronic musculoskeletal pain and sleep in postmenopausal women. J Clin Sleep Med 2019; 15(02):223–34.
61. Kupperman HS. Contemporary therapy of the menopausal syndrome. J Am Med Assoc 1959; 171(12):1627.
62. Chung F, Yegneswaran B, Liao P, et al. STOP questionnaire. Anesthesiology 2008;108(5):812–21.
63. Moudi A, Dashtgard A, Salehiniya H, et al. The relationship between health-promoting lifestyle and sleep quality in postmenopausal women. Biomedicine 2018;8(2):11.
64. Blümel JE, Fica J, Chedraui P, et al. Sedentary lifestyle in middle-aged women is associated with severe menopausal symptoms and obesity. Menopause 2016;23(5):488–93.
65. Falkingham J, Evandrou M, Qin M, et al. Chinese women's health and wellbeing in middle life: unpacking the influence of menopause, lifestyle activities and social participation. Maturitas 2021;143: 145–50.
66. Pereira N, Naufel MF, Ribeiro EB, et al. Influence of dietary sources of melatonin on sleep quality: a review. J Food Sci 2020;85(1):5–13.
67. The 2017 hormone therapy position statement of the North American Menopause Society. Menopause 2017;24(7):728–53.
68. Writing Group for the Women's Health Initiative Investigators. Risks and benefits of estrogen plus progestin in healthy postmenopausal women: principal results from the women's health initiative randomized controlled trial. JAMA, J Am Med Assoc 2002;288(3):321–33.
69. Hodis HN, Mack WJ, Henderson VW, et al. Vascular effects of early versus late postmenopausal treatment with estradiol. N Engl J Med 2016;374(13):1221–31.
70. Hachul H, Bittencourt LRA, Andersen ML, et al. Effects of hormone therapy with estrogen and/or progesterone on sleep pattern in postmenopausal women. Int J Gynecol Obstet 2008;103(3):207–12.
71. Teran-Perez G, Arana-Lechuga Y, Esqueda-Leon E, et al. Steroid hormones and sleep regulation. Mini-Rev Med Chem 2012;12(11):1040–8.
72. Guidozzi F. Sleep and sleep disorders in menopausal women. Climacteric 2013;16(2):214–9.
73. Cintron D, Lipford M, Larrea-Mantilla L, et al. Efficacy of menopausal hormone therapy on sleep quality: systematic review and meta-analysis. Endocrine 2017;55(3):702–11.
74. Lindberg E, Bonsignore MR, Polo-Kantola P. Role of menopause and hormone replacement therapy in sleep-disordered breathing. Sleep Med Rev 2020;49:101225.
75. Manetta IP, Ettlin D, Sanz PM, et al. Mandibular advancement devices in obstructive sleep apnea: an updated review. Sleep Science 2022;15: 398–405.
76. Kushida CA, Littner MR, Hirshkowitz M, et al. Practice parameters for the use of continuous and bilevel positive airway pressure devices to treat adult patients with sleep-related breathing disorders. Sleep 2006;29(3):375–80.
77. Qaseem A, Kansagara D, Forciea MA, et al. Management of chronic insomnia disorder in adults: a clinical practice guideline from the American college of physicians. Ann Intern Med 2016;165(2):125.

78. Attarian H, Hachul H, Guttuso T, et al. Treatment of chronic insomnia disorder in menopause. Menopause 2015;22(6):674–84.
79. Chung KF, Lee CT, Yeung WF, et al. Sleep hygiene education as a treatment of insomnia: a systematic review and meta-analysis. Fam Pract 2018;35(4):365–75.
80. Kline CE, Irish LA, Buysse DJ, et al. Sleep hygiene behaviors among midlife women with insomnia or sleep-disordered breathing: the SWAN sleep study. J Womens Health 2014;23(11):894–903.
81. Tandon V, Sharma S, Mahajan A, et al. Menopause and sleep disorders. J Midlife Health 2022;13(1):26.
82. Caretto M, Giannini A, Simoncini T. An integrated approach to diagnosing and managing sleep disorders in menopausal women. Maturitas 2019;128:1–3.
83. Joffe H, Guthrie KA, LaCroix AZ, et al. Low-dose estradiol and the serotonin-norepinephrine reuptake inhibitor venlafaxine for vasomotor symptoms. JAMA Intern Med 2014;174(7):1058.
84. Ensrud KE, Guthrie KA, Hohensee C, et al. Effects of estradiol and venlafaxine on insomnia symptoms and sleep quality in women with hot flashes. Sleep 2015;38(1):97–108.
85. Reed SD, LaCroix AZ, Anderson GL, et al. Lights on MsFLASH: a review of contributions. Menopause 2020;27(4):473–84.
86. Messina M, Hughes C. Efficacy of soyfoods and soybean isoflavone supplements for alleviating menopausal symptoms is positively related to initial hot flush frequency. J Med Food 2003;6(1):1–11.
87. Hachul H, Brandão LC, D'Almeida V, et al. Isoflavones decrease insomnia in postmenopause. Menopause 2011;18(2):178–84.
88. Shinjyo N, Waddell G, Green J. Valerian root in treating sleep problems and associated disorders—a systematic review and meta-analysis. J Evid Based Integr Med 2020;25. 2515690X2096732.
89. Poyares DR, Guilleminault C, Ohayon MM, et al. Can valerian improve the sleep of insomniacs after benzodiazepine withdrawal? Prog Neuro-Psychopharmacol Biol Psychiatry 2002;26(3):539–45.
90. Taavoni S, Ekbatani N, Kashaniyan M, et al. Effect of valerian on sleep quality in postmenopausal women. Menopause 2011;18(9):951–5.
91. Barnes PM, Bloom B, Nahin RL. Complementary and alternative medicine use among adults and children: United States, 2007. Natl Health Stat Report 2008;(12):1–23. https://doi.org/10.1037/-001.
92. National Center for Complementary and Integrative Health. Complementary, Alternative, or Integrative Health: What's In a Name? NCCIH. Available at: https://www.nccih.nih.gov/health/complementary-alternative-or-integrative-health-whats-in-a-name. Accessed November 22, 2022.
93. Hunt KJ, Coelho HF, Wider B, et al. Complementary and alternative medicine use in England: results from a national survey. Int J Clin Pract 2010;64(11):1496–502.
94. Cramer H, Lauche R, Klose P, et al. Yoga for improving health-related quality of life, mental health and cancer-related symptoms in women diagnosed with breast cancer. Cochrane Database Syst Rev 2017;2017(1). https://doi.org/10.1002/14651858.CD010802.pub2.
95. Yeung KS, Hernandez M, Mao JJ, et al. Herbal medicine for depression and anxiety: a systematic review with assessment of potential psycho-oncologic relevance. Phytother Res 2018;32(5):865–91.
96. Greenlee H, DuPont-Reyes MJ, Balneaves LG, et al. Clinical practice guidelines on the evidence-based use of integrative therapies during and after breast cancer treatment. CA Cancer J Clin 2017;67(3):194–232.
97. Garcia MC, Kozasa EH, Tufik S, et al. The effects of mindfulness and relaxation training for insomnia (MRTI) on postmenopausal women: a pilot study. Menopause 2018;25(9):992–1003.
98. Afonso RF, Hachul H, Kozasa EH, et al. Yoga decreases insomnia in postmenopausal women. Menopause 2012;19(2):186–93.
99. Oliveira DS, Hachul H, Goto V, et al. Effect of therapeutic massage on insomnia and climacteric symptoms in postmenopausal women. Climacteric 2012;15(1):21–9.
100. dos Reis Lucena L, dos Santos-Junior JG, Tufik S, et al. Lavender essential oil on postmenopausal women with insomnia: double-blind randomized trial. Complement Ther Med 2021;59:102726.
101. Härtel U, Volger E. Inanspruchnahme und Akzeptanz klassischer naturheilverfahren und alternativer heilmethoden in deutschland – ergebnisse einer repräsentativen bevölkerungsstudie. Complement Med Res 2004;11(6):327–34.
102. de Moraes Mello Boccolini P, Siqueira Boccolini C. Prevalence of complementary and alternative medicine (CAM) use in Brazil. BMC Complement Med Ther 2020;20(1):51.
103. Steel A, McIntyre E, Harnett J, et al. Complementary medicine use in the Australian population: results of a nationally-representative cross-sectional survey. Sci Rep 2018;8(1):17325.
104. Peng W, Adams J, Sibbritt DW, et al. Critical review of complementary and alternative medicine use in menopause. Menopause 2014;21(5):536–48.
105. Bair YA, Gold EB, Zhang G, et al. Use of complementary and alternative medicine during the menopause transition. Menopause 2008;15(1):32–43.
106. Gökbulut N, Ibici Akça E, Karakayali Ay Ç. The impact of foot massage given to postmenopausal

women on anxiety, fatigue, and sleep: a randomized-controlled trial. Menopause 2022; 29(11):1254–62.

107. Susanti HD, Sonko I, Chang P, et al. Effects of yoga on menopausal symptoms and sleep quality across menopause statuses: a randomized controlled trial. Nurs Health Sci 2022;24(2):368–79.
108. Avis NE, Legault C, Russell G, et al. Pilot study of integral yoga for menopausal hot flashes. Menopause 2014;21(8):846–54.
109. Rubio-Arias JÁ, Marín-Cascales E, Ramos-Campo DJ, et al. Effect of exercise on sleep quality and insomnia in middle-aged women: a systematic review and meta-analysis of randomized controlled trials. Maturitas 2017;100:49–56.
110. Rusch HL, Rosario M, Levison LM, et al. The effect of mindfulness meditation on sleep quality: a systematic review and meta-analysis of randomized controlled trials. Ann N Y Acad Sci 2019;1445(1):5–16.
111. Lin PC, Lee PH, Tseng SJ, et al. Effects of aromatherapy on sleep quality: a systematic review and meta-analysis. Complement Ther Med 2019;45: 156–66.
112. Cheong MJ, Kim S, Kim JS, et al. A systematic literature review and meta-analysis of the clinical effects of aroma inhalation therapy on sleep problems. Medicine 2021;100(9):e24652.
113. Hachul H, Garcia TKP, Maciel AL, et al. Acupuncture improves sleep in postmenopause in a randomized, double-blind, placebo-controlled study. Climacteric 2012;16(1):36–40.
114. Bezerra AG, Pires GN, Andersen ML, et al. Acupuncture to treat sleep disorders in postmenopausal women: a systematic review. Evid base Compl Alternative Med 2015;2015:1–16.
115. Hachul H, Tufik S. Hot flashes: treating the mind, body and soul. Menopause 2019;26(5):461–2.

The Effects of Hormonal Contraceptives on the Sleep of Women of Reproductive Age

Andréia Gomes Bezerra, PhD[a], Gabriel Natan Pires, PhD[a,b], Monica L. Andersen, PhD[a,b], Sergio Tufik, MD, PhD[a,b], Helena Hachul, MD, PhD[a,b,*]

KEYWORDS

• Sleep • Woman • Estrogen • Progestin • Reproductive age • Menstrual cycle • Insomnia

KEY POINTS

- Previous evidence from studies about sleep across the menstrual cycle, in postmenopausal women, and evaluating the effects of hormone replacement therapy suggests that sexual hormones have a role on the physiology of sleep and on the onset of sleep disorders and complaints. This has been the main rationale for the research about the relationship between sleep and hormonal contraceptives.
- Most of the studies available about contraceptives and sleep are based on observational designs, rather than on proper randomized controlled trials, and entail a substantial level of methodological heterogeneity both between and within studies. It includes variability on the types of contraceptives being tested, their composition, dosage, administration route, sleep assessment methods, and population under investigation. Therefore, the evidence level and the certainty of evidence in this field are typically low.
- Considering the available results, it is likely that hormonal contraceptives impact sleep, but the direction of this association is not clear. Positive effects on sleep are possibly due to a primary improvement on obstructive sleep apnea caused by progestins, which secondarily improves other sleep variables (such as arousal index and sleep efficiency). Negative effects are also attributed to progestins and include mainly increased sleepiness. Secondary effects such as insomnia symptoms, decreased total sleep time and sleep efficiency, or a reduced overall sleep quality are also observed, although less frequently.
- The evidence about the effects of different types of contraceptives is low. It is suggested that the intrauterine route (such as in levonorgestrel-releasing intrauterine devices) could lead to less negative outcomes, as its effects are more local than systemic. However, this should be confirmed by proper randomized controlled trials.
- Clinicians should be attentive to sleep complaints on patients initiating or changing their hormonal contraceptive therapy. If sleep-related signs, symptoms, or complaints are observed, it should be considered to change the contraceptive prescription.

[a] Departamento de Psicobiologia, Universidade Federal de São Paulo, Rua Napoleão de Barros, 925 – CEP: 04024-002, São Paulo, Brazil; [b] Sleep Institute, Rua Marselhesa, 500 - CEP: 04020-060, São Paulo, Brazil
* Corresponding author. Departamento de Psicobiologia, Universidade Federal de São Paulo, Rua Napoleão de Barros, 925 – CEP: 04024-002, São Paulo, Brazil
E-mail address: helena.hachul@gmail.com

Sleep Med Clin 18 (2023) 435–448
https://doi.org/10.1016/j.jsmc.2023.06.005

INTRODUCTION

The first hormonal contraceptive pill (norethindrone) was developed in the 1950s, and in 1960s, commercial presentations of oral contraceptives were already approved and available in the United States and Europe.[1–3] In the following decades, a surge in clinical research about hormonal contraceptives was observed, resulting in new formulations and an increasing availability of contraceptive pills.[3]

The development of hormonal contraception was one of the most important hallmarks on the history of modern women, impacting both their health and their positions on society. First, it proved to be an effective contraceptive method in comparison with those available at the time (such as barrier, behavioral, and surgical methods), as it was efficient, easy to use, inexpensive, and reversible. However, the true revolution came more from a social perspective. The development of contraceptive pills happened more or less simultaneously to several important women's social achievements (which were happening since suffrage movements), and contraception, which was once criminalized, was being gradually endorsed by the society.[4] With that, family planning became more effective, and women became protagonists on the decision of when or whether to have children. The possibility of preventing or delaying maternity is related to women's increasing educational attainment, growing presence in the workforce, increased social representativeness, among other results. Although gender parity still has not been assured in many social and economic realms, hormonal contraception is certainly an important feature of modern women empowerment.

Such importance can be attested by the frequency of use of hormonal contraceptives. According to the World Health Organization, oral contraception is the fourth most common contraceptive method worldwide, being used by 16% of women of reproductive age (following female sterilization: 24%, male condom: 21%, and intrauterine devices: 17%).[5] Different patterns are observed in the Europe and North America, in which oral contraceptives are the most common contraceptive method.[5] In the United States, oral contraceptives are used by 16% of women of reproductive age, being more frequently used than female sterilization (15.5%) and male condom (9.4%).[6] The proportion of use of different contraceptive methods is presented for the entire world in **Fig. 1** and for different world regions in **Fig. 2**.

With such frequent use, the investigation of noncontraceptive effects of hormonal contraceptives became more common, including side effects and other clinical uses. Hormonal contraceptives are currently considered as the choice therapy for polycystic ovary syndrome and dysmenorrhea,[7,8] are used as an effective adjuvant treatment for facial acne, alopecia, seborrhea, and hirsutism,[9] and have been associated with reduced incidence of ovarian, endometrial, and colorectal cancer.[10] All these conditions have in common a clear involvement of female sexual hormones on its pathophysiology, which justifies their use. Current research has been analyzing the effects of contraceptives on other areas, and their relationship with cognitive and behavioral outcomes has been studied,[11] including mood disorders and depression, memory, and others. It also includes their possible effects on sleep and the relationship with sleep disorders.

The relationship between hormonal contraceptive use and sleep in women of reproductive age has indeed been a growing focus of research. Early studies on the field have suggested that specific contraceptive formulations could be used as an adjuvant treatment for insomnia,[12] but more recent evidence suggests that the relationship is far more complex. Since then, this study field has been growing consistently. This review summarizes the literature about contraceptive use and sleep in women of reproductive age, including the rationale behind this relationship, practical points, analysis of the current level of evidence, and a research agenda for future studies.

RATIONALE

Women experience oscillations and changes in the pattern of sexual hormone production and activity at many moments throughout their life, such as in puberty, across the menstrual cycle, at pregnancy, and at the menopause.[12,13] All of them have been related to effects on sleep to some extent. The idea that hormonal contraceptives might impact sleep is based on indirect evidence coming from three main sources: the sleep alteration observed along the menstrual cycle, sleep in the postmenopausal period, and evidence generated from preclinical studies. These three aspects are briefly reviewed below.

Sleep Across the Menstrual Cycle

The premenopausal phase (ie, the reproductive age) begins at puberty concomitantly with the production of female sexual hormones estrogen and progesterone. From this moment onward, an average 28-day menstrual cycle is established, being characterized by hormonal oscillations that prepare the female reproductive system to ovulation, fertilization, and implantation or to the elimination of the oocyte through menstruation. During the follicular phase, the ovarian follicle develops due to the action of the follicle-stimulating

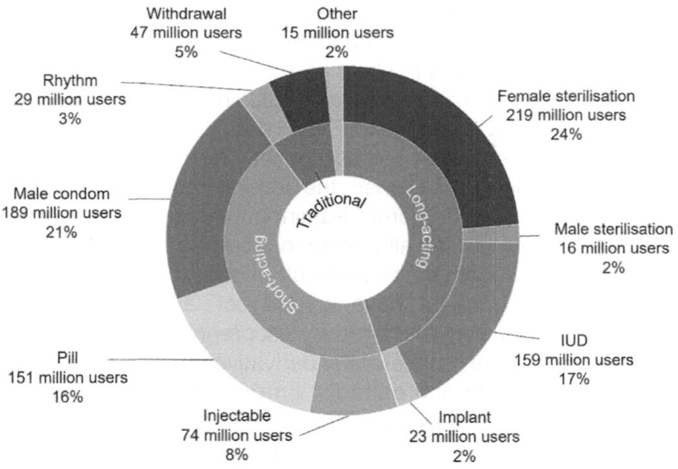

Fig. 1. Worldwide estimated number of women of reproductive age using different contraceptive methods (15–49 years). Oral contraceptive pills are the fourth most common contraceptive method worldwide (16%), followed by female sterilization (24%), male condom (21%), and intrauterine devices (17%). Hormonal contraceptive methods in general (contraceptive pills, injectables, and implants) are used by 26% of the population. (Figure extracted from the WHO Contraceptive Use by Method 2019 Data Booklet,[5] published under CC BY 3.0 IGO license.)

hormone. The level of estrogen rises progressively until a couple of days before ovulation, when it drops. On the days before ovulation, a peak on luteinizing hormone leads to the ovulation and to the conversion of the follicle into a *corpus luteum,* which corresponds to the beginning of the luteal phase. The *corpus luteum* produces high amounts of progesterone, which peaks at the mid-luteal phase, and a smaller peak of estrogen. The cyclic nature of the female sexual hormones, especially estrogen and progesterone, explains the variations on the function of several variables on women's physiology not only on the reproductive system but also in the whole body. It is important to note that several brain areas related to sleep regulation have estrogen and progesterone receptors, including the basal forebrain, hypothalamus, dorsal raphe nucleus, and locus coeruleus.[14,15] Therefore, it seems plausible to consider that sexual hormone fluctuations might have some impacts on sleep among women of reproductive age.

Self-reported sleep disturbances and complaints seem to rise during premenstrual and menstrual phases, comprising both the late luteal

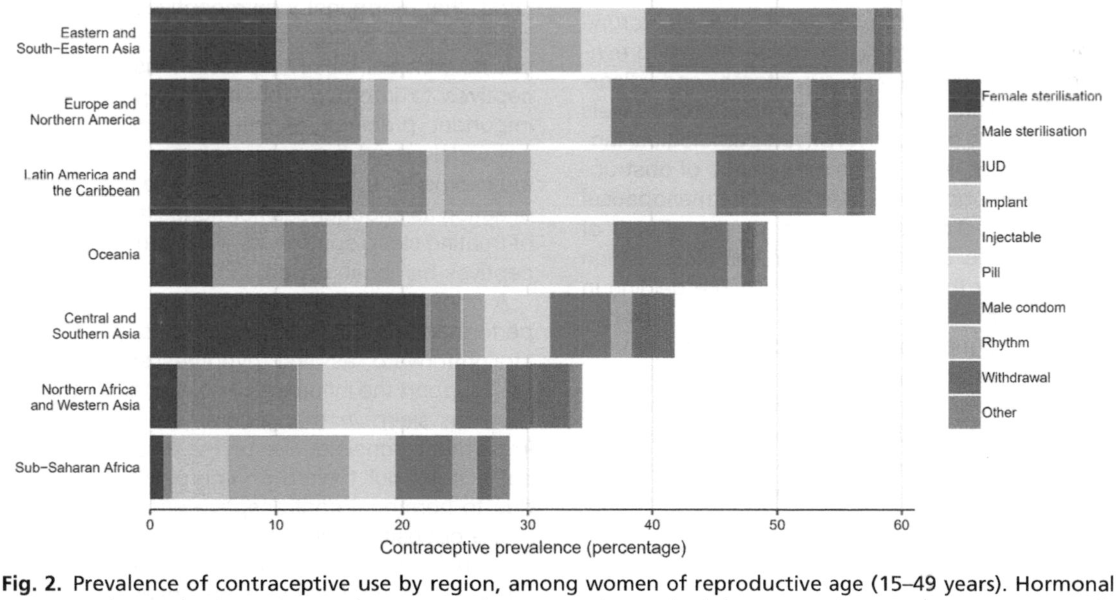

Fig. 2. Prevalence of contraceptive use by region, among women of reproductive age (15–49 years). Hormonal contraceptive methods are among the most used contraceptive methods in most regions. Oral contraceptive pills are the most common methods in Europe and North American (17.8%), Oceania (16.9%), Northern Africa, and Western Asia (10.5%) and the second most common method in Latin America and the Caribbean (14.9%), following female sterilization (16.0%). Injectables are the most common contraceptive methods in Sub-Saharan Africa (9.6%). (Figure extracted from the WHO Contraceptive Use by Method 2019 Data Booklet,[5] published under CC BY 3.0 IGO license.)

phase and the early follicular phase,[16,17] being usually worse in women with dysmenorrhea or premenstrual symptoms.[18] The symptoms can be attributed both to direct effect of the oscillations on sexual hormone levels or as a secondary consequence of other variables that oscillate across the menstrual cycle, such as anxiety and depression symptoms, headache, breast tenderness, among others. Some other profiles of self-reported sleep symptoms can be observed in women of reproductive age, with symptoms peaking at the periovulatory period, in the premenstrual phase, or cases in which the symptoms are spread all across the menstrual cycle with no clear relationship with any phase.[19] The regularity of the menstrual cycle also seems to be an important factor, as women with irregular cycles have more sleep complains, even when the analyses are controlled for dysmenorrhea and other premenstrual symptoms.[20] Regarding objective sleep variables, it has been observed decrease in the duration of rapid eye movements (REM) sleep episodes and in increase in the number of sleep spindles in the luteal phase in comparison to the follicular phase, which has been considered as an effect of progesterone.[18]

Sleep in Menopausal Women

The onset of menopause has been one of the most important proofs of the relationship between sleep and sexual hormones, as the decline on the levels of both estrogen and progesterone are concomitant to the increase on the prevalence of sleep-related symptoms and disorders.[21,22] The reduction on progesterone levels is considered as a critical physiopathological factor on the increase in the prevalence of obstructive sleep apnea (OSA) in postmenopausal women.[23,24] This is explained by the effects of progesterone as a respiratory stimulant, which ceases after the menopause.[23,24] The decline in estrogen levels is associated with the onset of insomnia symptoms and an overall impairment on the sleep pattern.[22]

Corroborating the importance of the hormonal influence to the incidence of sleep disorders and complaints in the perimenopausal period, studies have demonstrated that hormone replacement therapy leads to a reduction in sleep complaints and an overall improvement in the sleep pattern, which includes reduction in the severity of OSA and insomnia symptoms.[25–31]

Preclinical Evidence

Preclinical studies performed with rodent models reinforce the possible hypnotic effect of sexual hormones, especially progesterone. It is demonstrated that the administration of progesterone in rats leads to sleep effects similar to those caused by benzodiazepines, including reduced sleep latency, increased REM latency, reduced wakefulness after sleep onset, and reduced REM sleep.[32] Likewise, the administration of picrotoxin, a GABA (gamma-aminobutyric acid) antagonist, attenuates all effects induced by progesterone.[33] Altogether, these results suggest that progesterone might have an indirect GABAergic effect, possibly mediated by allopregnanolone, a neuroactive progesterone derivative.[34] The effects of estrogen and estradiol on preclinical sleep models are less evident. They are reported to be responsible for the sex-dependent sleep differences on baseline recordings.[35,36] Estradiol is argued to promote a more regular sleep following sleep deprivation, especially by matching awake periods with dark phase in rats (which corresponds to rodent's active phase), although not related to changes in total sleep time.[35–38]

HORMONAL CONTRACEPTIVES AND SLEEP

Altogether, the evidence from studies on the menstrual cycle, menopause, hormone replacement therapy, and preclinical research indicate and reinforce the relevance of female sexual hormones to sleep and to the incidence of sleep disorders and related symptoms. Based on that, studies speculated that hormonal contraceptives could also have positive effects on the sleep of premenopausal women.[12,13] The possible use of contraceptives to improve women's sleep could have important practical benefits. As contraceptives are widely used by women of reproductive age, are inexpensive, and share the same mechanisms of action as endogenous hormones, the possibility of treating sleep complaints with hormonal contraceptives has been raised.[12,13]

A considerable number of studies have been performed so far, and the results are not so straightforward as first hypothesized. Although they support the influence of hormonal contraceptives on sleep in the general sense, there are important inconsistencies on the results. Although some point out toward an improvement in sleep due to hormonal contraceptive use, others point in the opposite direction, showing a worse sleep pattern in this population. The overall body of knowledge is marked by a substantial heterogeneity on the types of contraceptives, sleep-related outcomes, population characteristics, and research design being implemented, which explain the variation on the results. **Table 1** summarizes the most important results of the studies

Table 1
Description of studies evaluating the relationship between hormonal contraceptives and sleep

	Experimental Design	Sample Size	Age Range	Type	Composition	Administration Route	Sleep-Related Outcomes	Summary of Effects
Albuquerque et al,[46] 2015	Before-after	30	25–44	COMB	EE (20 μg) + drospirenone (3 mg)	Oral	PSQI	No effects of contraceptive use on sleep quality score.
Baker et al,[51] 2001a	Cohort	19	N/A	COMB	Multiple	Oral	PSG	More N2 sleep and less N3 sleep.
Baker et al,[47] 2001b	Cohort	18	N/A	COMB	Multiple	Oral	PSG	Less N3 sleep.
Bezerra et al,[13] 2020	Cross-sectional	1286	18–40	Multiple	Multiple	Multiple	ESS and ISI	More insomnia symptoms and daytime sleepiness. Lower TST in users of progestogen-only therapies. Lower TST and higher ISI score in users of third-generation contraceptives. Lower ESS score in users of LNG-IUS.
Burdick et al,[45] 2002	Cross-sectional	37	14–46	N/A	N/A	Oral	PSG	Shorter REM latency, increased total REM time, and reduced slow-wave sleep.
Costa et al,[52] 2017	Cross-sectional	169	23.1 ± 5.4	N/A	N/A	Oral	PSQI	No effects of contraceptive use on PSG variables.
Guida et al,[49] 2019	Cross-sectional	125	20–50	Multiple	Multiple	Multiple	Sleep diary and PSQI	Longer TST in users of progestogen-only contraception and LNG-IUS
Guillermo et al,[53] 2010	Cohort	40	18–30	N/A	N/A	Oral	KSQ	No effects of contraceptive use on PSG variables.
Hachul et al,[39] 2010	Cross-sectional	524	N/A	N/A	N/A	N/A	PSG	Reduced AHI and SpO_2 > 90%. Shorter REM latency and fewer arousals.

(*continued on next page*)

Table 1
(*continued*)

	Experimental Design	Sample Size	Age Range	Type	Composition	Administration Route	Sleep-Related Outcomes	Summary of Effects
Hachul et al,[20] 2013	Cross-sectional	275	20–80	N/A	N/A	N/A	PSG, PSQI, ESS and ISI	Reduced AHI. No effect on sleep architecture and subjective sleep assessment.
Hachul et al,[13] 2020	Cross-sectional	235	19–45	N/A	N/A	Multiple	PSQI	Reduced sleep efficiency and PSQI scores
Hicks & Cavanaugh,[54] 1982	Cohort	49	20.5	COMB	N/A	Oral	Self-reported TST	No effects of contraceptive use on PSG variables.
Kalleinen et al,[40] 2008a	Cross-sectional	31	45–51	COMB	EE (20 μg) + desogestrel (0.15 mg)	Oral	PSG, SSS, BNSQ	Increased TST, sleep efficiency, REM latency, SWS, reduced WASO, stage transitions, and arousals.
Kalleinen et al,[26] 2008b	RCT	15	45–51	COMB	EV (2 mg) + norethisterone (1 mg)	Oral	PSG, BNSQ	More awakenings from N1.
Morssinkhof et al,[42] 2021	Retrospective cohort	1205	35.6 ± 9.0	N/A	N/A	Oral	WHI-IRS	More insomnia symptoms.
Plamberger et al,[44] 2021	Cross-sectional	62	21.4 ± 2.1	COMB	N/A	Oral	PSQI, MEQ, PSG	Reduced REM sleep time and higher density of sleep spindles.
Whitney et al,[41] 2022	Cross-sectional	1970	18–44	N/A	N/A	Multiple	Self-reported TST and sleep disturbances	Higher TST and higher prevalence of self-reported sleep disturbances

"Summary of effects" refers to the effects of hormonal contraceptives on sleep in comparison with non-users, unless otherwise indicated.

Abbreviations: AHI, apnea–hypopnea index; BNSQ, basic nordic sleep questionnaire; COMB, combined contraceptives; EE, ethinylestradiol; ESS, Epworth Sleepiness Scale; EV, estradiol valerate; ISI, insomnia severity index; KSQ, Karolinska Sleepiness Questionnaire; LNG-IUD, levonorgestrel-releasing intrauterine devices; MEW, morningness eveningness questionnaire; PSG, polysomnography; PSQI, Pittsburgh Sleep Quality Index; TST, total sleep time; WHI-IRS, Women's Health Initiative Insomnia Rating Scale.

Adapted and updated from **Bezerra et al., 2022.**[48]

currently available that evaluate the effects of hormonal contraceptives on sleep.

Observational data from epidemiologic studies in Brazil demonstrate that users of hormonal contraceptives have a reduced arousal index, reduced apnea–hypopnea index (AHI), and better sleep efficiency when compared with women not taking any hormonal interventions,[20,39] but no significant effects on subjective sleep-related variables (such as sleep quality, daytime sleepiness, and insomnia symptoms). The effects on the AHI calls attention, as it resembles the effects observed in postmenopausal women under hormone replacement therapy, usually attributed to progesterone and progestins. The reduced number of obstructive respiratory events in turn allows a more stable favorable sleep architecture, justifying the reduced arousal index, increased sleep efficiency, and the overall positive sleep profile in these studies. Positive effects have been corroborated by another study demonstrating increased total sleep time and sleep efficiency among contraceptive users.[40] Likewise, a study based on a large telephone-based survey in the United States demonstrated that a longer sleep time among contraceptive users, although also presenting a 6% higher prevalence of self-reported sleep disturbances.[41]

Opposite to the original hypothesis, most of the observational studies have demonstrated negative effects of hormonal contraceptives on sleep. A large online survey about sleep among women of reproductive in Brazil shown that women taking oral contraceptives had more insomnia symptoms and an increased daytime sleepiness score (as measured by the Insomnia Severity Index [ISI] and the Epworth Sleepiness Scale [ESS]).[13] Similarly, other studies have associated contraceptive use with an increase in insomnia symptoms[42] and decrease in sleep quality and sleep efficiency.[43] Negative results on polysomnographic recordings have also been reported including reduced REM percentage.[44,45] Finally, some studies have concluded that contraceptives and hormonal interventions in general have only marginal or no effects on sleep both on objective and subjective outcomes.[26,46,47]

Considering the inconsistency on the results among these studies, a systematic review and meta-analysis about the overall effects of contraceptives on sleep have been performed.[48] Systematic reviews and meta-analysis are appropriate approaches for cases in which heterogeneity on the results of a given intervention is observed, as it allows analyzing the available evidence in a comprehensive way, statistically combining the results of each study into a weighted measure of effect. This systematic review comprised a final sample of 2775 individuals from 13 studies about contraceptives and sleep in women of reproductive age, reporting either objective or subjective sleep outcomes. The only statistically significant results were observed on wake after sleep onset, which was 7 minute shorter among contraceptive users. No other effects were observed neither on polysomnographic outcomes nor sleep questionnaire scores. Based on these results, this meta-analytical study concluded that hormonal contraceptives are not associated with clinically relevant changes in sleep among women (**Fig. 3**).

Although the highest level of evidence available point toward no effect of contraceptives on sleep,[48] these results should be contextualized and scrutinized considering the heterogeneity of the results and the certainty of the generated evidence. Those results shall be understood as an average conclusion arising from the combination of all the available results so far and is likely to reflect more the heterogeneity of the studies, rather than the actual effects of contraceptives. Therefore, it probably does not override the possibility that one specific contraceptive formulation could lead into significant effects on sleep. Some possible confusion factors and methodological bias are listed below, which should be properly discussed in order to understand the results available.

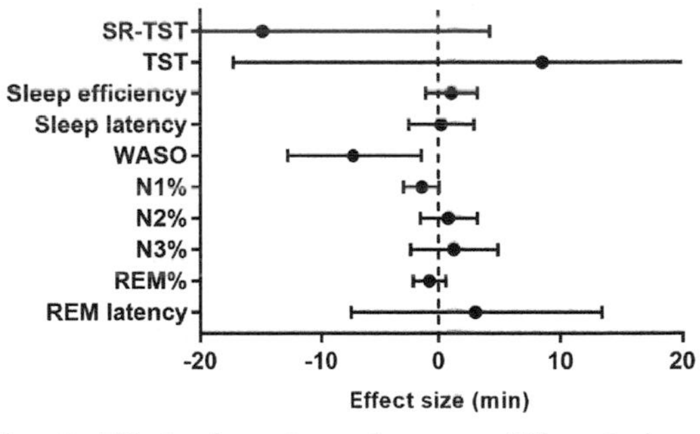

Fig. 3. Effect of contraceptives on different sleep-related outcomes. These data are based on and adapted from a meta-analysis published by Bezerra and colleagues[48] including results from 13 studies and a combined sample size of 2775 individuals. The central dot in each line represents the effect size of contraceptives on each sleep variable, in comparison with nonusers of hormonal contraceptives, whereas the horizontal error bars represent the 95% confidence interval. Statistical significance is marked by the confidence interval bar not crossing the central vertical axis. All effect sizes are presented in minutes. The only statistically significant effect of contraceptives was observed on WASO, which was reduced in 7 minutes, in average. SR-TST, self-reported total sleep time; TST, total sleep time; WASO, wake after sleep onset.

Heterogeneity on the Types of Contraceptives

The presentation of hormonal contraceptives varies considerably, and these variations are likely to affect the potential effects of hormonal contraceptives on sleep. Among the sources of variability are the type of progestin, composition (combined or progestin-only), administration route, and dosage. Although they all could theoretically influence the effects, very few studies allow such inference, because they are usually based on convenience samples in which very few (if none) restrictions to the type of contraceptives are implemented. Most of these convenience sample studies are restricted to oral contraceptives only, with no further information on the composition of the contraceptive being take (such as combined or progestin-only, or the type and dose of the progestin used). Even among the few that provide some stratification regarding the type of contraceptives being taken, the classification varies, hindering a proper comparison among studies. As an example, Bezerra and colleagues[13] categorizes contraceptives into generations, with stratified analyses for progestin-only and for levonorgestrel-releasing intrauterine devices (LNG-IUD). Hachul and colleagues[43] analyzed three groups: the first composed by users of combined oral contraceptives and monthly injectable contraceptives, the second composed by users of quarterly injectable contraceptives, and the third composed by users of progestin-only contraceptives and LNG-IUD. Guida and colleagues[49] analyzed 11 independent groups according to the type of contraceptive being used, which includes five groups for different combined contraceptive formulations, two groups for different LNG-IUD formulations, and an independent group for each of the following: progestin-only, natural estrogens, subcutaneous contraceptives, and vaginal ring.

The type of the progestin is one important source of variation, because their effects vary considerably according to their pharmacologic characteristics and generations.[50] An online survey with 1286 women of reproductive age performed a comparison among users of different contraceptive generations.[13] The results point out that users of third generation contraceptives have a higher score of insomnia symptoms and a reduced total sleep time. On the same study, users of progestin-only contraceptives presented an impaired sleep profile, with more self-reported sleep problems, more insomnia symptoms, and reduced total sleep time in comparison with both nonusers and users of combined therapy.

These results are mostly opposite to those observed by Guida and colleagues,[49] which reported positive outcomes in users of progestin-only hormones, including increased total sleep time and sleep quality, reduced sleep latency, and less sleep disturbances (although more sleep dysfunctions). However, it shall be noticed that this study includes a very low sample of progestin-only users ($n = 5$) and bases its outcome assessment on subscores of the Pittsburgh Sleep Quality Index (PSQI) and on a nonstandard PSQI score calculation.

Regarding the route of administration, most studies restrict the analyses to oral contraceptives. However, there are reports of different effects observed in users of LNG-IUD, which present more favorable sleep-related outcomes. Guida and colleagues[49] analyzed two different formulations of LNG-IUD (levonorgestrel at either 13.5 mg or at 20 mg/24 h), and in both cases, the overall sleep profile was better than in controls. The first formulation was associated with a 30-minute increase in total sleep time, less self-reported sleep disturbances, and better overall sleep quality. The second formulation had more self-reported sleep disturbances but also reduced daytime sleepiness and better overall sleep quality. The study by Bezerra and colleagues[13] demonstrated a significantly reduced sleepiness score among LNG-IUD user in comparison with users of other progestin-only contraceptives[13] (**Fig. 4**).

Altogether, these results seem to point out to a negative effect of progestins on overall sleep pattern and on inducing sleepiness. However, the results are more positive in case of users of LNG-IUD. The possible explanation lies in the fact that the intrauterine route of administration leads to more local and milder systemic effects.

Observational Research

Most of the studies available about contraceptives and sleep are based on observational designs, rather than on proper randomized controlled trials (RCTs). According to a traditional evidence-based medicine approach, RCTs are associated to a higher level of medical evidence than observational studies, which always possess an increased risk of methodological biases, random error, and uncertainties.

In general, these studies are based on two types of sampling methods common to observation studies: random or convenience samples. Random samples are used in the epidemiologic studies[20,39,41] and usually provide a reliable accounting of the number of individuals using hormonal contraceptives on a population as well as its association with sleep-related outcomes. However, it cannot be used to establish causal

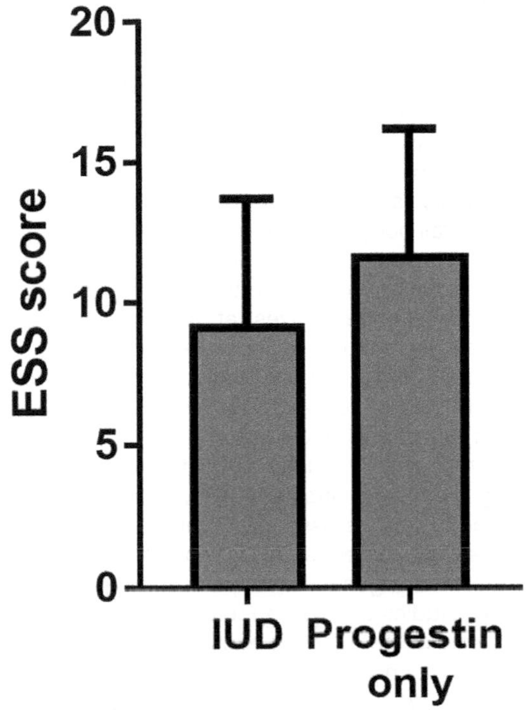

Fig. 4. Effect of levonorgestrel-releasing intrauterine devices on daytime sleepiness score, in comparison with progestin-only contraceptive users. ESS, Epworth Sleepiness Scale; IUD, intrauterine devices. (*Adapted from* Bezerra and colleagues.[13])

inference, in a way that whatever sleep pattern observed in contraceptive users (either positive or negative) cannot be attributed as a direct cause of hormonal contraception. Convenience samples refer to studies based on a group of participants easy to reach in a nonrandomized way. Studies like these include analyzing contraceptive users on a clinical database or from a specific medical service. Although easy to perform, this method increases the risk of sampling error, as the individuals might be prone to have a certain background condition, eventually collinear with the outcomes to be measured. Open-call online surveys (which are a type of convenience sampling study) refer to studies in which participants are invited to fill out an online questionnaire. It leads to important problems related to selection bias and interest bias. In open-call online surveys about sleep and contraceptives, women who have background sleep complaints might feel more interested in participating, therefore leading to an overestimation of the prevalence of sleep-related outcomes.

In addition, there are some problems that are common to most observational studies about sleep and contraceptives. First, most of them group contraceptive users altogether in a single group, regardless of the type and characteristics of the contraceptive being used. Second, they usually do not allow properly controlling the intervention/exposition factor, especially regarding for how long a woman has been taking contraceptives, nor the regularity of using it. Although questions about these items are usually added to these studies, answering it always entails a risk of recall bias.

Most of these methodological drawbacks could be surpassed by properly performed RCTs. This research design is the most appropriate to establish causal relations as well as to isolate the specific effect of the intervention from confounding factors and covariates. It also usually entails a more strictly defined population and more rigid inclusion and exclusion criteria. Finally, it would allow a more precise control of the intervention characteristics, focusing on one specific contraceptive, rather than grouping several types of contraceptives on a single analysis, therefore, increasing the internal validity of the results.

To the best of our knowledge, only one RCT has been performed to analyze the effects of contraceptives on sleep.[26] It was a study with 17 women, in which 9 took a cyclic combined oral estrogen–progestin therapy, and the sleep-related outcomes were measured both with polysomnography and the Basic Nordic Sleep Questionnaire (BNSQ). The only statistically significant result observed was an increase in the number of awakening from N1. Although the certainty of evidence generated by this single RCT is higher than those generated by any of the other observational studies, their effects cannot be extrapolated to all possible contraceptives. The types, combinations, dosage, and route of administration of contraceptives vary considerably, and all these other presentations are not covered in this RCT. Therefore, new RCTs are necessary, investigating the effects of one type of contraceptive at a time (including composition, dosage, and route of administration).

Ceiling and Floor Effects

As most studies about contraceptives and sleep are based on convenience samples, they do not have strict inclusion criteria or parameters for the background sleep condition. In other words, most of them does not restrict recruitment to patients with a clinically diagnosed condition (eg, clinically defined chronic insomnia) or to the presentation of a given symptom or characteristic (eg, ESS score >10 or sleep efficiency < 85%). Rather, most convenience sample studies simply collect data on a large population regardless of proper clinical diagnosis or baseline sleep-related complaints.

This procedure seems to be a methodological bias due to a mismatch between the study hypothesis and the background characteristics of the population, leading to either ceiling or floor effects. As an example, if a study is based on the hypothesis that oral contraceptives could improve sleep efficiency, the study population should have been composed by individuals with reduced sleep efficiency on the baseline. If the population had normal average sleep efficiency on the baseline, the intended intervention does not have room to work, because the largest possible effect size is not clinically relevant. In other words, an intervention cannot improve a parameter if it is not impaired in the baseline, denoting a case of ceiling effect. On the other hand, if a study is based on the hypothesis that oral contraceptives would decrease daytime sleepiness score, the sample should have been preselected for individuals with increased daytime sleepiness. If the daytime sleepiness score is already low in the baseline, there is no room for decreasing it even more, therefore denoting a case of floor effect.

Matching the recruitment methods and inclusion criteria to the hypothesis of a study is a simple methodological aspect that has been surprisingly overlooked in most of the studies in this area, which reduces the likelihood of detecting significant results, especially on observational studies.

Time of Contraceptive Use

The time of the day a woman takes her oral contraceptive pills usually follows her own preferences. It could be at waking up, together with a meal, at bedtime, or at whatever other time she is likely to remember, assuring regular use with no missing days. Currently, there is no clinical data or formal recommendation that support saying that one specific time is better than the other and the only concern is that a woman takes its pills regularly. However, thinking about the possible effects of contraceptives on sleep, chronotherapeutics might be an important issue. Considering that sexual hormones (mainly progesterone) might impact sleep, the time someone takes any hormonal intervention might have clinical effects. If a specific hormonal contraceptive has hypnotic effects, taking it by the morning would lead to increased daytime sleepiness. In such a case, it would be preferable to take it by bedtime. To date, this concern is based on theoretic reasoning only, as to the best of our knowledge, no study has evaluated the effect of contraceptive use timing on sleep.

RESEARCH AGENDA

The number of studies on the relationship between contraceptive use and sleep has been increasing on the previous years, but the publication output encompasses a remarkable heterogeneity related to both methods and results. New studies are necessary, as long as they are able to increase the overall body of knowledge. Although observational studies based on convenience samples were important to explore the potential effects of hormonal contraceptives at an early research phase, they should be no longer encouraged, as they are likely to increase the overall heterogeneity on this field of research, rather than to properly generate applicable evidence.

Instead, future studies should focus on generating robust and unbiased data, ideally based on research designs associated with the high levels of medical evidence. Also, more than trying to establish the general effect of contraceptives on sleep, studies should be more specific, intending to disclose the effect of each type of contraceptive, on each different sleep outcome, for each different type of patient. A tentative research agenda is disclosed below.

- *Population-based studies:* Although convenience sample studies are discouraged is most cases (especially those based on online surveys), population-based studies are still valid, as they are a reliable way to analyze the profile of contraceptive use and its association with sleep. A couple of them have already been performed, being important to generate initial evidence on the field.[20,39] New population-based studies are still valid as long as they can provide information on the use of different types and formulations of contraceptives (rather than on contraceptive use in general, as done before). This might be useful to evaluate in a representative way if the sleep profile of oral contraceptive is different from used of LNG-IUD, for example,
- *Randomized controlled trials:* This is the most important research design to properly evaluate the effects of a given contraceptive formulation on sleep. Further RCTs are strongly encouraged, as long as they are able to reduce methodological heterogeneity. It is suggested that these trials have strict inclusion and exclusion criteria and focus on evaluating the effects of a single contraceptive formulation at a time. Evaluating both objective (eg, polysomnography and actigraphy) and subjective (eg, sleep questionnaires) is equally important. Therefore, these studies will be able to analyze whether

and how each specific type of contraceptives influence sleep.

- *Meta-analysis of randomized controlled trials:* Although a meta-analysis about contraceptives and sleep have already been performed,[48] it is based only on observational data, therefore dragging with it all the methodological biases typically observed in these studies. A meta-analysis of RCTs would generate a higher level of evidence regarding a given hormonal contraceptive on sleep, with both good internal and external validity. However, this would only become feasible if a good number of RCTs are performed and made available.
- *Network meta-analysis:* This type of meta-analysis allows the comparison of multiple interventions for a same condition and outcome. In cases like the current one, in which there are multiple variations on the possible interventions, a network meta-analysis might be useful to compare the effects among the different types of contraceptives, therefore evaluating which formulation has the biggest effect size on a given sleep outcome. This would be the best way to disclose which is the contraceptive that leads to the best or worse clinical effects on sleep, therefore being able to drive and shape clinical practice. However, it would also require a good number of RCTs to become suitable.

SUMMARY

The evidence on the relevance of female sexual hormones on the onset of sleep disorders and complaints is robust, mainly coming from studies about sleep across the menstrual cycle, after the menopausal transition and evaluating the effects of hormone replacement therapy. However, when it comes to the research about the effects of hormonal contraceptives on sleep among reproductive age women, it is still on its early and exploratory phase.

By the currently available results, it is possible to conclude that oral contraceptives are associated with changes on the sleep pattern in both objective and subjective assessment methods. However, the direction of this association is not clear, as some studies points out toward an improvement in sleep-related outcomes among contraceptive users, and others point out to impairment.

The possible reason for such inconsistencies relies on the methodological heterogeneity both between and within studies. It includes variability on the types of contraceptives being tested, their composition, dosage, and administration route. The types of sleep assessment methods and population under investigation also vary among studies. Considering all the available evidence, there is no specific contraceptive formulation that has been evaluated consistently. It is also remarkable that no large RCTs have been performed regarding the effects of contraceptives on sleep, and all current publication outputs on this area are composed by observational trials, most of them entailing an important risk of methodological biases. New RCTs are encouraged intending to leverage the level of evidence in this field of research and circumvent the limitations of the observational studies currently performed. In the current condition, the process of synthesis of evidence is impaired and all possible conclusions on the actual effects of contraceptives entail some level of uncertainty and speculation.

The effects of hormonal interventions on protecting against OSA exist in women of reproductive age and were observed in a couple of studies, resembling the effect observed in postmenopausal women. This might be an intermediate factor explaining cases in which hormonal contraceptives are associated with a better sleep profile, as by preventing obstructive events, sleep naturally becomes less fragmented, therefore leading to a more consolidated sleep with reduced arousal index, increased sleep efficiency, and a more favorable sleep architecture. However, such effects were observed only in a few studies, which might be explained by two factors: first, the possible effects of hormones (especially progestins) on respiratory parameters would depend on high and supraphysiologic doses. Second, the prevalence of OSA in women of reproductive age is substantially lower than what is observed after menopause, which decreases its potential to improve sleep.

Regardless of OSA, the most likely effects of progestins are causing or increasing sleepiness. Secondary effects such as insomnia symptoms, decreased total sleep time and sleep efficiency, or a reduced overall sleep quality are also observed, although less frequently. In any case, all these possible effects are subjected to variations on administration route, type of progestin, route of administration, and timing in which contraceptives are taken. Interestingly, some studies suggest that LNG-IUD leads to a reduced effect of sleep, possibly because there is more local than systemic effects.

Considering the current data, its limitations, and under an evidence-based medicine approach, it is not possible to establish any formal recommendation for or against the use of hormonal contraceptives in what regards sleep-related outcomes. No specific contraceptive formulation seems to promote a more favorable sleep pattern, and there is no evidence that it could be used as a treatment for insomnia or other sleep disorders in women of reproductive age. In any case, clinicians and practitioners should be attentive to the onset or worsening of sleep-related signals, symptoms, complaints, or disorders, especially in cases in which hormonal contraceptive therapy has been initiated or recently changed. In these cases, if the sleep-related symptoms can be attributed to the contraceptive therapy by either the patient or the clinician, changing the prescription could be considered.

CLINICS CARE POINTS

- There is no evidence that hormonal contraceptives could be used as a treatment (either alone or combined) for insomnia or other sleep disorders in premenopausal women.
- It is likely that hormonal contraceptives impact sleep, but the direction of this association is not clear.
- Although some studies have demonstrated an improvement in sleep-related outcomes among contraceptive users, most studies point toward impairment in both objective and subjective sleep variables.
- The heterogeneity among available data can be explained by the observational nature of the studies and by the great methodological variability on the formulation, administration route, dosage, and timing of use of contraceptives.
- Clinicians should be attentive to sleep complaints on patients initiating or changing their hormonal contraceptive therapy. If sleep-related signs, symptoms, or complaints are observed, it should be considered to change the contraceptive prescription.
- The intrauterine route (such as in LNG-IUD) could lead to less negative sleep outcomes, as its effects are more local than systemic. However, this should be confirmed by proper randomized controlled trials.
- Despite the possibility of negative effects of hormonal contraceptives on sleep, it benefits still surpasses the harms. There is no formal recommendation to discontinue hormonal contraception because of incident sleep complaints. Doing so can be considered in individual cases, when the symptoms can be attributed to the hormonal contraception, and the patient should be informed and advised of the risks of discontinuing the use of hormonal contraceptive.

DISCLOSURE

G.N. Pires is a shareholder at SleepUp and founder of P&P Metanálises. The other authors have no conflicts of interest to disclose. Our studies are supported by the Associação Fundo de Incentivo à Pesquisa, Brazil (AFIP). M.L. Andersen is a recipient of a *Conselho Nacional de Desenvolvimento Científico e Tecnológico* (CNPq) fellowship.

REFERENCES

1. Pletzer BA, Kerschbaum HH. 50 years of hormonal contraception-time to find out, what it does to our brain. Front Neurosci 2014;8:256.
2. Christin-Maitre S. History of oral contraceptive drugs and their use worldwide. Best Pract Res Clin Endocrinol Metab 2013;27(1):3–12.
3. Dhont M. History of oral contraception. Eur J Contracept Reprod Health Care 2010;15(Suppl 2):S12–8.
4. Leininger WM, Gupta P. One hundred years of Women's suffrage: health care advocacy, and why we vote. Obstet Gynecol 2020;136(2):349–53.
5. United Nations, Department of Economic and Social Affairs, Population Division (2019). Contraceptive Use by Method 2019: Data Booklet. https://www.un.org/development/desa/pd/sites/www.un.org.development.desa.pd/files/files/documents/2020/Jan/un_2019_contraceptiveusebymethod_databooklet.pdf.
6. Daniels K, Daugherty J, Jones J. Current contraceptive status among women aged 15-44: United States, 2011-2013. NCHS Data Brief 2014;173:1–8.
7. Bonny AE, Appelbaum H, Connor EL, et al. Clinical variability in approaches to polycystic ovary syndrome. J Pediatr Adolesc Gynecol 2012;25(4):259–61.
8. Strowitzki T, Kirsch B, Elliesen J. Efficacy of ethinylestradiol 20 µg/drospirenone 3 mg in a flexible extended regimen in women with moderate-to-severe primary dysmenorrhoea: an open-label, multicentre, randomised, controlled study. J Fam Plann Reprod Health Care 2012;38(2):94–101.
9. Arowojolu AO, Gallo MF, Lopez LM, et al. Combined oral contraceptive pills for treatment of acne. Cochrane Database Syst Rev 2012;7:CD004425.
10. Schindler AE. Non-contraceptive benefits of oral hormonal contraceptives. Int J Endocrinol Metab 2013;11(1):41–7.
11. Giatti S, Melcangi RC, Pesaresi M. The other side of progestins: effects in the brain. J Mol Endocrinol 2016;57(2):R109–26.
12. Bezerra AG, Andersen ML, Pires GN, et al. Effects of hormonal contraceptives on sleep - a possible treatment for insomnia in premenopausal women. Sleep Sci 2018;11(3):129–36.

13. Bezerra AG, Andersen ML, Pires GN, et al. Hormonal contraceptive use and subjective sleep reports in women: an online survey. J Sleep Res 2020;29(6): e12983.
14. Shughrue PJ, Lane MV, Merchenthaler I. Comparative distribution of estrogen receptor-alpha and -beta mRNA in the rat central nervous system. J Comp Neurol 1997;388(4):507–25.
15. Curran-Rauhut MA, Petersen SL. The distribution of progestin receptor mRNA in rat brainstem. Brain Res Gene Expr Patterns 2002;1(3–4):151–7.
16. Baker FC, Driver HS. Self-reported sleep across the menstrual cycle in young, healthy women. J Psychosom Res 2004;56(2):239–43.
17. Baker FC, Driver HS. Circadian rhythms, sleep, and the menstrual cycle. Sleep Med 2007;8(6):613–22.
18. Baker FC, Lee KA. Menstrual cycle effects on sleep. Sleep Med Clin 2022;17(2):283–94.
19. Van Reen E, Kiesner J. Individual differences in self-reported difficulty sleeping across the menstrual cycle. Arch Womens Ment Health 2016; 19(4):599–608.
20. Hachul H, Andersen ML, Bittencourt L, et al. A population-based survey on the influence of the menstrual cycle and the use of hormonal contraceptives on sleep patterns in Sao Paulo, Brazil. Int J Gynecol Obstet 2013;120(2):137–40.
21. Hachul H, Bittencourt L, Haidar M, et al. Sleep disturbance prevalence in postmenopausal women. Rev Bras Ginecol Obstet 2005;27(12):6.
22. Mong JA, Cusmano DM. Sex differences in sleep: impact of biological sex and sex steroids. Philos Trans R Soc Lond B Biol Sci 2016;371(1688): 20150110.
23. Popovic RM, White DP. Upper airway muscle activity in normal women: influence of hormonal status. J Appl Physiol (1985) 1998;84(3):1055–62.
24. Andersen ML, Bittencourt LRA, Antunes IB, et al. Effects of progesterone on sleep: a possible pharmacological treatment for sleep-breathing disorders? Curr Med Chem 2006;13(29):3575–82.
25. Anttalainen U, Saaresranta T, Vahlberg T, et al. Short-term medroxyprogesterone acetate in postmenopausal women with sleep-disordered breathing: a placebo-controlled, randomized, double-blind, parallel-group study. Menopause 2014;21(4):361–8.
26. Kalleinen N, Polo O, Himanen SL, et al. The effect of estrogen plus progestin treatment on sleep: a randomized, placebo-controlled, double-blind trial in premenopausal and late postmenopausal women. Climacteric 2008;11(3):233–43.
27. Wesstrom J, Ulfberg J, Nilsson S. Sleep apnea and hormone replacement therapy: a pilot study and a literature review. Acta Obstet Gynecol Scand 2005; 84(1):54–7.
28. Saaresranta T, Polo-Kantola P, Rauhala E, et al. Medroxyprogesterone in postmenopausal females with partial upper airway obstruction during sleep. Eur Respir J 2001;18(6):989–95.
29. Saaresranta T, Aittokallio T, Polo-Kantola P, et al. Effect of medroxyprogesterone on inspiratory flow shapes during sleep in postmenopausal women. Respir Physiol Neurobiol 2003;134(2):131–43.
30. Saaresranta T. Female hormones and sleep-disordered breathing. Kumar VM, Mallick HN, editors, 2005. 17-23 p.
31. Saaresranta T, Aittokallio T, Utriainen K, et al. Medroxyprogesterone improves nocturnal breathing in postmenopausal women with chronic obstructive pulmonary disease. Respir Res 2005;6.
32. Lancel M, Faulhaber J, Holsboer F, et al. Progesterone induces changes in sleep comparable to those of agonistic GABAA receptor modulators. Am J Physiol 1996;271(4 Pt 1):E763–72.
33. Lancel M, Faulhaber J, Holsboer F, et al. The GABA(A) receptor antagonist picrotoxin attenuates most sleep changes induced by progesterone. Psychopharmacology (Berl) 1999;141(2):213–9.
34. Lancel M, Faulhaber J, Schiffelholz T, et al. Allopregnanolone affects sleep in a benzodiazepine-like fashion. J Pharmacol Exp Ther 1997;282(3): 1213–8.
35. Paul KN, Losee-Olson S, Pinckney L, et al. The ability of stress to alter sleep in mice is sensitive to reproductive hormones. Brain Res 2009;1305: 74–85.
36. Choi J, Kim SJ, Fujiyama T, et al. The role of reproductive hormones in sex differences in sleep homeostasis and arousal response in mice. Front Neurosci 2021;15:739236.
37. Schwartz MD, Mong JA. Estradiol modulates recovery of REM sleep in a time-of-day-dependent manner. Am J Physiol Regul Integr Comp Physiol 2013;305(3):R271–80.
38. Deurveilher S, Rusak B, Semba K. Female reproductive hormones alter sleep architecture in ovariectomized rats. Sleep 2011;34(4):519–30.
39. Hachul H, Andersen ML, Bittencourt LR, et al. Does the reproductive cycle influence sleep patterns in women with sleep complaints? Climacteric 2010; 13(6):594–603.
40. Kalleinen N, Polo-Kantola P, Himanen SL, et al. Sleep and the menopause - do postmenopausal women experience worse sleep than premenopausal women? Menopause Int 2008;14(3): 97–104.
41. Whitney MA, Schultz DN, Huber LRB, et al. The effects of hormonal contraceptive use on sleep patterns in women of reproductive age. Ann Epidemiol 2022;74:125–31.
42. Morssinkhof MWL, Lamers F, Hoogendoorn AW, et al. Oral contraceptives, depressive and insomnia symptoms in adult women with and without depression. Psychoneuroendocrinology 2021;133:105390.

43. Hachul H, Bisse AR, Sanchez ZM, et al. Sleep quality in women who use different contraceptive methods. Sleep Sci 2020;13(2):131–7.
44. Plamberger CP, Van Wijk HE, Kerschbaum H, et al. Impact of menstrual cycle phase and oral contraceptives on sleep and overnight memory consolidation. J Sleep Res 2021;30(4):e13239.
45. Burdick RS, Hoffmann R, Armitage R. Short note: oral contraceptives and sleep in depressed and healthy women. Sleep 2002;25(3):347–9.
46. Albuquerque RG, Dias da Rocha MA, Hirotsu C, et al. A randomized comparative trial of a combined oral contraceptive and azelaic acid to assess their effect on sleep quality in adult female acne patients. Arch Dermatol Res 2015;307(10):905–15.
47. Baker FC, Waner JI, Vieira EF, et al. Sleep and 24 hour body temperatures: a comparison in young men, naturally cycling women and women faking hormonal contraceptives. Journal of Physiology-London 2001;530(3):565–74.
48. Bezerra AG, Andersen ML, Pires GN, et al. The effects of hormonal contraceptive use on sleep in women: a systematic review and meta-analysis. J Sleep Res 2022;e13757.
49. Guida M, Rega A, Vivone I, et al. Variations in sleep associated with different types of hormonal contraceptives. Gynecol Endocrinol 2020;36(2):166–70.
50. Vigo F, Lublanca JN, Corleta HvE. Progestagens: pharmacology and clinical use. Femina 2011;39(3):11.
51. Baker FC, Mitchell D, Driver HS. Oral contraceptives alter sleep and raise body temperature in young women. Pflueg Arch Eur J Physiol 2001;442(5):729–37.
52. Costa R, Costa D, Pestana J. Subjective sleep quality, unstimulated sexual arousal, and sexual frequency. Sleep Sci 2017;10(4):147–53.
53. Guillermo CJ, Manlove HA, Gray PB, et al. Female social and sexual interest across the menstrual cycle: the roles of pain, sleep and hormones. BMC Wom Health 2010;10:19.
54. Hicks RA, Cavanaugh AM. Oral-contraceptive use, the menstrual-cycle, and the need for sleep. Bull Psychonomic Soc 1982;19(4):215–6.

Dysmenorrhea and Sleep
A Review

Isabela A. Ishikura, MSc[a], Helena Hachul, MD, PhD[b], Sergio Tufik, MD, PhD[a], Monica L. Andersen, PhD[a,*]

KEYWORDS

• Sleep • Dysmenorrhea • Women • Menstrual cycle • Insomnia • Daytime sleepiness • Obstructive sleep apnea • Menstrual pain

KEY POINTS

- Women are constantly affected by dysmenorrhea during the reproductive phase of life, which causes pain, discomfort, headache, and sleep complaints during the menstrual period.
- The consequences of this dysfunction lead to work and school absenteeism, resulting in social and life routine impairments.
- The inflammatory component in dysmenorrhea dysfunction results in pain that has an impact in sleep.
- Poor sleep quality or sleep-related disorders can negatively influence the inflammatory response of the dysmenorrhea condition, worsening the clinical symptoms reported in this dysfunction.

INTRODUCTION

Dysmenorrhea is a gynecologic condition that affects women during their reproductive phase of life. It is characterized by painful cramps that occur during the menstruation period of the menstrual cycle. In addition to the presence of pain, other symptoms can be accompanied, such as fatigue, nausea, vomiting, diarrhea, headache, lower backache,[1] and sleep complaints.[2] Although dysmenorrhea is a common and prevalent dysfunction, its etiology is still unknown.

Definitions

Dysmenorrhea is considered when woman reports painful menstruation, varying according to its severity. There are 2 different types of this dysfunction: primary dysmenorrhea (PD) and secondary dysmenorrhea (SD). PD is defined as painful cramps during menstruation without any alteration in pelvic image examinations.[3] It is based on the clinical symptoms reported by the patient that leads to underestimated diagnosis of this dysfunction. This type of dysmenorrhea is known to be initiated within the menarche of the adolescent, and depending on its severity, it can lead to school absenteeism and difficult to social relation during the painful menstruation days.[3]

The SD is determined when other pathology is present in combination with the painful menstruation.[3] Endometriosis is one of the most referenced pathologies linked to SD, but other pathologies can be related, including adenomyosis, myomas, and pelvic inflammatory disease. The painful menstruation is associated with other preexistent pathology, and pelvic image examinations can help confirming it, such as ultrasound, laparoscopy, cystoscopy, colonoscopy, and sigmoidoscopy.[3]

Both types of the dysfunction bring on disability in daily activities, being the leading cause of absenteeism in work and school for women with this condition.[4,5]

[a] Departamento de Psicobiologia, Universidade Federal de São Paulo (UNIFESP), Rua Botucatu, 862 - Vila Clementino - 04023062 - São Paulo - SP - Brazil; [b] Departamento de Ginecologia, Universidade Federal de São Paulo (UNIFESP), Rua Botucatu, n° 740 - Vila Clementino - 04023-062 - São Paulo - SP - Brazil

* Corresponding author. Departamento de Psicobiologia, Universidade Federal de São Paulo (UNIFESP), Rua Botucatu, 862 - Vila Clementino - 04023062 - São Paulo - SP - Brazil.

E-mail address: ml.andersen12@gmail.com

Sleep Med Clin 18 (2023) 449–461
https://doi.org/10.1016/j.jsmc.2023.06.006

sleep.theclinics.com

Background

One of the preliminary and important reports focused on dysmenorrhea is dated from 1987. In this study, Dawood[1] approached the incidence and clinical features of both types of dysmenorrhea, with a detailed description of the potential etiology of this dysfunction. Coco in 1999[6] delineated the main possible factors that can be involved in these 2 types of dysmenorrhea. According to their reports, dysmenorrhea has inflammatory elements that induce the release of prostaglandins by endometrial cells, causing pain prior or during the menstruation days.[1,6] This fact had been commented a long time ago in a paper of Pickles in 1979, when he resumed studies performed in women with dysmenorrhea that found evidence of increased prostaglandins during the pain menstruation condition.[7]

Women with PD exhibits alterations in intrauterine activity compared to women without dysmenorrhea.[1] It has been demonstrated that women with PD showed increases in uterine resting tone, activity pressure, and in the number of contractions. The activity in uterus may appear incoordinate and dysrhythmic, resulting in reduction in blood flow.[1] Corroborating with this, studies have identified higher levels of prostaglandins in women with dysmenorrhea when compared to the noncondition women.[7,8] In SD the increase in prostaglandins was associated with the use of the intrauterine device.[1]

The presence of anovulatory cycles seems to preserve women from dysmenorrhea symptoms, but not in all women,[1] which leads the researchers to believe that there is a hormonal implication in dysmenorrhea scenario. Recent studies have confirmed this relation between progesterone and prostaglandins. Prostaglandins are increased when progesterone levels drop before menstruation.[9,10] In addition to the inflammatory and hormonal factors, PD has been discussed to be triggered by behavioral and psychologic conditions.[1,11]

Prevalence

PD has been manifested by many women in different countries. Although the prevalence varies according to population studied, it has been considered the most common gynecologic dysfunction in women during reproductive life.[11] The risk factors related to the development of this condition are family history of dysmenorrhea, heavy and long menstrual bleeding, and psychologic conditions, such as anxiety and depression.[11] Severity of the dysmenorrhea symptoms may differ according to women and each menstrual cycle, as women with depression, anxiety, and stress are under higher risk to dysmenorrhea symptoms.[12,13]

The absence of a specific examination that detects PD increases the prevalence of underdiagnosed women with this condition. Studies around the world noticed that up to 96% of women present dysmenorrhea during their reproductive life (**Table 1**). As it is a recurrent dysfunction that occurs in a monthly basis, it is understandable that its symptoms might affect the routine and social life of these women. The severity of dysmenorrhea has been correlated with high stress levels and less working hours.[14] School absenteeism was stated by 20% to 24% of students with dysmenorrhea[15,16] and 37% had reported reduction in social and sports activities.[16] Other studies have indicated that dysmenorrhea is the cause of lost 1 to 2 working days per month for 10% to 30% of women in this condition.[17,18] The consequences of all this absence have serious implication in global economic aspect, reaching a cost of USD 2 billion in the United States.[19]

Clinical outcomes

The most relevant and markable symptom of the PD is the painful menstruation, which can start 2 to 3 days before the first menstrual day. In SD the pain can starts 1 to 2 weeks before menstruation lasting up to few days after cessation of the menstruation. The cramps can have different severities depending on the menstrual cycle and the women per se, being classified as mild, moderate, or severe. It can be accompanied by other symptoms previously mentioned, which contribute to worsening the clinical condition of the women. During the menstruation days, women with dysmenorrhea are more prone to experience sleep disturbances since painful conditions can interfere in the sleep pattern by increasing the time to fall asleep, inducing night awakenings and stimulating the early morning awakenings.[20] Inversely, a bad night of sleep provokes impairments in cognition, immune system, hormonal release, and in many other physiologic aspects[21–23] (**Fig. 1**). Homeostasis is strongly related to a good quality of sleep and is essential for the well-functioning of the body[22]; thus, it is crucial to consider sleep when treating painful diseases to avoid imbalance of the organic body mechanisms.

Clinical relevance

Sleep is an essential behavior for humans to maintain their survival and well-being.[24] Being awake night along has been adopted to modern routines by many societies especially due to workload, social and economic demands. Studies have

Table 1
Studies with dysmenorrhea and sleep collected for discussion in this review

1st Author/Year Location	Sample Size (N) Groups Studied	Dysmenorrhea Prevalence	Sleep Measures	Sleep Findings in Dysmenorrhea
Abdel-Salam et al,[49] 2018 Saudi Arabia	366 students Dysmenorrhea Non-dysmenorrhea	88%	Study specific questionnaire	↑ Sleep disturbances
Araújo et al,[30] 2011 Brazil	24 women Dysmenorrhea Dysmenorrhea + medication Non-dysmenorrhea	66.6%	PSG	No significant statistical findings
Atta,[42] 2016 Pakistan	200 students Dysmenorrhea	86.5%	Study specific questions about hours of sleep and issue related to sleepiness	↓Total sleep time (associated with severity of dysmenorrhea)
Bahrami et al,[41] 2017 Iran	897 adolescents Dysmenorrhea Non-dysmenorrhea PMS	68.8%	ISI, Epworth Sleepiness Scale, Stop-Bang questionnaire	↑ Insomnia ↑ Daytime sleepiness ↑ OSA
Baker[28] 1999 South Africa	18 women Primary dysmenorrhea Non-dysmenorrhea	Not reported	PSG	↓ REM sleep ↓ Sleep quality ↑ % stage 1 sleep
Chen[45] 2021 United States	678 women Dysmenorrhea + acetomiphen Dysmenorrhea + combined OC Dysmenorrhea + NSAID	Not reported	PROMIS Sleep Disturbance 8-item Short Form	No significant statistical findings
Çaltekin/2020[33] Turkey	102 students PD Non-dysmenorrhea	Not reported	Epworth Sleepiness Scale, Berlin questionnaire, ISI, PSQI	↑ Insomnia ↑ Daytime sleepiness ↓ Sleep quality
Gagua[43] 2012 Georgia	2561 students Dysmenorrhea Non-dysmenorrhea	Not reported	Study specific questions	↓ Total sleep time
Hamzekhani[33] 2019 Iran	280 students Severities of dysmenorrhea	Not reported	PSQI	↓ Sleep quality

(*continued on next page*)

Table 1
(*continued*)

1st Author/Year Location	Sample Size (N) Groups Studied	Dysmenorrhea Prevalence	Sleep Measures	Sleep Findings in Dysmenorrhea
He[35] 2021 Libanon	2260 women Dysmenorrhea Menstrual blood volume Menstrual regularity	Not reported	Study specific e-questionnaire	↓ Sleep quality
Iacovides/2009[29] South Africa	10 women PD + placebo PD + diclofenac PD control	Not reported	PSG PSQI	Diclofenac treatment: ↑ Sleep efficiency ↑ % REM ↓ % stage 1 sleep
Kazama[44] 2015 Japan	1018 adolescents Moderate-severe dysmenorrhea	46.8% (moderate dysmenorrhea) 17.7% (severe dysmenorrhea)	Specific questions about time awaking and time going to bed	↓ Total sleep time (<6 h) (associated with dysmenorrhea prevalence)
Kannan[46] 2019 New Zealand	70 women Primary dysmenorrhea Aerobic exercise Primary dysmenorrhea Control	Not reported	Brief Pain Inventory, Women's Health Initiative Insomnia Rating Scale	No significant statistical findings
Keshavarzi[31] 2018 Iran	14 women First menstruation baseline dysmenorrhea Second menstruation melatonin dysmenorrhea Third menstruation meloxicam dysmenorrhea	Not reported	PSQI, Actigraphy	Melatonin and meloxicam improved subjective sleep quality and objectively sleep efficiency and shortened sleep latency. Melatonin induced the most improvements.
Kirmizigil[48] 2020 Turkey	28 participants Dysmenorrhea Combined exercise Dysmenorrhea Control	Not reported	PSQI	↑ Sleep quality with combined exercise
Liu[2] 2017 China	**5800 girls** Menstrual problems (length, regularity, pain, interval)	**61.7%**	**PSQI adapted,** Adolescent Health Quest (AHQ), Questions about DIS, DMS and EMA related to insomnia	**↑ Insomnia** ↓ Sleep quality

Polat[36] 2021 Turkey	250 students Dysmenorrhea Non-dysmenorrhea	82.4%	PSQI	↓ Sleep quality (according to severity of dysmenorrhea) Difficulty falling asleep
Sahin[37] 2014 Turkey	520 students Dysmenorrhea Non-dysmenorrhea	69%	PSQI	↓ Sleep quality
Wang[32] 2019 China	5813 girls Menstrual pain Menstrual irregularity Control	Not reported	Chinese Adolescent Daytime Sleepiness Scale (CADSS), Adolescent Health Questionnaire (AHQ), Study specific questions	↑ Daytime sleepiness
Weng et al,[38] 2019 Taiwan	120 women Dysmenorrhea Non-dysmenorrhea	Not reported	PSQI, ISI, Epworth Sleepiness Scale, Sleep Diary	↑ Insomnia ↑ WASO ↑ Daytime sleepiness ↓ Sleep quality
Woosley[39] 2014 United States	89 students Dysmenorrhea with insomnia Dysmenorrhea without insomnia	Not reported	ISI, ICSD-2, Consensus Sleep Diary, PSQI	↑ Insomnia ↑ Sleep onset latency ↓ Sleep efficiency ↓ Sleep quality rating (related to dysmenorrhea severity)
Xing[40] 2020 China	1006 students Menstrual problems (pain, length, regularity, interval)	Not reported	PSQI, ISI	↑ Insomnia related to severe pain ↓ Sleep quality

DIS, difficult to initiate sleep; DMS, difficult to maintain sleep; EMA, early morning awakening; ICSD, International Classification of Sleep Disorders; ISI, Insomnia Severity Index; NSAID, nonsteroidal anti-inflammatory drug; OC, oral contraceptive; OSA, obstructive sleep apnea; PD, primary dysmenorrhea; PSG, polysomnography; PSQI, Pittsburgh Sleep Quality Index; REM, rapid eye movement; WASO, wake after sleep onset.

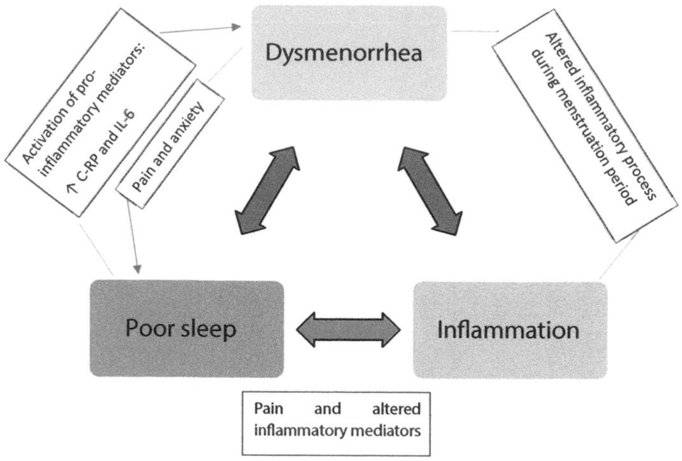

Fig. 1. Relationship among dysmenorrhea, inflammation, and sleep.C-RP = C-reactive protein, IL-6 = interleukin 6.

confirmed the positive influence of a good quality sleep on improving the body response to a disease/inflammation[21] and its protective effect on the development of psychologic disorders, such as anxiety and depression.[23]

The literature is still controversial in establishing the sleep pattern of women, especially those with dysmenorrhea. The hormonal oscillations presented during the menstrual cycle can affect a variety of physiologic elements triggering feedbacks and mechanisms that might result in a sleep different from each woman and from that observed in males.[25,26] Animal studies have verified that sleep deprivation causes disruption in estrous cycle of the female rats and can affect cardiovascular blood parameters.[25,26] Women with dysmenorrhea is known to experience inflammatory circumstances that lead to painful menstruation,[27] and may interfere in sleep and vice versa.

GOALS

This study brought together the relevant studies in the literature that investigated the sleep of women with dysmenorrhea. We tried to compile the most interesting studies and develop a discussion about the possible mechanisms involved in the relation between dysmenorrhea and sleep. It is important to emphasize that we included studies that used subjective and objective methods to evaluate sleep, such as questionnaires, actigraphy, and polysomnography (PSG). Our objective was to group all the results in a narrative review with all aspects of sleep for dysmenorrhea conditions.

OVERVIEW OF THE STUDIES SELECTED

As expected, the majority of the studies that we collected from the literature about dysmenorrhea and sleep had used questionnaires to evaluate sleep (see **Table 1**). The number of studies published using objective methods, like PSG or actigraphy is scarce for this topic. It is understandable, as PSG is an expensive examination that demands physical space, time, trained technicians, and technology to be applied. Questionnaires became easier to be implemented and embrace a greater sample size, in addition to be dynamic for clinical research.

Table 1 depicts all the 22 studies selected to be discussed in this review. Three of them used PSG for sleep evaluation[28–30] and one used actigraphy.[31] Pittsburgh Sleep Quality Index (PSQI) was the most applied questionnaire to analyze sleep in women with dysmenorrhea. A variety of sample size could be seen among the studies, with Wang's study presenting the greater sample size, which included 5813 participants.[32] The prevalence of dysmenorrhea found in the studies was higher than 45%, reaching 96.1%.[33]

The sleep variable that was most explored and which had more significant results was sleep quality. Of the 22, 9 studies identified worse sleep quality in women with dysmenorrhea according to questionnaires.[2,33–40] Insomnia in women with dysmenorrhea was observed in 5 studies,[2,34,38,39,41] followed by increased daytime sleepiness presented in 4 studies[32,34,38,41] (**Table 2**). Three studies have described a reduction in total sleep time in dysmenorrhea condition,[42–44] whereas 3 studies have not observed significant findings in any sleep variables of this population,[30,45,46] being one of them based on PSG data.[30]

PSQI is recommended to analysis of the sleep quality. Scores greater than 5 indicates sleep disturbance related to poor sleep quality. Half of the studies included in this review have used PSQI to evaluate sleep of women with dysmenorrhea.[2,31,33,34,36–40,47,48] The 3 studies

Table 2
Number of studies for each sleep variable found altered in women with dysmenorrhea

Findings	Sleep Variables	Number of Studies
↓	Sleep quality	9
	Sleep efficiency	2
	% REM sleep	2
	Total sleep time	3
↑	Daytime sleepiness	4
	Insomnia	5
	Sleep onset latency	2
	% Stage 1	2
	Wake after sleep onset	1
	OSA	1
	Sleep disturbances	1
No findings		3

OSA, obstructive sleep apnea; REM, rapid eye movement.

that adopted PSG in their sample reported controversial results.[28–30] Only 1 of them noted poor sleep quality in women with dysmenorrhea,[28] whereas the other 2 studies have not detected significant results associated with sleep quality.[29,30]

Insomnia was the second variable to have more significant results among the studies. The Insomnia Severity Index (ISI) was the questionnaire used by 5 studies,[34,38–41] and 4 of them observed positive scores for insomnia from women with dysmenorrhea.[34,38,39,41] One study was performed with the Women's Health Initiative Insomnia Rating Scale in 70 women and did not refer to significant outcomes.[46] In respect to daytime sleepiness, only 3 studies had implemented the Epworth Sleepiness Scale with all results positive for daytime sleepiness.[34,38,41] Six of the studies developed or conducted their own specific study questionnaires, with their own questions and interpretations.[32,35,42–44,49] This strategy is not welcome to clinical research studies being strongly recommended a validation of the questionnaire before its utilization in a clinical study.

The analysis of sleep by actigraphy was done by 1 study.[31] It involved groups of women with dysmenorrhea treated with melatonin and meloxicam during menstruation days and compared to baseline. They mentioned significative improvements in sleep efficiency with both treatments. Curiously, only 2 studies used sleep diary in their study procedures,[38,39] which is strongly suggested to complement data about sleep routine.

Obstructive sleep apnea (OSA) has been poorly investigated in this population, according to our review. Berlim and Stop-Bang questionnaires, commonly used to evaluate the risk of OSA, were adopted by 2 studies,[34,41] demonstrating positive result for OSA by dysmenorrhea group in the study that used Stop-Bang questionnaire.

Five studies consisted of interventions as attempts to improve dysmenorrhea symptoms.[29,31,38,46,48] The interventions comprised medication or physical exercises. Three of them stated better results with the interventions,[29,31,48] and 2 of them did not report any significant improvement with the interventions.[38,46]

DISCUSSION

The main proposal of this review was to discuss the most interesting studies published in literature about sleep and dysmenorrhea. As previously revealed, few studies have used objective tools to measure sleep quality and its parameters, which includes PSG and actigraphy. The majority of them applied sleep specific questionnaires or developed its own study questionnaire.

One of the most complete and detailed study with dysmenorrhea was accomplished by Baker and colleagues in 1999.[28] In this investigation, the authors collected PSG data of women with mild-to-moderate PD in 3 different phases of the menstrual cycle: follicular, luteal, and menstrual.[28] The same was done to women with no complaints of dysmenorrhea. Women with dysmenorrhea rated their sleep quality statistically worse than the control group during menstruation day. In respect to PSG findings, women with dysmenorrhea had lower sleep efficiency (88% × 95%) and less rapid eye movement (REM) sleep (65 minutes × 79 minutes) than control group during menstruation.[28] Women with dysmenorrhea presented less REM sleep throughout the menstrual cycle than the controls. The sleep efficiency in women with dysmenorrhea was also lower during menstruation compared with the other phases of the menstrual cycle (M = 88%, F = 96%, L = 96%).[28] Although the results are intriguing, the sample size was small and would be more reliable to augment the sample size to confirm the findings.

Another study with PSG evaluated the sleep of women with PD pre- and post-treatment. The study from Iacovides and colleagues[29] explored the effect of diclofenac potassium treatment for menstrual pain in the sleep parameters of women with PD.[29] Ten women with severe dysmenorrheic pain had their sleep recordings in 3 moments: (1) in the mid follicular phase of the menstrual cycle treated with diclofenac (no menstrual pain/diclofenac), (2) in the first menstruation day treated with placebo (menstrual pain/placebo intervention), and the (3) in the first menstruation day of another menstrual cycle treated with diclofenac (menstrual pain/diclofenac). The results evidenced that women in the moment of menstrual pain treated with placebo had reduced sleep efficiency, less REM sleep, and higher stage 1 sleep when compared with the no pain/diclofenac moment. The diclofenac intervention in the third moment of the menstrual cycle restored these sleep variables.[29]

In Brazil, Araujo and colleagues[30] distributed 24 women with dysmenorrhea in 3 groups: no menstrual pain, menstrual pain without medication, and menstrual pain with medication to alleviate painful cramping. The women undergone one-night PSG and had their sleep variables analyzed, but no statistical differences in these parameters were observed among the groups.[30]

PSG is the gold standard method to assess the sleep variables and to diagnose most of the sleep disorders. In these studies, the use of PSG could not confirm the interference of dysmenorrhea symptoms in sleep due to inconsistent findings among them. Two of them found reduced sleep efficiency and REM sleep in dysmenorrhea condition,[28,29] whereas the third one did not find any significant differences, although the sample size was higher.[30] Included in the objective sleep methods is the actigraphy, which is a portable device that measures periods of time in activity and sleeping. This method restrains obtaining data about sleep stages and sleep disorders. A study with 14 women with PD and PSQI score greater than 5 demonstrated that melatonin and meloxicam were effective to improve the subjective sleep and the menstrual pain of this population.[31] Positive results were detected in actigraphy data, which was related to the reduction in sleep onset latency after both treatments, being the larger effect size with melatonin treatment.[31] This study is interesting as meloxicam is a pain reliever and was effective in improving the subjective and objective sleep of women with PD.

As pain is the main symptom of dysmenorrhea and is deeply connected to sleep,[50] it seems predictable that women with this condition would present more sleep complaints. The bidirectional relation between sleep and pain is still under discussion as most data published in this topic are more conclusive in respect to the effects of sleep on pain and not the inverse.[51] A painful day predicts a worse night of sleep and the inverse was also perceived.[52] The experience of pain is amplified with a sleep deprivation condition, with enhancement of nociceptive behavior.[53] Low pain threshold has been observed in sleep deprived patients,[54] as well as difficulties to fall asleep, night and early awakenings were reported by patients with painful condition.[20] Sleep loss can activate the inflammatory system especially for women, which is more vulnerable to the effects of sleep on inflammatory parameters.[21] C-reactive protein and IL-6 are augmented in conditions of poor sleep quality, sleep duration less than 7 hours, and long sleep duration[21] (see **Fig. 1**).

We can hypothesize that the inflammatory aspect sustained in dysmenorrhea promotes the release of prostaglandins causing pain in every menstruation of the menstrual cycle. This menstrual pain disturbs sleep, provoking activation of the inflammatory system. Altered inflammatory parameters lead to worsening dysmenorrhea symptoms that impact negatively in women's quality of life and the sleep becomes affected again. This cycle is ceased when the dysmenorrhea is successfully treated, with no sleep and pain complaints.

It becomes relevant to obtain firstly the sleep information of women with dysmenorrhea during the medical appointment that can be done with subjective methods, such as questionnaires or questions related to sleep. It helps health professionals understand if the sleep complaints are associated with the dysmenorrhea condition. Untreated women with dysmenorrhea that have to deal with this menstrual pain at every month might be more susceptible to anxiety symptoms that can influence the sleep quality.[55]

Nine studies of this review identified a reduction in the subjective sleep quality due to dysmenorrhea symptoms.[2,33–40] Eight of them evaluated this variable by applying the PSQI,[2,33,34,36–40] which is the most used sleep questionnaire to evaluate quality of sleep.[56] The remaining 2 studies had their subjective sleep quality based on a study specific questionnaire and sleep diary.[35,38] In addition to the studies mentioned above, 2 studies with application of the PSQI in the dysmenorrhea population verified an improvement in sleep quality/efficiency with exercise and intervention of melatonin and meloxicam.[31,48]

A Chinese study involving 5800 girls (age 12–18 years) investigated menstrual problems, including length, regularity, pain, and interval of the menstrual cycles.[2] The researchers applied an adapted PSQI to acquire information about sleep and insomnia symptoms. The dysmenorrhea was present in 61.7% of the participants included in the study, and its severity was associated with a higher risk to insomnia symptoms and poor sleep quality.[2] Other more recent study conducted in China with 1006 university students who filled the PSQI and ISI found that severe period pain was associated with poor sleep quality and insomnia symptoms, with an odds ratio of 1.91.[40] The findings could not clarify if the menstrual pain was triggered by sleep problems, or if sleep was affected by menstrual problems.

Two studies performed with Turkish students observed different prevalence of dysmenorrhea condition between years of 2012 and 2016.[36,37] In 2012, dysmenorrhea was experienced by 69% of the 520 students included in the study. The PSQI revealed a reduced sleep quality in those students presenting dysmenorrhea.[37] Four years later, Polat and Mucuk[36] reported a prevalence of 82.4% of dysmenorrhea in 250 university students with and without dysmenorrhea. Dysmenorrhea was significantly correlated with difficulty to fall asleep and its severity was linked to poor sleep quality, according to the questionnaires applied. All the studies confirmed the high prevalence of dysmenorrhea in women in different countries.

In a high number of studies, the sleep quality was the parameter that showed the most significant alterations in women with dysmenorrhea (see **Table 1**), especially when it is related to the severity of dysmenorrhea condition.[33] Poor sleep quality can interfere in daytime routine, causing sleepiness in these women that affects their social and professional lives.[32,34,41] Insufficient sleep time leads to difficulty to maintain adequate levels of wakefulness and alertness[57] resulting in daytime sleepiness and fatigue.[58,59] Three studies of our review described reduced total sleep time in women with dysmenorrhea.[42–44] Reduced sleep time predicts the frequency and severity of pain,[60,61] and it can be an important matter to approach in women with dysmenorrhea.

Although daytime sleepiness is a frequently complaint of insomnia condition and poor sleep quality, few studies have examined this outcome in dysmenorrhea scenario. Four studies of our review have explored this factor in women with dysmenorrhea, and all of them found the presence of sleepiness in these women.[32,34,38,41] Associated with daytime sleepiness, 3 of the studies have detected insomnia symptoms in women with dysmenorrhea.[32,34,41] This fact is commonly expected as insomnia disturbs sleep by reducing the total sleep time or disrupting the sleep cycle, which leads to inefficiency sleep or poor sleep quality.[62] In one of these studies, aggressive behavior and depression was also significantly higher and correlated with severity of dysmenorrhea than the control group.[34,41] Anxiety behavior was also statistically higher in dysmenorrhea women compared with non-dysmenorrhea, according to Beck Anxiety Index.[34]

Women are more prone to develop insomnia due to the changes in hormones and life cycle events, especially with an increasing age.[63] Insomnia is characterized by the difficulty to fall asleep, to maintain the sleep at night and/or getting up too early for more than 3 months.[64] Women with dysmenorrhea may be at a higher risk to experience insomnia symptoms due to the effects of pain in sleep.[65] Five studies of our review have observed an increase in insomnia symptoms in women with dysmenorrhea when compared with control women (without dysmenorrhea).[2,34,38,40,41] Woosley and Lichstein[39] inspected the association of dysmenorrhea symptoms in women with or without insomnia. The findings indicated that women with insomnia are more susceptible to severe dysmenorrhea than women without insomnia. Difficulty to falling asleep was higher in women with dysmenorrhea when compared with non-dysmenorrhea women.[36] In other study that applied the PROMIS Sleep Disturbance 8-item Short Form for women with dysmenorrhea in treatment with acetomiphen, combined oral contraceptive or nonsteroidal anti-inflammatory drugs (NSAIDs), no significant findings were reported in respect to insomnia symptoms.[45]

It should be noted that insomnia per se causes a variety of symptoms that depending on the severity they can jeopardize the quality of life, interfering with attention, focus, memory, mood, and physical detriment.[66,67] Insomnia is related to increased risk of inflammatory diseases[68] and pain conditions.[69] It is expected that women with dysmenorrhea and insomnia are under higher risk to develop more intense clinical symptoms and lack of success in treatment of this gynecologic condition.

Other considerable sleep disorder that affects a high number of people and leads to injuries in cardiovascular and immune systems is the OSA. According to an epidemiologic study developed in Brazil, this sleep-breathing disorder is present in 30% of the population.[70] In women, OSA is more prevalent after menopause transition, when their sexual hormones decrease, and they become similar to men in respect to hormonal profile.[70] OSA comprises young women although it is less frequent. Two studies of our review have investigated the OSA in women with dysmenorrhea whose findings were controversial,[34,41] with a positive association between these 2 conditions in 1 of the studies.[41]

THERAPEUTIC OPTIONS

The first-line treatment for dysmenorrhea is the therapy with NSAIDs. This type of drugs acts blocking the production of prostaglandins relieving menstrual pain.[71,72] In the study of Iacovides and colleagues,[29] they found a significant improvement in pain after administration of diclofenac potassium when compared with placebo administration in PD women. Painful menstruation without treatment had reduced sleep efficiency and REM sleep and increased stage 1 sleep when compared with a non-pain moment of the menstrual cycle. The administration of diclofenac potassium restored these values demonstrating that treating women with dysmenorrhea can impact positively in their sleep.[29] The side effects of using NSAIDs are gastrointestinal symptoms, edema, nephrotoxicity, and hematologic abnormalities; however, these effects seem to be more frequently detected when the use of NSAIDs exceeds 72 hours per treatment in health young woman.[73] The indication to use NSAIDs for treating dysmenorrhea starts 1 to 2 days before menstruation (ACOG, 2018).

Hormonal contraceptive is another option to treat dysmenorrhea[73] and it is effective in approximately 70% to 80% of women with dysmenorrhea.[74] The main purpose to use hormonal contraceptive is to inhibit ovulation that will avoid endometrial proliferation. Preventing ovulation and endometrial proliferation, there will be a cessation of prostaglandins that is known to cause pain in dysmenorrhea condition.[73] Different hormonal contraceptive methods, such as combined hormonal contraceptive, progesterone-only contraceptive, and levonorgestrel intrauterine device, have shown to reduce the symptoms of dysmenorrhea[74–76]; however, they may have side effects that interfere in the cardiovascular risk, especially related to deep vein thrombosis.[77]

Nonpharmacologic treatments may improve dysmenorrhea symptoms in some women. Acupuncture,[78,79] yoga,[80] exercise,[81,82] continuous heat therapy in suprapubic region,[83] and transcutaneous electrical nerve stimulation[84,85] are some of the nonpharmacologic options to reduce dysmenorrhea symptoms.

The choice of the better treatment for each woman with dysmenorrhea may be based on the clinical findings reported during the medical appointment. The dysmenorrhea symptoms should improve with the proposed treatment and without success, a new choice of treatment should be recommended. It is essential to observe if the cessation of dysmenorrhea symptoms will lead to improvement in sleep complaints. If there is no improvement in sleep, a PSG should be prescribed to exclude sleep disorders or to propose new approaches to treat the sleep complaints.

Health professionals should have knowledge of the factors that may affect sleep routine and if any gap in sleep hygiene is identified, it should be discussed with the patient to ameliorate the sleep complaints. Sleep diary is strongly recommended to obtain sleep information regarding time of sleep and awakening, and eventually the presence of naps during the day. As already mentioned above, it is important to maintain a good sleep quality in these women as poor sleep is associated with inflammatory outcomes, which could interfere in enhancement of the dysmenorrhea symptoms.

SUMMARY

Our review pointed out the prevalence of dysmenorrhea in different countries, the tools used to investigate sleep characteristics and its related disorders, and the results found in all studies included in this survey. Sleep quality exhibited the most significant results for dysmenorrhea condition, followed by insomnia. Except for 3 studies, the remaining 19 studies of this review have reported alterations in sleep of women with dysmenorrhea, such as alteration in percentage of sleep stages, poor sleep quality, insomnia, and daytime sleepiness. These findings indicate that dysmenorrhea symptoms can be triggered not only by inflammatory factors, but also by consequences of a poor sleep quality. Poor sleep quality and sleep deprivation, both caused by reduced total sleep time or insomnia or other sleep disorder, are known to interfere negatively in anxiety, mood, memory, physical capability, and others. The monthly events occurred in dysmenorrhea condition encompass a variety of manifestations that compromise women's life and their health.

CLINICS CARE POINTS

- Sleep quality is affected in some women with dysmenorrhea, especially those with severe dysmenorrhea symptoms.
- Insomnia can be present in woman with dysmenorrhea, affecting their daily routine.
- Treating dysmenorrhea symptoms seem to be effective in improving sleep complaints.
- Patient's sleep report should be taken during the gynecologic medical appointment, as poor sleep can interfere with the progress of the dysmenorrhea treatment.
- Choose the better treatment for dysmenorrhea symptoms and without success in improving sleep complaints, a PSG may be recommended to exclude possible sleep disorders.
- For health professionals, it is important to discuss with the patient the importance to maintain a sleep hygiene routine.
- Treating sleep complaints may have benefits in the inflammatory outcomes present in dysmenorrhea condition, ameliorating the symptoms and improving women's quality of life.

FUNDING

Our studies are supported by the Associação Fundo de Incentivo à Pesquisa (AFIP). M.L. Andersen receives CNPq and FAPESP (2020/13467-8) fellowships. No funding or sponsorship was received for the publication of this review. This research did not receive any specific grant from funding agencies in the public, commercial, or not-for-profit sectors.

DISCLOSURE

The authors have nothing to disclose.

REFERENCES

1. Dawood MY. Dysmenorrhea and prostaglandins. Gynecologic Endocrinology 1987;405–21.
2. Liu X, Chen H, Liu ZZ, et al. Early menarche and menstrual problems are associated with sleep disturbance in a large sample of Chinese adolescent girls. Sleep 2017;40(9). https://doi.org/10.1093/sleep/zsx107.
3. ACOG COMMITTEE OPINION Dysmenorrhea and Endometriosis in the Adolescent. Available at: http://journals.lww.com/greenjournal. Accessed October 20, 2022.
4. Zannoni L, Giorgi M, Spagnolo E, et al. Dysmenorrhea, absenteeism from school, and symptoms suspicious for endometriosis in adolescents. J Pediatr Adolesc Gynecol 2014;27(5):258–65.
5. Chen CX, Kwekkeboom KL, Ward SE. Beliefs about dysmenorrhea and their relationship to self-management. Res Nurs Health 2016;39(4):263–76.
6. Coco AS. Primary Dysmenorrhea Menstrual Fluid Prostaglandin Levels. Vol 60.; 1999.
7. Pickles VR. Prostaglandins and dysmenorrhea: historical survey. Acta Obstet Gynecol Scand 1979;58(87 S):7–12.
8. Bieglmayer C, Hofe G, Kainz C, et al. Concentrations of various arachidonic acid metabolites in menstrual fluid are associated with menstrual pain and are influenced by hormonal contraceptives. Gynecol Endocrinol 1995;9(4):307–12.
9. Wong CL, Farquhar C, Roberts H, et al. Oral contraceptive pill as treatment for primary dysmenorrhoea. Cochrane Database Syst Rev 2009;(2). https://doi.org/10.1002/14651858.CD002120.pub2.
10. Iacovides S, Avidon I, Baker FC. What we know about primary dysmenorrhea today: a critical review. Hum Reprod Update 2015;21(6):762–78.
11. Patel V, Tanksale V, Sahasrabhojanee M, et al. The burden and determinants of dysmenorrhoea: a population-based survey of 2262 women in Goa, India. BJOG 2006;113(4):453–63.
12. Tavallaee M, Joffres MR, Corber SJ, et al. The prevalence of menstrual pain and associated risk factors among Iranian women. J Obstet Gynaecol Res 2011;37(5):442–51.
13. Bajalan Z, Moafi F, Moradibaglooei M, et al. Mental health and primary dysmenorrhea: a systematic review. J Psychosom Obstet Gynecol 2019;40(3):185–94.
14. Al-Husban N, Odeh O, Dabit T, et al. The influence of lifestyle variables on primary dysmenorrhea: a cross-sectional study. Int J Womens Health 2022;14:545–53.
15. Ortiz MI, Rangel-Flores E, Carrillo-Alarcón LC, et al. Prevalence and impact of primary dysmenorrhea among Mexican high school students. Int J Gynecol Obstet 2009;107(3):240–3.
16. Armour M, Parry K, Manohar N, et al. The prevalence and academic impact of dysmenorrhea in 21,573 young women: a systematic review and meta-analysis. J Womens Health 2019;28(8):1161–71.
17. Sundell G, Milsom T, Andersch B. Factors influencing the prevalence and severity of dysmenorrhoea in young women. Br J Obstet Gynaecol 1990;97(7):588–94.
18. Burnett MA, Antao V, Black A, et al. Prevalence of primary dysmenorrhea in Canada. J Obstet Gynaecol Can 2005;27(8):765–70.
19. Sharghi M, Mansurkhani SM, Ashtary-Larky D, et al. An update and systematic review on the treatment of primary dysmenorrhea. J Bras Reprod Assist 2019;23(1):51–7.
20. National Sleep Foundation. Gallup Poll on Adult public's experiences with night-time pain. Published online 1996.
21. Irwin MR. Sleep and inflammation: partners in sickness and in health. Nat Rev Immunol 2019;19(11):702–15.
22. Nollet M, Wisden W, Franks NP. Sleep deprivation and stress: a reciprocal relationship. Interface Focus 2020;10(3). https://doi.org/10.1098/rsfs.2019.0092.
23. Simon EB, Vallat R, Barnes CM, et al. Sleep loss and the socio-emotional brain. Trends Cogn Sci 2020;24(6):435–50.
24. Schmidt MH. The energy allocation function of sleep: a unifying theory of sleep, torpor, and continuous wakefulness. Neurosci Biobehav Rev 2014;47:122–53.
25. Antunes IB, Andersen ML, Baracat EC, et al. The effects of paradoxical sleep deprivation on estrous cycles of the female rats. Horm Behav 2006;49(4):433–40.
26. Antunes IB, Andersen ML, Alvarenga TAF, et al. Effects of paradoxical sleep deprivation on blood parameters associated with cardiovascular risk in intact and ovariectomized rats compared with male rats. Behav Brain Res 2007;176(2):187–92.
27. Ma H, Hong M, Duan J, et al. Altered cytokine gene expression in peripheral blood monocytes across

the menstrual cycle in primary dysmenorrhea: a case-control study. PLoS One 2013;8(2). https://doi.org/10.1371/journal.pone.0055200.
28. Baker FC, Driver HS, Rogers GG, et al. High nocturnal body temperatures and disturbed sleep in women with primary dysmenorrhea. Am J Physiol Endocrinol Metabolism 1999;277(6):E1013–21.
29. Iacovides S, Avidon I, Bentley A, et al. Diclofenac potassium restores objective and subjective measures of sleep quality in women with primary dysmenorrhea. Sleep 2009;32(8):1019–26.
30. Araujo P, Hachul H, Santos-Silva R, et al. Sleep pattern in women with menstrual pain. Sleep Med 2011;12(10):1028–30.
31. Keshavarzi F, Mahmoudzadeh F, Brand S, et al. Both melatonin and meloxicam improved sleep and pain in females with primary dysmenorrhea—results from a double-blind cross-over intervention pilot study. Arch Womens Ment Health 2018;21(6):601–9.
32. Wang ZY, Liu ZZ, Jia CX, et al. Age at menarche, menstrual problems, and daytime sleepiness in Chinese adolescent girls. Sleep 2019;42(6). https://doi.org/10.1093/sleep/zsz061.
33. Hamzekhani M, Gandomani SJ, Tavakol Z, et al. The relation between sleep quality and primary dysmenorrhea students university of medical sciences shahroud. J Adv Pharmacy Education & Res 2019;9(4):100–4.
34. Çaltekin İ, Hamamcı M, Demir Çaltekin M, et al. Evaluation of sleep disorders, anxiety and depression in women with dysmenorrhea. Sleep Biol Rhythms 2021;19(1):13–21.
35. He H, Yu X, Chen T, et al. Sleep status and menstrual problems among Chinese young females. BioMed Res Int 2021;2021. https://doi.org/10.1155/2021/1549712.
36. Polat CD, Mucuk S. The relationship between dysmenorrhea and sleep quality. Cukurova Medical Journal 2021;46(1):352–9.
37. Sahin S, Ozdemir K, Unsal A, et al. Review of frequency of dysmenorrhea and some associated factors and evaluation of the relationship between dysmenorrhea and sleep quality in university students. Gynecol Obstet Invest 2014;78(3):179–85.
38. Weng M, Tu CH, Lin CL, et al. A. Basic and Translational Sleep Science XIII. Sleep and Aging, Sleep and Gender sleep loss may mess with premesntrual syndromes in dysmenorrheic women Hsing. Vol 42. Abstract Supplement; 2019. https://academic.oup.com/sleep/article/42/Supplement_1/A111/5451659
39. Woosley JA, Lichstein KL. Dysmenorrhea, the menstrual cycle, and sleep. Behav Med 2014;40(1):14–21.
40. Xing X, Xue P, Li SX, et al. Sleep disturbance is associated with an increased risk of menstrual problems in female Chinese university students. Sleep Breath 2020;24(4):1719–27.
41. Bahrami A, Sadeghnia H, Avan A, et al. Neuropsychological function in relation to dysmenorrhea in adolescents. Eur J Obstet Gynecol Reprod Biol 2017;215:224–9.
42. Atta K, Jawed S, Zia S. Correlating primary dysmenorrhea with stressors: a cross sectional study investigating the most likely factors of primary dysmenorrhea and its effects on quality of life and general well being. J University Medical & Dental College 2016;7(4).
43. Gagua T, Tkeshelashvili B, Gagua D. Primary dysmenorrhea: prevalence in adolescent population of Tbilisi, Georgia and risk factors. Journal of the Turkish German Gynecology Association 2012;13(3):162–8.
44. Kazama M, Maruyama K, Nakamura K. Prevalence of dysmenorrhea and its correlating lifestyle factors in Japanese female junior high school students. Tohoku J Exp Med 2015;236(2):107–13.
45. Chen CX, Carpenter JS, Lapradd M, et al. Perceived ineffectiveness of pharmacological treatments for dysmenorrhea. J Womens Health 2021;30(9):1334–43.
46. Kannan P, Chapple CM, Miller D, et al. Effectiveness of a treadmill-based aerobic exercise intervention on pain, daily functioning, and quality of life in women with primary dysmenorrhea: a randomized controlled trial. Contemp Clin Trials 2019;81:80–6.
47. Shaver JL, Iacovides S. Sleep in women with chronic pain and autoimmune conditions: a narrative review. Sleep Med Clin 2018;13(3):375–94.
48. Kirmizigil B, Demiralp C. Effectiveness of functional exercises on pain and sleep quality in patients with primary dysmenorrhea: a randomized clinical trial. Arch Gynecol Obstet 2020;302(1):153–63.
49. Abdel-Salam DM, Alnuman RW, Alrwuaili RM, et al. Epidemiological aspects of dysmenorrhea among female students at Jouf University, Saudi Arabia. Middle East Fertil Soc J 2018;23(4):435–9.
50. Moldofsky H. Sleep and pain. Sleep Med Rev 2001;5(5):385–96.
51. Tang NKY, Goodchild CE, Sanborn AN, et al. Deciphering the temporal link between pain and sleep in a heterogeneous chronic pain patient sample: a multilevel daily process study. Sleep 2012;35(5):675–87.
52. O'brien EM, Waxenberg LB, Atchison JW, et al. Intraindividual Variability in Daily Sleep and Pain Ratings Among Chronic Pain Patients: Bidirectional Association and the Role of Negative Mood.; 2011. www.clinicalpain.com
53. Stroemel-Scheder C, Kundermann B, Lautenbacher S. The effects of recovery sleep on pain perception: a systematic review. Neurosci Biobehav Rev 2020;113:408–25.
54. Krause AJ, Prather AA, Wager TD, et al. The pain of sleep loss: a brain characterization in humans. J Neurosci 2019;39(12):2291–300.

55. Alonso C, Coe CL. Disruptions of social relationships accentuate the association between emotional distress and menstrual pain in young women. Health Psychol 2001;20(6):411–6.
56. Yu L, Buysse DJ, Germain A, et al. Development of Short forms from the PROMIS™ sleep disturbance and sleep-related impairment item banks. Behav Sleep Med 2011;10(1):6–24.
57. American Academy of Sleep Medicine. International Classification of Sleep Disorders. 3rd ed.; 2014.
58. Hillman DR, Lack LC. Public health implications of sleep loss: the community burden. Med J Aust 2013;199:s7–10.
59. Chattu VK, Sakhamuri SM, Kumar R, et al. Insufficient sleep syndrome: is it time to classify as a major noncommunicable disease? Sleep Sci 2018;11(2):56–64.
60. Edwards RR, Almeida DM, Klick B, et al. Duration of sleep contributes to next-day pain reporting the general population. Pain 2008;137(1):202–7.
61. Salwen JK, Smith MT, Finan PH. Mid-treatment sleep duration predicts clinically significant knee osteoarthritis pain reduction at 6 months: effects from a behavioral sleep medicine clinical trial. Sleep 2017;40(2):zsw064.
62. American Academy of Sleep Medicine. Sleep Education: Insomnia. Available at: https://sleepeducation.org/sleep-disorders/insomnia/. Accessed October 14, 2022.
63. Mong JA, Cusmano DM. Sex differences in sleep: impact of biological sex and sex steroids. Philos Trans R Soc Lond B Biol Sci 2016;371(1688). https://doi.org/10.1098/rstb.2015.0110.
64. American Academy of Sleep Medicine. Practice guidelines. Available at: https://aasm.org/clinical-resources/practice-standards/practice-guidelines/. Accessed October 14, 2022.
65. Andersen ML, Araujo P, Frange C, et al. Sleep disturbance and pain: a tale of two common problems. Chest 2018;154(5):1249–59.
66. Ohayon M. Prevalence and correlates of nonrestorative sleep complaints. Arch Intern Med 2005;165(1):35–41.
67. Morin CM, Benca R. Chronic insomnia. Lancet 2012;379(9821):1129–41.
68. Irwin M, Olmstead R, Carrillo C, et al. Cognitive behavioral therapy vs. Tai Chi for late life insomnia and inflammatory risk: a randomized controlled comparative efficacy trial. Sleep 2014;37(9):1543–52.
69. Generaal S, Torkzahrani S, Akbarzadeh A, et al. Insomnia, sleep duration, depressive symptoms, and the onset of chronic multisite musculoskeletal pain. Sleep 2017;40(1).
70. Tufik S, Santos-Silva R, Taddei J, et al. Obstructive sleep apnea syndrome in the são paulo epidemiologic sleep study. Sleep Med 2010;11(5):441–6.
71. Zahradnik H, Hanjalic-Beck A, Groth K. Nonsteroidal anti-inflammatory drugs and hormonal contraceptives for pain relief from dysmenorrhea: a review. Contraception 2010;81(3):185–96.
72. Marjoribanks J, Ayeleke R, Farquhar C, et al. Nonsteroidal anti-inflammatory drugs for dysmenorrhoea. Cochrane Database Syst Rev 2015;7:CD001751.
73. Ferris-Rowe E, Corey E, Archer J. Primary dysmenorrhea: diagnosis and therapy. Obst Gynecol 2020;136(5):1047–58.
74. ACOG - The American Academy of College of Obstetricians and Gynecologists. Noncontraceptive uses of hormonal contraceptives. practice bulletin n. 110. Obstet Gynecol 2010;115:206–18.
75. Croxatto H. Clinical profile of Implanon: a single-rod etonogestrel contraceptive implant. Eur J Contracept Reprod Health Care 2000;5(suppl 2):21–8.
76. Morrow C, Naumburg E. Dysmenorrhea. Prim Care 2009;36:19–32.
77. Gomes M, Deitcher S. Risk of venous thromboembolic disease associated with hormonal contraceptives and hormone replacement therapy: a clinical review. Arch Intern Med 2004;164:1965–76.
78. Gharloghi S, Torkazahrani S, Akbarzadeh A. The effects of acupressure on severity of primary dysmenorrhea. Patient Prefer Adherence 2012;6:137–42.
79. Wang Y, Hsu C, Yeh M, et al. Auricular acupressure to improve menstrual pain and menstrual distress and heart rate variability for primary dysmenorrhea in youth with stress. Evid Based Complement Alternat Med 2013;2013.
80. Kim SD. Yoga for menstrual pain in primary dysmenorrhea: a meta-analysis of randomized controlled trials. Complement Ther Clin Pract 2019;36:94–9.
81. Israel R, Sutton M, O'Biren K. Effects of aerobic training on primary dysmenorrhea symptomatology in college females. J Am Coll Health 1985;33:241–4.
82. Carroquino-Garcia P, Jiménez-Rejano J, Medrano-Sanchez E, et al. Therapeutic exercise in the treatment of primary dysmenorrhea: a systematic review and meta-analysis. Phys Ther 2019;99(10):1371–80.
83. Jo J, Lee SH. Heat therapy for primary dysmenorrhea: a systematic review and meta-analysis of its effects on pain relief and quality of life. Sci Rep 2018;8(1). https://doi.org/10.1038/s41598-018-34303-z.
84. Proctor M, Smith C, Farquhar C, et al. Transcutaneous electrical nerve stimulation and acupuncture for primary dysmenorrhoea. Cochrane Database Syst Rev 2002;1:CD002123.
85. Igwea S, Tabansi-Ochuogu C, Abaraogu U. TENS and heat therapy for pain relief and quality of life improvement in individuals with primary dysmenorrhea: a systematic review. Complement Ther Clin Pract 2016;24:86–91.

Yoga Nidra, a Nonpharmacological Technique in Management of Insomnia and Overall Health in Postmenopausal Women

Kamalesh K. Gulia, PhD[a,*], Sapna Erat Sreedharan, MD, DM[b]

KEYWORDS

- Menopause • Yoga nidra • Nonpharmacological technique • Well-being • Insomnia • Sleep • Yoga • Walking

KEY POINTS

- Yoga nidra is a potential nonpharmacological technique to improve sleep quality in postmenopausal women.
- This technique can be practiced in home setting after a brief training.
- There are no documented side effects of this practice.
- Improvement in sleep influences overall well-being of postmenopausal women.

INTRODUCTION

Menopause is a natural and gradual transition from reproductive to a nonreproductive phase of women's life confirmed by a complete absence of menstrual cycle for a year (amenorrhea). It is noted that several women across globe also undergo surgical menopause due to surgical removal of uterus (hysterectomy due to various underlying condition of endometrial polyps, fibroids, inflammation, prolapse, dysplasia or intraepithelial neoplasia, cancer or postpartum complications) or ovaries (oophorectomy due to benign tumor or cancer, cysts, endometriosis, and so forth).[1–6] There are increasing evidences of early menopause termed as premature menopause occurring due to premature ovarian failure before the age of 40 years) in the current life styles.[7–11] Life after menopause (premature, normally occurring or surgical) is marked insomnia, anxiety, depression, increased risk of cardiovascular diseases, osteoporosis, poor health, reduced quality of life affecting overall well-being.[12–15] A longer life span in women compared with men[16,17] also needs attention as more years will be spent in poor health. Definitely, there is increased vulnerability of women in menopausal phase to poor sleep quality and overall deterioration in health for nearly more one-third of their life.

As the length of menopausal process is variable and range in years, a uniform staging system for reproductive aging through menopause, provided in executive summary for the Stages of Reproductive Aging Workshop (termed as STRAW)[18,19] are useful to comprehend complex changes. It is widely used now wherein the final menstrual period is taken as zero point on a 7-point staging. The postmenopause is described into an Early (+1 stage) for the initial 1 year of amenorrhea followed

[a] Division of Sleep Research, Department of Applied Biology, Biomedical Technology Wing, Sree Chitra Tirunal Institute for Medical Sciences and Technology, Trivandrum, Kerala 695012, India; [b] Department of Neurology, Comprehensive Centre for Sleep Disorders, Sree Chitra Tirunal Institute for Medical Sciences and Technology, Trivandrum, Kerala 695011, India
* Corresponding author.
E-mail address: kkguliak@hotmail.com

Sleep Med Clin 18 (2023) 463–471
https://doi.org/10.1016/j.jsmc.2023.06.007

by another 4 years while Late (+2 stage) is the stage thereafter until the last breath. The perimenopausal period is also variable and defined as an Early (−2 stage) and Late (−1 stage). It is real challenge in the current era to adapt to a revised life style amid altered hormonal profile, physiologic functions, and neurologic effects. Decline in sleep quantity and quality directly and indirectly disrupts every function of a person. The third sustainable developmental goal formulated by the United Nations to attain Good Health and Well-being is a timely goal to achieve globally. In recent years, yoga is increasingly recognized as a universally accepted science to achieve physical, emotional, and mental well-being.[20–23] In postmenopausal women, studies indicate promising effects of various forms of yoga, exercise (such as walking), and so forth on health parameters.[24–29] There is persistent need to carry out large-scale randomized clinical trials to strengthen the evidence-based medicine. Our recent report also provided the therapeutic potential of Yoga Nidra (yogic sleep) in the postmenopausal age in a longitudinal pilot study.[30]

In this review, various viable treatment strategies for the management of insomnia to improve well-being are discussed. This is followed by a comprehensive discussion on the technique of Yoga Nidra as a nonpharmacological intervention during menopause.

MENOPAUSE-RELATED HEALTH CONCERNS AND PLAUSIBLE TREATMENT OPTIONS (HORMONAL REPLACEMENT THERAPY/ COGNITIVE BEHAVIORAL THERAPY/YOGA)

During perimenopause and postmenopause, multifactorial changes in the central and endocrine system (drop in estradiol, increased follicle stimulating hormone [FSH], increased testosterone, and hot flashes) contribute to sleep disorders, anxiety, depression with comorbid illnesses such as obesity, gastroesophageal reflux, chronic pain, and fibromyalgia, thereby affecting the overall health.[31] Frequent early morning awakenings are the hallmark in this age as shown in the actigraphy-derived actogram of a postmenopausal subject (**Fig. 1**). It is often accompanied by pain, headache, low mood, anxiety, and a feeling of nonrestorative sleep in postmenopausal women[30,32] A change in the quantity and quality of sleep is an underlying factor to cause these psycho-behavioral changes.[33,34] Further, sedentary life and reduced mobility aggravate sleep and mental health.[35] Additional discomforts due to accompanying headaches and pain, which usually occur during the postmenopausal stage, only worsen the general health conditions.

During perimenopause, prolonged vasomotor symptoms contribute significantly to hot flashes, night sweats, sedentary life, and early morning awakenings leading to overall poor sleep quality.[35–38] There are no clear evidences to show that yoga interventions alone can completely alleviate the vasomotor symptoms; however, it is beneficial in the management of insomnia and well-being during post-menopause.[24,25,39,40]

Regarding treatment therapy, the cognitive behavioral therapy (CBT-I) is a gold standard for the treatment of insomnia during menopause[41,42] but lack of sufficient numbers of trained experts and easily accessible centers in most of the developing and underdeveloped nations make it a limiting factor. Moreover, expenses involved in CBT-I might make it less approachable to the general population. Another option is the hormonal replacement therapy (HRT) but prolonged HRT increases the risk for endometrial and breast cancer[43,44] report LANCET, 2019.[45] Thus, HRT also cannot be considered a viable treatment for a long term. Further, the classic yoga asanas (Hatha yoga) may be difficult and impractical for postmenopausal subjects who are struggling with central obesity, osteoporosis, muscle stiffness, and high basal metabolic rate (BMI). Postmenopause is a prolonged phase in women's life lasting for 2 to 4 decades, thus it is a challenge to identify a suitable nonpharmacological intervention to improve their sleep, health, and well-being. Yoga nidra is one such profound technique with reported therapeutic potential for various ailments in different age groups (**Table 1**). These studies indicated that in spite of variable duration of practice of Yoga nidra, ranging from few minutes to several weeks, alleviation of stress, anxiety, depression, pain, and improvement of physiologic parameters of sleep and menstrual cycle were evident that were measured objectively or subjectively.[30,46–60] Scientific studies are aimed to capture more objective measures especially the complex brain waves and sleep to understand the underlying mechanism for the effects of the Yoga nidra.

WHAT IS YOGA NIDRA TECHNIQUE?

The word Yoga Nidra, termed as psychic sleep or yogic sleep, is derived from Sanskrit word yoga, means or one-pointed awareness and Nidra denoting sleep.[61–63] It is a profound technique by which a deep relaxation of the body and mind is consciously achieved by specific meditation practice lying in a corpse position (Shavasana)

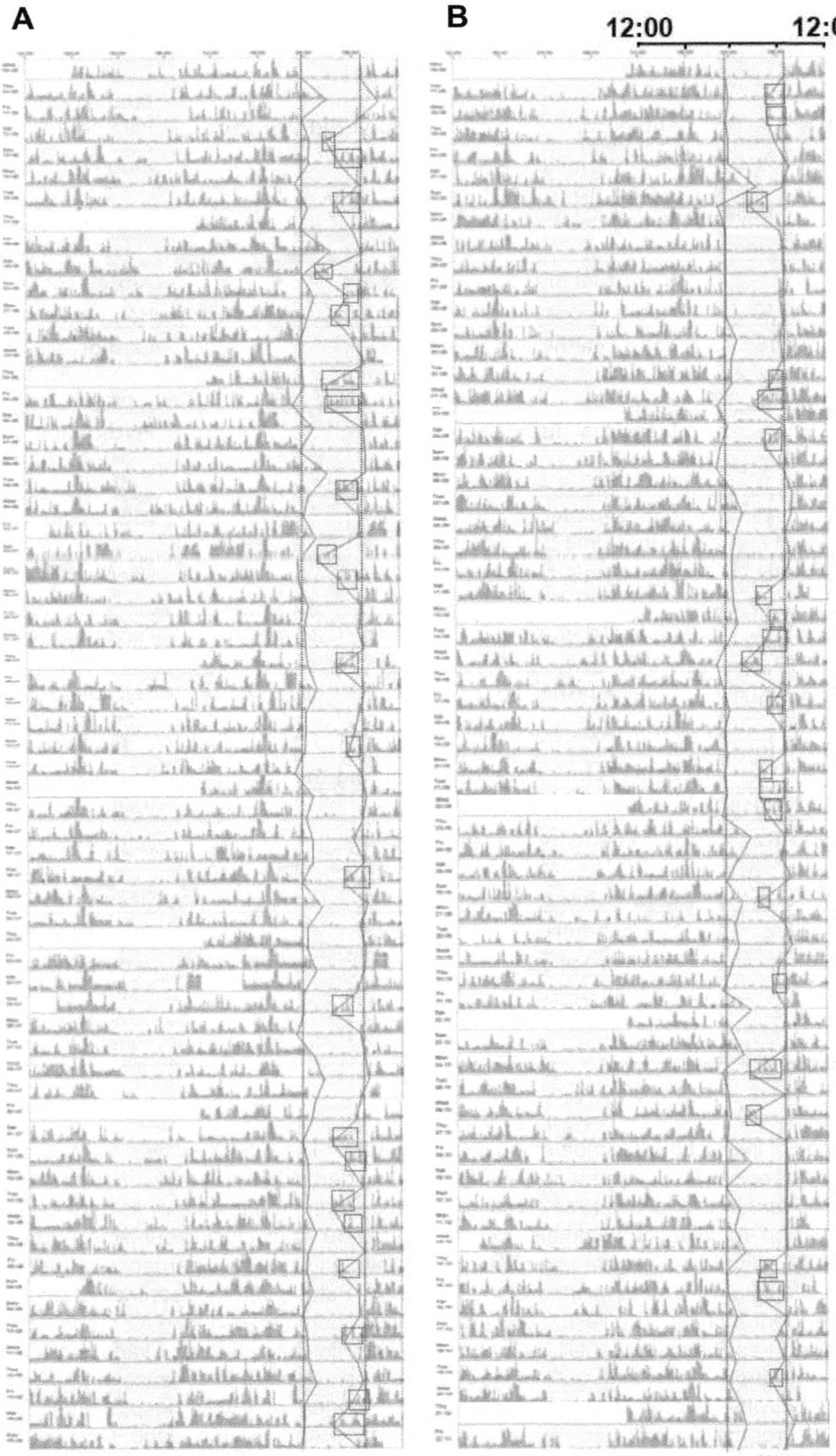

Fig. 1. Sleep-wakefulness pattern of a normal menopausal woman showing early morning awakenings in actigraph (raster plot). Raster plot showing 19 weeks' activity pattern (*A* and *B*) where each row in panel A/B is depicting the daily activity. Red vertical lines are providing outline of 8 hours ideal sleep while blue zig-zag lines are showing the actual sleep across 134 days. Red dotted line-boxes are depicting early morning awakenings.

Table 1
Reported therapeutic effects of Yoga Nidra on various health conditions in different age groups

Study Group	Subjects	Yoga Nidra Practice	Studied Outcomes/ Parameters
Amita et al,[46] 2009	Diabetic middle-age patients	13 wk	Blood glucose
Kamakhya and Joshi,[47] 2009	Young healthy adult	7 wk	EEG and galvanic skin response (GSR)
Rani et al,[48] 2012	Menstrual disorders	24 wk	Anxiety, depression
Markil et al,[50] 2012	Adults	30 min	Herat rate variability
Bajpai et al,[51] 2015	Yong healthy students	12 wk	Cardiovascular hyper-reactivity to cold pressor test
Rani et al,[49] 2016	Menstrual disorders	24 wk,	Psycho-biological well-being, hormonal profile
Anand et al,[52] 2015	Cancer patients, insomnia	2 wk	PSQI based sleep
Chaudhary and Pal,[53] 2016	Spondylitis, backache	5 wk	Stress
Datta et al,[54] 2017	Male archer, chronic insomnia	4 wk, Case report	Performance
Ferriera-Vorkapic et al,[57] 2018	College professors	12 wk	Psychological variables: anxiety, stress, depression
Li et al,[58] 2019	Patients for colonoscopy	During the procedure	Pain management
Vaishnav et al,[59] 2018	Adolescent	4 wk	Well-being
Ozdemir and Saritas,[60] 2019	Burn patients	4 wk	Self-esteem, body image
Datta et al,[55] 2021	Chronic insomnia	2 wk	Sleep by PSG
Datta et al,[56] 2022	Young adults	2 wk	19 EEG channel PSG
Gulia and Sreedharan,[30] 2022	Postmenopausal Woman	24 wk, Case report	Actigraphy-based sleep quality and quantity, self-reported mood, well-being

following a series of instruction. To understand the Yoga Nidra, one needs to first understand the science of sleep. A natural sleep consists of 2 distinct states, that is, non–rapid eye movement sleep (NREM) and REM sleep that alternate in a distinct pattern across each night in a state of unconscious in an age-dependent manner. The NREM state is further subdivided into 3 substages, N1, N2, and N3, which occur in progression and are regulated by a complex interplay of brain networks. Even though the neurophysiological correlates of NREM and REM sleep are documented to a certain extent,[14,64–66] the purpose, functional significance of each substate, optimal duration of these substates and significance of alternation into a consolidated sleep in health and disease still remain some of the unanswered mysteries of the nature. The alpha waves in cortical EEG are considered the hallmark of relaxation processes that attain prominence while getting into relaxation procedures by closing our eyes. Further slowing of brain activity with emergence of theta waves during N1 stage, and appearance of peculiar spindles and K complexes during N2 stage have been subject of investigations for various cognitive regulatory processed in disease and health. The N3 component of NREM sleep, marked by prominent delta waves, is the deep state of sleep when thalamo-cortical networks elicit very slow oscillations. This state is associated with glymphatic clearance, and memory consolidation etc.[67–69] Further, the REM sleep with prominent theta waves mimics a state similar to wakefulness but without conscious awareness of it.

The Yoga Nidra practice aims to achieve an internal state of profound relaxation of body, mind, and emotions without going into actual sleep but attaining a state of awareness of his/her conscious.[61] In the field of yoga, it is achieved through *Pratyahara*, the fifth element of Ashtanga yoga as per Patanjali Yoga involving disassociation of consciousness/senses from the outside environment other than the auditory one. Yoga Nidra intervention developed by Swami Satyananda Saraswati from Bihar School of Yoga (Munger, India) for beginners is practiced every morning using instructions from audio CD. It was practiced for 27 minutes on working days, and for 48 minutes on weekends and holiday (audio CD session). Basically, Yoga Nidra technique involves systematic observation of several steps while lying down in shavasana (in corpse pause with eyes closed) beginning with preparation involving internalization, taking resolve (sankalpa), rotation of consciousness, breathing awareness, manifestations of opposites, image visualization, resolve and externalization, or return to full awareness at the end. A conscious systematic control of brain makes this technique more special and powerful to attain enhanced relaxed state by integrating body and mind.

As postmenopausal age is marked by sleep disorders and related health issues, there is need to pay attention to sleep health and bringing in appropriate management measures in place.[70] In one of our study, effects of 24 week's Yoga Nidra practice in a postmenopausal woman (age 56 years) showed promising results.[30] Before the practice, a baseline recording of 4 weeks of sleep–wake activity was carried out using actigraphy that was worn during the entire study period of 28 weeks. In this longitudinal study, the effects of 24 weeks of Yoga Nidra practice were measured parameters such as sleep latency, total sleep time, early morning awakenings, activity rhythm of body using 24-hour actigraphy, and sleep diary. Everyday mood on waking and during day were also noted. In the evening, the subject was motivated to walk for 25 to 30 minutes. After administering the dual protocol (Yoga nidra in morning and walking in evening), there was remarkable elevation in mood both on waking-up and entire day from fifth week onward. Mood shifted toward a happier state. Latency to sleep decreased after 4 weeks while total sleep time improved only after 16 weeks of dual management strategy. The BMI was also reduced to 28.4 from initial value of 30.3. Morning awakening patterns did not change but it was not accompanied by pain or headache.

DISCUSSION

There is continuous search for a viable nonpharmacological treatment options to derive adaptive changes to modern era for improving sleep and physiology. It is ideal to cherish natural age-matched recuperative sleep but that becomes a challenge during menopause associated physiologic changes in women. Practice of Yoga Nidra offers a doable nonpharmacological promising technique in improving the emotional state of a subject by relaxing the brain and strengthening self-determination component (resolve). Through relaxation techniques of simple shavasana, mere relaxation of physical body (muscles) may be achieved. However, Yoga Nidra carried out in the shavasana position has profound effect calming of mind by internalization, rotating of consciousness. Increasing numbers of studies are substantiating the therapeutic potential of this technique in achieving deep relaxation of mind, stress reduction, alleviation of anxiety, depression, menstrual disorders, insomnia, blood pressure, and for attaining overall mental health.[30,54,56,60,71–73,]

It is pointed that a regular practice is the key to get the beneficial effects of Yoga Nidra for insomnia in menopausal age. It is shown that sleep duration was increased only after regular practice of 16 weeks while reduction in latency were achieved faster (after 4 week).[30] This indicated that effects on the sleep initiation network were faster than the maintenance networks. However, 2 to 4 weeks practice of Yoga Nidra improved sleep in young subjects with chronic insomnia.[55] Moreover, 24 week's practice was also found optimal for the improvement of anxiety, depression, and symptoms of the menopausal syndrome.[48,49] Probably, 24 week's practice may be ideal in aging-related insomnia.

Another crucial concern is regarding the ideal time to practice the Yoga Nidra. From our experience, it is suggested that the early morning is the best time for several reasons: (1) postmenopausal subjects are generally experiencing early morning awakening thus it is an ideal time to practice Yoga Nidra because no special effort is required to get up, (2) low noise levels with minimal disturbances, and (3) it will make for the proper utilization of morning hours to relax brain. It is emphasized that Yoga Nidra alone might not be sufficient to lower the menopause-related increased BMI. However, the evening activity including walking would help in strengthening the circadian rhythm of body for improving sleep quality. It is understood that walking alone helps in burning calories and thereby would contribute in improving the BMI. However, it remains a challenge to involve people in activities in postmenopausal stage due to fatigue, lethargy, and reduced self-drive. Thus, the dual strategy of practicing Yoga Nidra in morning and walking in evening would have synergistic effects in improving sleep during night and maintaining the overall mood during the day.[26,30] The insomnia is a risk factor for the cardiovascular diseases especially women undergoing menopause, thus management of sleep may help in improving the heart health.[74]

Effects of Yoga Nidra are multifaceted, that is, self-control on mind can help in reducing anxiety and fills confidence and affirmation to carry out work each day. Thus, the dual strategy (Yoga Nidra and walking) complemented each other for overall health outcomes. It is likely that a long-term practice may be required to contain the morning awakenings as 24 weeks of Yoga Nidra did not significantly reduce the postmenopausal age-related organic changes.[30] However, even the short practice of Yoga Nidra alleviated pain and headache associated with the morning awakenings.

In Yoga Nidra practice, one accomplishes sleep-like state consciously but actually without getting into the unconscious sleep and without waking up. It is mentioned that the experienced Yoga practitioner (Swami Veda) reportedly achieved the classic Yoga Nidra state, state of deep sleep marked by the delta and theta waves in EEG in the conscious state.[75,76] However, it would be great to have the objective documentation of such extraordinary phenomenon of consciousness, which are so unique and intriguing. In a recent polysomnography study conducted in healthy subjects wherein the EEG was monitored during the Yoga Nidra (after 2 weeks of practice), reported an increase in the total delta power in the central area and a decrease in the prefrontal area when compared with the preyoga values.[56] It is shown that controlled sleep deprivation in the rat model resulted in appearance of slow wave sleep in the local population of cortical neurons.[77] It is similar to the getting into local sleep while staying in the wake state wherein some areas of brain will get into slow mode (similar to NREM deep sleep). It is so interesting from the homeostatic perspective of sleep regulation, as electrical activity of the neurons in brain is influenced by the prior activities carried out by the subject, and the sleep and waking profiles in addition to the effects of momentary indulgence in various task and activities.[77,78] Thus, the homeostatic changes in sleep EEG are the results of dynamic alterations in neuronal firing and synchrony arising from changes in functional neuronal connectivity in healthy aging.[78–80] The study of EEG phenomenology of local sleep in the science of Yoga Nidra is like opening a Pandora box of mysteries of consciousness. In future, the relevance of isolated local sleep versus consolidated deep sleep during N3 (recuperative sleep) will possibly help us in understanding neural substrates of deep relaxation that is crucial for maintaining good health and also in the management of disease in different age groups.

The preliminary results obtained from this report[30] clearly indicate the therapeutic potential of Yoga Nidra and exercise package based on this actigraphy-based longitudinal pilot study. A large randomized trial with EEG correlates will definitely will amplify on the evidence in a larger population.

The Indian ancient literature gave importance to sleep as one of the foundation pillars of good health other than nutrition and exercise, and holistic approaches to improve sleep are described in the traditional School of Indian Medicine.[81] Yoga is a comprehensive science consisting of processes of restraining various states of mind (chitta) from any fluctuation. Recent meta-analysis also showed that yoga improves the sleep quality in women without any documented side effects.[23]

SUMMARY

It is emphasized that Yoga Nidra is a powerful technique to consciously achieve a complete physical, mental, and emotional relaxation of brain and body. It derives strength from the naturally occurring deep sleep that plays a crucial role in every night recuperation processes. It is a nonpharmacological intervention to simulate such a state by practicing several minutes of Yoga Nidra in the wee hours that is marked by frequent early morning awakening during postmenopausal life (aging). Moreover, it can be practiced easily at home lying in simple comfortable shavasan position thus making it a viable technique with a tremendous potential for a self-regulation of mind and body. Under current sedentary metropolitan digital era stressful lifestyles, there is dire need of revisiting this practice in a big randomized controlled trial so that can be used by larger set of aging population. Restorative and good quality sleep helps in uplifted mood during the day for effectively carrying out the daily work.

CLINICS CARE POINTS

- Yoga Nidra is a potential nonpharmacological technique to improve sleep quality and well-being during menopause.

- Yoga Nidra in mornings and exercise (walking, and so forth) during evening will derive robust effect.

Pitfalls

- Wash out effect period need to be assessed with EEG markers.
- A large randomized clinical trial for the Yoga Nidra frequency and time years will provide more answers.

DISCLOSURE

The authors have nothing to disclose

REFERENCES

1. Schottenfeld D. Epidemiology of endometrial neoplasia. J Cell Biochem Suppl 1995;23:151–9.
2. Tortolero-Luna G, Mitchell MF. The epidemiology of ovarian cancer. J Cell Biochem Suppl 1995;23: 200–7.
3. Permuth-Wey J, Sellers TA. Epidemiology of ovarian cancer. Methods Mol Biol 2009;472:413–37.
4. Neis KJ, Zubke W, Fehr M, et al. Hysterectomy for Benign Uterine Disease. Dtsch Arztebl Int 2016 Apr 8;113(14):242–9.
5. Kallianidis AF, Maraschini A, Danis J, et al. Epidemiological analysis of peripartum hysterectomy across nine European countries. Acta Obstet Gynecol Scand 2020;99(10):1364–73.
6. Kumari P, Kundu J. Prevalence, socio-demographic determinants, and self-reported reasons for hysterectomy and choice of hospitalization in India. BMC Women's Health 2022;22(1):514.
7. Jewelwicz R, Schwartz M. Premature ovarian failure. Bull N Y Acad Med 1986;62:219–36.
8. Menopause, premature menopause and post menopausal bleeding. In: Padubidri VG, Daftary SN, editors. Shaw's Textbook of Gynecology. 13th edition. New Delhi: Elsevier; 2004. p. 56–67.
9. Shuster LT, Rhodes DJ, Gostout BS, et al. Premature menopause or early menopause: long-term health consequences. Maturitas 2010;65(2):161.
10. Okeke TC, Anyaehie UB, Enzenyeaku CC. Premature Menopause. Ann Med Health Sci Res 2013; 3(1):90–5.
11. Peycheva D, Sullivan A, Hardy R, et al. Risk factors for natural menopause before the age of 45: evidence from two British population-based birth cohort studies. BMC Womens Health 2022;22(1): 438.
12. Ohayon MM. Epidemiology of insomnia: what we know and what we still need to learn. Sleep Medicine Reviews 2002;6:97–111.
13. Whiteley J, daCosta DiBonaventura M, Wagner JS, Shah S. The Impact of Menopausal Symptoms on Quality of Life, Productivity, and Economic Outcomes. J Women's Health (Larchmt). 2013;22(11): 983–90.
14. Gulia KK, Kumar VM. Sleep disorders in the elderly: A growing challenge. Psychogeriatrics 2018;18: 155–65.
15. Vitale SG, Riemma G, Mikuš M, et al. Quality of Life, Anxiety and Depression in Women Treated with Hysteroscopic Endometrial Resection or Ablation for Heavy Menstrual Bleeding: Systematic Review and Meta-Analysis of Randomized Controlled Trials. Medicina (Kaunas) 2022;58(11):1664.
16. Zarulli V, Jones JAB, Oksuzyan A, et al. Women live longer than men even during severe famines and epidemics. Proc Natl Acad Sci U S A 2018;115(4): E832–40.
17. Arias E, Tajada-Vera B, Kochanek KD, Ahmad FB. Provisional Life Expectancy Estimates for 2021, Vital Statistics Rapid Release. Report No. 23, 2022. Available at: https://www.cdc.gov/nchs/data/vsrr/vsrr023.pdf
18. Soules MR, Sherman S, Parrott E, et al. Stages of Reproductive Aging Workshop (STRAW). Journal of Women's Health & Gender-Based Medicine 2001;10:843–8.
19. Harlow SD, Gass M, Hall JE, et al. Executive summary of the Stages of Reproductive Aging Workshop + 10: addressing the unfinished agenda of staging reproductive aging. Menopause 2012; 19(4):387–95.
20. Woodyard C. Exploring the therapeutic effects of yoga and its ability to increase quality of life. Int J Yoga 2011;4(2):49–54.
21. Balasubramaniam M, Telles S, Doraiswamy PM. Yoga on Our Minds: A Systematic Review of yoga for neuropsychiatric disorders. Front Psychiatry 2012;3:117.
22. Jeter PE, Slutsky, Singh N, Khalsa SB. Yoga as a therapeutic intervention: a bibliometric analysis of published work studies from 1967 to 2013. The J of Alternative and Complementary Medicine 2015; 21:586–92.
23. Wang W, Chen K, Pan Y, et al. The effect of yoga on sleep quality and insomnia in women with sleep problems: a systematic review and meta-analysis. BMC Psychiatry 2020;20:195.
24. Afonso RF, Hachul H, Kozasa EH, et al. Yoga decreases insomnia in postmenopausal women: a randomized clinical trial. Menopause 2012;19(2): 186–93.
25. Jorge MP, Santaella DF, Pontes IMO, et al. Hatha Yoga practice decreases menopause symptoms and improves quality of life: A randomized controlled trial. Complement Ther Med 2016;26:128–35.
26. Tadayon M, Abedi P, Farshadbakht F https://pubmed.ncbi.nlm.nih.gov/26757356/. Impact of pedometer-based walking on menopausal women's sleep quality: a randomized controlled trial.

Climacteric 2016;19:364-368.https://pubmed.ncbi.nlm.nih.gov/26757356/
27. Buchanan DT. Landis CA , Hohensee C, et al. Effects of yoga and aerobic exercise on actigraphic sleep parameters in menopausal women with hot flashes. J Clin Sleep Med 2017;13:11–8. https://pubmed.ncbi.nlm.nih.gov/27707450/.
28. Duman M, Taşhan ST. The effect of sleep hygiene education and relaxation exercises on insomnia among postmenopausal women: A randomized clinical trial. Int J Nurs Pract 2018;24:e12650.
29. Sydora BC, Turner C, Malley A, et al. Can walking exercise programs improve health for women in menopause transition and postmenopausal? Findings from a scoping review. Menopause 2020;27: 952–63.
30. Gulia KK, Sreedharan SE. Yogic sleep and walking protocol induced improvement in sleep and well-being in postmenopausal subject: A longitudinal case study during COVID lockdown. Sleep and Vigilance 2022;6:229–33.
31. Baker FC, Joffe, Lee KA. Sleep and Menopause. Chapter 159, Principles and practice of sleep Medicine. 6th Ed Edited by Meir Kryger, Thomas Roth, William C Dement, Elsevier. Part II, Sleep in Women. 1553-1563. ISBN 978-0-323-24288-2, 2015
32. Monteleone P, Mascagni G, Giannini A, et al. Symptoms of menopause - global prevalence, physiology and implications. Nat Rev Endocrinol 2018;14: 199–215.
33. Moreno-Frías C, Figueroa-Vega N, Malacara JM. Relationship of sleep alterations with perimenopausal and postmenopausal symptoms. Menopause 2014;21:1017–22.
34. Li DX, Romans S, De Souza MJ, et al. and self-reported sleep quality in women: associations with ovarian hormones and mood. Sleep Med 2015;16: 1217–24. https://pubmed.ncbi.nlm.nih.gov/26429749/Actigraphic.
35. Creasy SA, Crane TE, Garcia DO, et al. Higher amounts of sedentary time are associated with short sleep duration and poor sleep quality in postmenopausal women. Sleep 2019;42:zsz093.
36. Avis NE, Crawford Greendale G, et al. Duration of menopausal vasomotor symptoms over the menopause transition. JAMA Intern Med 2015;175(4): 531–9.
37. Lampio L, Polo-Kantola, Himanen SL, et al. Sleep During Menopausal Transition: A 6-Year Follow-Up. Sleep 2017;40(7).
38. Pengo MF, Won CH, Bourjeily G. Sleep in Women Across the Life Span. Chest 2018;154(1):196–206.
39. Avis NE, Legault C, Russell G, et al. A pilot study of integral Yoga for menopausal hot flashes. Menopause 2014;21(8):846–54.
40. Reed SD, Guthrie KA, Newton KM, et al. Menopausal quality of life: RCT of yoga, exercise, and omega-3 supplements. Am J Obstet Gynecol 2014;210(3):244.e1-11.
41. Nowakowski S, Meers JN. CBT-I and women's health: Sex as a biological variable. Sleep Med Clin 2019;14(2):185–97.
42. Meers JM, Dawson DB, Nowakowski S. CBT-I for perimenopause and postmenopause (Chapter 16), Editor(s): Sara Nowakowski, Sheila N. Garland, Michael A. Grandner, Leisha J. Cuddihy, Adapting Cognitive Behavioral Therapy for Insomnia, Academic Press, 2022, Pages 333-346, ISBN 9780128228722, https://doi.org/10.1016/B978-0-12-822872-2.00011-6.
43. Beral V, Bull D, Reeves G, et al. Endometrial cancer and hormone-replacement therapy in the Million Women Study. Lancet 2005;365(9470):1543–51.
44. Collaborative Group on Hormonal Factors in Breast Cancer. Type and timing of menopausal hormone therapy and breast cancer risk: individual participant meta-analysis of the worldwide epidemiological evidence. The LANCET 2019;394:1159–68.
45. Liang Y, Jiao H, Qu L, Liu H. Association Between Hormone Replacement Therapy and Development of Endometrial Cancer: Results from a Prospective US Cohort Study. Front. Med. 2022;8:802959.
46. Amita S, Prabhakar S, Manoj I, et al. Effect of yoga-nidra on blood glucose level in diabetic patients. Indian J Physiol Pharmacol 2009;53(1):97–101.
47. Kamakhya K, Joshi B. Study on the effect of *Pranakarshan pranayama* and *Yoga nidra* on alpha EEG & GSR. Indian J of Traditional Knowledge 2009;8:453–4.
48. Rani K, Tiwari SC, Singh U, et al. Yoga Nidra as a complementary treatment of anxiety and depressive symptoms in patients with menstrual disorder. Int J Yoga 2012;5(1):52–6.
49. Rani K, Tiwari SC, Kumar S, et al. Psycho-Biological Changes with Add on Yoga Nidra in Patients with Menstrual Disorders: a Randomized Clinical Trial. J Caring Sci 2016;5(1):1–9.
50. Markil N, Whitehurst M, Jacobs PL, Zoeller R. Yoga Nidra relaxation increases heart rate variability and is unaffected by a prior bout of Hatha yoga. J Altern Complement Med 2012;18(10):953–8.
51. Bajpai R, Rajak S, Rampalliwar S. Effect of Bhramari Pranayama and Yoga Nidra on cardiovascular hyper-reactivity to cold pressor test. International J of Med Sci Res and Practice 2015;2:24–6.
52. Anand DN, George LS, Raj A. Effectiveness of Yoga Nidra on quality of sleep among cancer patients. Manipal Journal of Nursing and Health Sciences 2015;1:30–3.
53. Chaudhary N, Pal VK. A study on the effect of Yoga Nidra on stress level of the patients suffering with spondolitis and backache. International Journal of Yoga and Allied Sciences (ISSN: 2278 – 5159) 2016;5:24–6.
54. Datta K, Tripathi, Mallick HN. Yoga Nidra: An innovative approach for management of chronic insomnia – A case report. Sleep Sci and Practice 2017;1:7–11.

55. Datta D, Tripathi M, Verma M, et al. Yoga nidra practice shows improvement in sleep in patients with chronic insomnia: A randomized controlled trial. The National Medical Journal of India 2021;34: 143–50.
56. Datta K, Mallick HN, Tripathi M, Ahuja N, Deepak. Electrophysiological Evidence of Local Sleep During Yoga Nidra Practice. Front Neurol 2022;13:910794.
57. Ferriera-Vorkapic C, Borba-Pinheiro CJ, Marchioro M, Santana D. The Impact of *Yoga Nidra* and Seated Meditation on the Mental Health of College Professors. Int J Yoga 2018;11(3):215–23.
58. Li L, Shu W, Li Z, et al. Using Yoga Nidra Recordings for Pain Management in Patients Undergoing Colonoscopy. Pain Management Nursing 2019;1:39–46.
59. Vaishnav BS, Vaishnav SV, Vaishnav VS, Varma JR. Effect of Yoga-nidra on Adolescents Well-being: A Mixed Method Study. Int J Yoga 2018;11(3):245–8.
60. Ozdemir A, Saritas S. Effect of yoga nidra on the self-esteem and body image of burn patients. Complement Ther Clin Pract 2019;35:86–91.
61. Saraswati SS. Yoga Nidra. Bihar, India: Yoga Publishing Trust. Munger; 1998.
62. Parker S, Bharati SV, Fernandez M. Defining yoganidra: traditional accounts, physiological research, and future directions. Int J Yoga Therap 2013; 23(1):11–6.
63. Parker S. Yoga Nidrā: an opportunity for collaboration to extend the science of sleep states. Sleep Vigil 2017.
64. Brown RE, Basheer R, McKenna J, et al. Control of Sleep and Wakefulness. Physiol Rev 2012;92: 1087–187.
65. Porkka-Heiskanen T, Zitting KM, Wigren HK. Sleep, its regulation and possible mechanisms of sleep disturbances. Acta Physiol 2013;208:311–28.
66. Eban-Rothschild, Appelbaum L, de Lecea L. Neuronal mechanisms for sleep/wake regulation and modulatory drive. Neuropsychopharmacology 2018;43:937–57.
67. Diekelmann S, Born J. The memory function of sleep. Nat Rev Neurosci 2010;11:114–26.
68. Eugene AR, Masiak J. The neuroprotective aspects of sleep. MEDtube Sci 2015;3:35–40.
69. Benveniste H, Liu X, Koundal S, et al. The glymphatic system and waste clearance with brain aging: A Review. Gerontology 2019;65:106–19.
70. Caretto M, Giannini A, Simoncini T. An integrated approach to diagnosing and managing sleep disorders in menopausal women. Maturitas 2019;128: 1–3.
71. Saraswati SS, Nidra Yoga. Yoga. 6th Edition. Bihar, India: Publishing Trust, Munger; 2001.
72. Rani K, Tiwari S, Singh U, et al. Impact of Yoga Nidra on psycho-biological general wellbeing in patients with menstrual irregularities: a randomized controlled trial. Int J Yoga 2011;4:20–5.
73. Sang-Dol K. Psychological effects of yoga nidra in women with menstrual disorders: A systematic review of randomized controlled trials. Complement Ther Clin Pract 2017;28:4–8.
74. Gulia KK, Kumar VM. Sleep is vital for brain and heart: Post COVID-19 assessment by World Health Organization and the American Heart Association. Sleep and Vigilance 2022. https://doi.org/10.1007/s41782-022-00221-4.
75. Parker S. Training attention for consious non-REM sleep: the yogic practice of yoga-nidra and its implicationsfor neuoscience research. Prog Brain Res 2019;244:255–72.
76. Bharti SV. Yogi in the Lab: Future Directions of Scientific Research in Meditation. Rishikesh, India: AHMSIN Publishers; 2006.
77. Vyazovskiy VV, Olcese U, Hanlon EC, et al. Local sleep in awake rats. Nature 2011;472(7344):443–7.
78. Gulia KK. Dynamism in activity of the neural networks in brain is the basis of sleep-wakefulness oscillations. Front Neurol 2012;3:38.
79. Vyazovskiy VV, Cirelli C, Tononi G. Electrophysiological correlates of sleep homeostasis in freely behaving rats. Prog Brain Res 2011b;193:17–38.
80. McKillop LE, Fisher SP, Cui N, et al. Effects of Aging on Cortical Neural Dynamics and Local Sleep Homeostasis in Mice. J Neurosci 2018;38(16):3911–28.
81. Gulia KK, Radhakrishnan A, Kumar VM. Approach to Sleep Disorders in the Traditional School of Indian Medicine: Alternative Medicine II. In: Sleep Disorders Medicine: Basic Science, Technical Considerations and Clinical Aspects. (4th Edition) Chapter 57, 2017 ISBN 978-1-4939-6578-6, pp 1221-1232.

The Cardiovascular Impact of Obstructive Sleep Apnea in Women
Current Knowledge and Future Perspectives

Barbara K. Parise, PhD[a,b], Naira Lapi Ferreira, RN[a,b], Luciano F. Drager, MD, PhD[a,b,c,*]

KEYWORDS

• Gender • Sex • Sleep apnea • Cardiovascular disease

KEY POINTS

- As observed in several fields, women are underrepresented in clinical studies addressing the cardiovascular impact of obstructive sleep apnea (OSA).
- The contribution of OSA to hypertension (HTN) appears to be lower in female than in male patients, but in patients with HTN, OSA is associated with nondipping blood pressure and increased arterial stiffness regardless of sex.
- It is unclear whether the blood pressure response to continuous positive airway pressure (CPAP) is different in women and men with OSA. Current evidence suggests that the incidence of arrhythmias was similar in women and matched men with OSA.
- Whether the impact of OSA on heart remodeling is modulated by gender is unclear, considering inconsistent findings from the literature. Data from a historical cohort study revealed that the association between the percentage of sleep time spent with oxygen saturation less than 90% and cardiovascular events was more substantial for women.
- An observational study showed that women with severe OSA had a higher risk of cardiovascular mortality as compared with women without OSA, and CPAP mitigates this risk; randomized studies are lacking.

INTRODUCTION

In the last 3 decades, a considerable amount of evidence from basic, translational, and clinical research demonstrated with reasonable consistency the impact of obstructive sleep apnea (OSA) on several cardiovascular conditions and endpoints.[1] However, OSA has been predominantly observed in men: Epidemiologic studies in community samples report a 2:1 male:female ratio,[2] but women represent only one-eighth to one-quarter of patients in OSA clinics.[3] Among the potential explanations for this male predominance, women have anatomic and functional differences in the upper airways and adiposity distribution.[4] However, because women might have distinct sleep

Statement disclosure: None.
Funding sources: L.F. Drager receives funding support from FAPESP, Brazil (2019/234496–8).
[a] Center of Clinical and Epidemiologic Research (CPCE), University of Sao Paulo, Sao Paulo, Sao Paulo, Brazil; [b] Unidade de Hipertensão, Disciplina de Nefrologia, Hospital das Clínicas HCFMUSP, Faculdade de Medicina, Universidade de Sao Paulo, Sao Paulo, Sao Paulo, Brazil; [c] Unidade de Hipertensão, Instituto do Coração (InCor) do Hospital das Clínicas HCFMUSP, Faculdade de Medicina, Universidade de Sao Paulo, Sao Paulo, Sao Paulo, Brazil
* Corresponding author. Av., Enéas de Carvalho Aguiar, 44, 2° andar, bloco 2, sala 8, São Paulo CEP 05403-900, Brazil.
E-mail address: luciano.drager@incor.usp.br

Sleep Med Clin 18 (2023) 473–480
https://doi.org/10.1016/j.jsmc.2023.06.008
1556-407X/23/

complaints and significant influences of menopause and hormone replacement therapy on OSA severity,[4] it is conceivable that women are also frequently underrepresented in clinical studies. Unfortunately, the underrepresentation of women is not a specific limitation in the Sleep field but is commonly observed in the literature.[5] Understanding the varying characteristics of disease manifestation and outcomes is warranted for a prompt and tailored treatment for both men and women (beyond the "one-size-fits-all" paradigm).

In this review article, the authors critically evaluate the literature examining the influence of gender on the potential impact of OSA on several cardiovascular conditions. They also propose a research agenda for shedding light on this important research area.

HYPERTENSION

Previous studies have shown that hypertension (HTN) is responsible for about 1 out of 5 deaths of women in the United States[6] and HTN is among the most important risk factors for the development of cardiovascular disease.[7] Women with HTN seem to be more susceptible than men to the development of related pathophysiologic changes, such as left ventricular hypertrophy, diastolic dysfunction, increased arterial stiffness, diabetes, chronic kidney disease, and heart failure (HF).[8,9] This susceptibility seems to have multiple contributors, such as progressive impairment of endogenous estrogen stimulation of NO synthesis,[10] sympathetic nervous system[11] activation, in addition to pregnancy complications, such as preeclampsia.[12]

OSA and HTN are multifactorial diseases sharing similar risk factors, such as obesity, male sex, and advanced age.[13] However, there is a significant amount of evidence suggesting that OSA is associated with prevalent[14] and incident HTN,[15,16] as well as target-organ damage in these patients.[17,18] However, what is the current evidence exploring potential sex differences on the impact of OSA in the HTN scenario?

Cross-Sectional Studies

In a population-based case-control study, Hedner and colleagues[19] found that the prevalence of severe OSA (apnea-hypopnea index [AHI] ≥30 events/h) was higher in hypertensive men than in women (47% vs 26%, respectively). Moreover, the odds ratio (OR) for HTN increased across AHI tertiles from 1.0 to 2.1 (95% confidence interval [CI]: 0.9–4.5) and 1.0 to 3.7 (95% CI: 1.7–8.2) in men but not in women.

Another study evaluating 95 consecutive patients with HTN (56% women) found that the presence of OSA was independently associated with nondipping blood pressure (BP) and arterial stiffness in both men and women.[20] Pedrosa and colleagues[21] reported a higher frequency of HTN among 277 perimenopause women with OSA as compared with the control group (no OSA). Despite the lack of a sex-related comparison, the investigators reported that women with moderate to severe OSA versus those without OSA had a higher prevalence of HTN, were prescribed more medications for HTN, had higher awake BP, had higher nocturnal BP, and had higher values of arterial stiffness. The investigators found that oxygen desaturation during the night was independently associated with increased 24-hour BP and arterial stiffness.

Longitudinal Studies

In a prospective study, Cano-Pumarega and colleagues[22] explored the association of untreated OSA and incident stage 2 HTN (BP ≥ 160/100 mm Hg) based on gender differences in 1155 normotensive subjects (650 of them women, 56%) at baseline. The presence of moderate to severe OSA was higher in men than in women (18.6% vs 8.6%). After a mean follow-up of 7.5 years, the investigators found that 23% of the hypertensive patients developed stage 2 HTN with significant differences between men and women (13.7% vs 3.2%, $P<.001$). A respiratory disturbance index ≥14/h (comprising moderate and severe OSA) was independently associated with incident stage 2 HTN in men (OR, 2.54; 95% CI: 1.09–5.95) but not in women. The neutral results observed in women may be related to the relatively small sample size of women with severe OSA (N = 48). Supporting this argument, the OR for women with OSA to develop stage 2 HTN was more than 2-fold, but the CI was large (0.40–11.36).[23]

Interventional Studies

Overall, the impact of continuous positive airway pressure (CPAP) on BP in patients with OSA is modest (~2–3 mm Hg).[24] There are several potential reasons for these disappointing findings, including the heterogeneity of patients studied (normotensive patients, controlled and uncontrolled patients with HTN), nonideal CPAP compliance, clinical presentation, and the multifactorial nature of HTN. To date, no single study was specifically designed to compare the effects of OSA treatment on BP/HTN in women and men. Available meta-analyses did not stratify the BP response according to sex, probably because of the underrepresentation of women in most of the interventional studies.[25–27] However, a multicenter, randomized trial conducted in 304 women with moderate to severe OSA revealed that 12 weeks of CPAP promoted similar (again modest) effects on BP than observed in meta-analysis with predominantly male patients (diastolic BP: −2.04 mm Hg, 95% CI: −4.02 to −0.05; $P=.045$; systolic BP: −1.54 mm Hg, 95% CI: −4.58–1.51; $P=.32$; **Fig. 1**).[28]

CARDIAC REMODELING AND HEART FAILURE

Previous studies indicated significant sex- and race/ethnicity differences in the risk of developing HF throughout life, with white men and black women being the most susceptible profile of patients.[29] HF is an important cause of morbidity and mortality in women, who tend to develop the disease at an older age than men.[30] It is estimated that the incidence of HF approximately doubles every 10 years in the male population aged 65 to 85 years, whereas in women, the incidence triples between the ages of 65 to 74 years and 75 and 84 years.[30,31]

In the OSA scenario, repetitive obstructive respiratory episodes during sleep elicit negative intrathoracic pressure and increases venous return, consequently increasing the filling of the vena cava leading to right ventricular distention and a deviation of the intraventricular septum to the left, causing an impaired filling of the ventricle. The reduction in preload and increase in afterload reduce systolic volume and cardiac output. In the long term, all these factors can contribute to the development of heart remodeling and ventricular dysfunction.[17,32,33] To date, few investigations addressed the potential effect of sex on heart remodeling and HF in patients with OSA. In a community-based study, Roca and colleagues[34] studied 1645 participants (54.3% women) without cardiovascular disease at baseline. The participants were submitted to echocardiogram after 15.2 years of follow-up. Among surviving participants without incident cardiovascular events, OSA was independently associated with higher left ventricle mass index only among women. In contrast, Javaheri and colleagues[35] found that left ventricular mass (evaluated by cardiac MRI) was significantly increased with increasing AHI category in both men and women younger than 65 years from 1412 participants from the Multi-Ethnic Study of Atherosclerosis. In terms of the risk of developing HF, a population-based cohort study, namely Sleep and Health in Women, showed that symptoms of OSA were associated with an increased risk of developing HF in women.[36] Lebek and colleagues[37] identified that in patients with respiratory disorders, diastolic dysfunction and HF with preserved ejection fraction were more frequent in women than in men, with the severity of respiratory disorders associated with the degree of cardiac dysfunction only in women.

In a prospective evaluation from Sleep Heart Health Study, predicted incident HF was significant in men but not in women (adjusted hazard ratio [HR], 1.13; 95% CI: 1.02–1.26 per 10-unit increase in AHI). Men with AHI greater than or equal to 30 were 58% more likely to develop HF than those with AHI less than 5 (**Fig. 2**).[38] The relatively low number of women with severe OSA may partially explain the neutral results in women.

ARRHYTHMIAS

Cardiac arrhythmias affect men and women differently, and this is due to differences in heart size, hormonal effects on ion channels, autonomic tone, and a combination of both.[39,40] The implications caused by the menstrual cycle, pregnancy, and menopause can also predispose women to electrocardiographic changes.[41] Physiologically, women have a higher sinus frequency than men,

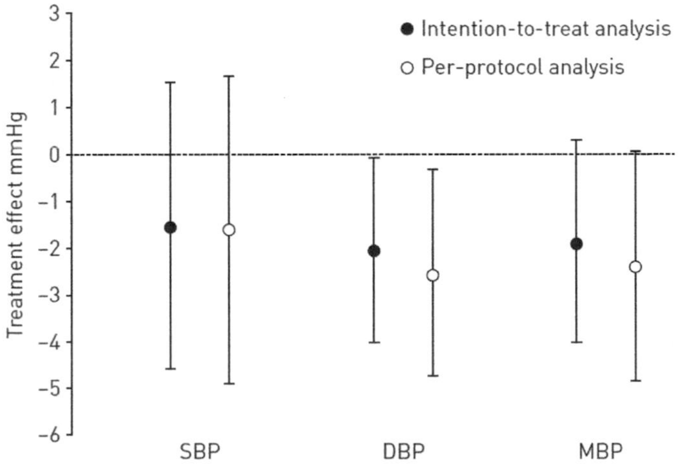

Fig. 1. Effect of CPAP treatment on BP measurements. DBP, diastolic blood pressure; MBP, mean blood pressure; SBP, systolic blood pressure. Adjusted treatment effects and 95% CIs (adjusted by baseline values, age, body mass index, and antihypertensive medication) of CPAP versus conservative treatment at the end of follow-up compared with baseline. (Reproduced with permission of the © ERS 2023: European Respiratory Journal Aug 2017, 50 (2) 1700257; https://doi.org/10.1183/13993003.00257-2017.)

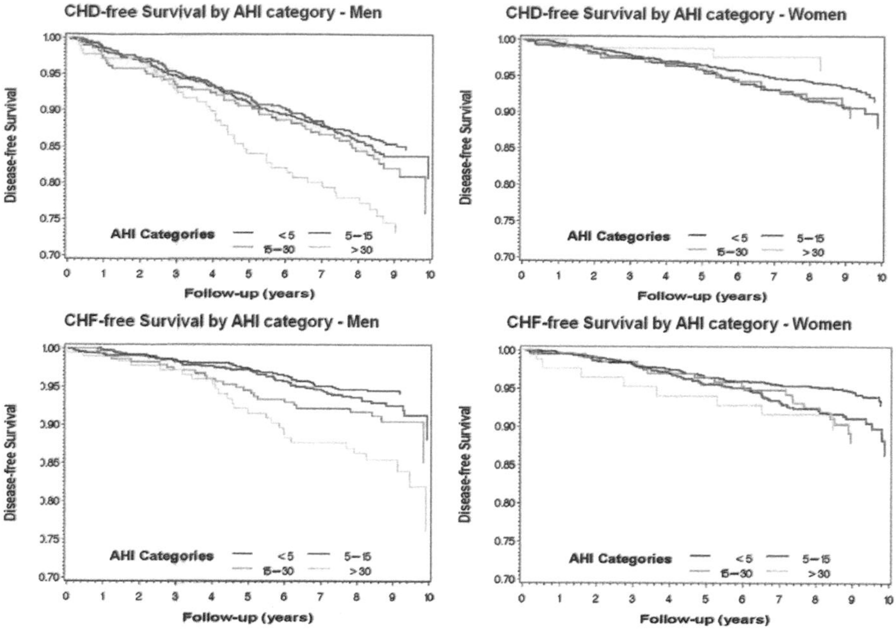

Fig. 2. Unadjusted Kaplan-Meier survival curves for AHI clinical categories by sex and event type. CHD, coronary heart disease; CHF, congestive heart failure. (Reproduced with permission from reference.[38])

with an increase of 3 to 5 beats per minute in periods with higher levels of estrogen circulating in the blood.[42] Studies indicate that women have a longer QT interval than men, especially during menstruation, because of the effects of female hormones on sodium and potassium channels, a smaller QRS complex, a shorter P wave, and a shorter PR interval.[39] These differences play a role in the prevalence of types of arrhythmias in each sex, although it is still not well understood how such changes are manifested in arrhythmias.[43]

Atrial fibrillation (AF) is the most common supraventricular arrhythmia and affects mainly men, approximately 23.2 million men and 23.1 million women worldwide, but the incidence approaches in both genders after 70 years of age.[39,42,44,45] A survey found differences between sex and skin color with the risk of developing AF during life, whereby white women had rates of 30%, a value higher than black women and men, which were 22% and 21%, respectively. The group composed of white men had the highest risk among the others, at 36%.[46] The association between AF and all-cause death was also greater among women than men.[47] Other arrhythmic disorders, such as supraventricular tachycardia (SVT), present heterogeneously between genders. A study with premenopausal women with a clinical history of SVT showed that in the luteal phase of the menstrual cycle, where estrogen levels decrease and progesterone levels increase, longer-lasting episodes of tachyarrhythmia occur, whereas another study identified that tachycardia owing to nodal reentry affects women twice as often,[41,43] and atrioventricular reentrant tachycardia involving accessory pathways is more commonly present in men.[42]

Physiologic stress caused by respiratory events predicts changes in heart rhythm. Intermittent hypoxia, hypercapnia, negative intrathoracic pressure oscillations, and activation of the sympathetic nervous system during OSA are the primary mechanisms that influence the development of cardiac arrhythmias. OSA can also lead to cardiac remodeling, increasing the risk of developing arrhythmias.[48,49] The prevalence of arrhythmias in patients with OSA is greater than in those without the disorder. It has been estimated that in patients with AF, the frequency of OSA varies from 21% to 74%, in contrast to 3% to 49% in patients without OSA.[50] The presence of sleep-disordered breathing doubles the chances of developing AF,[45] and alterations, such as prolonged P-wave dispersion, interatrial and intra-atrial electromechanical delays, have been observed in patients with moderate and severe OSA; these are risk factors for the development of AF.[49]

Although several studies have found an association between OSA and AF, there is limited information on differences between women and men. A large US nationwide health insurance database found a significant increase in several relevant comorbidities in women with OSA compared with controls, including a higher incidence of

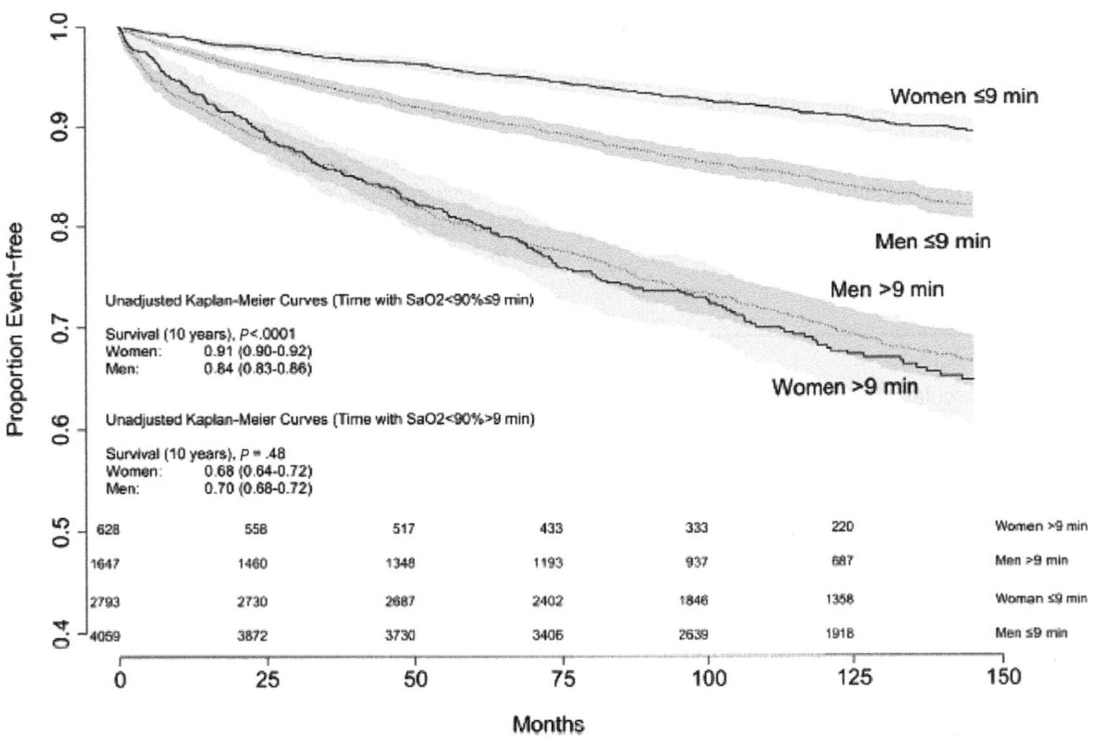

Fig. 3. Unadjusted Kaplan-Meier survival curves stratified by sex in individuals: (i) without OSA (AHI < 5 events per hour); (ii) with severe OSA (AHI > 30 events per hour). The numbers at risk are presented above the x-axis. (Reproduced with permission from reference.[55])

arrhythmias and stroke. However, compared with matched male patients, the incidence of arrhythmias was similar.[51]

CARDIOVASCULAR EVENTS

Cross-sectional studies suggest that markers of subclinical atherosclerosis are independently related to OSA in women, providing biological relevance for exploring cardiovascular events in this population.[52,53]

In a cohort of 2 sleep clinics in Spain, Campos-Rodriguez and colleagues[54] evaluated 1116 women for a median follow-up of 72 months. The investigators found a lower cardiovascular mortality in the control group (no OSA: 0.28 per 100 person-years [95% CI: 0.10–0.91]) than in the untreated groups with mild to moderate OSA (0.94 per 100 person-years [CI: 0.10–2.40]; *P* = .034) or severe OSA (3.71 per 100 person-years [CI: 0.09–7.50]; *P*<.001). Compared with the control group, the fully adjusted HRs for cardiovascular mortality were 3.50 (CI: 1.23–9.98) for the untreated, severe OSA group; 0.55 (CI: 0.17–1.74) for the CPAP-treated, severe OSA group; 1.60 (CI: 0.52–4.90) for the untreated, mild to moderate OSA group; and 0.19 (CI: 0.02–1.67) for the CPAP-treated, mild to moderate OSA group.[54]

Direct sex comparisons addressing the impact of OSA on cardiovascular events are limited. In a large cohort of adults who underwent a sleep study at a large urban academic hospital in Toronto, the association between the percentage of sleep time spent with oxygen saturation less than 90% and cardiovascular outcomes was stronger for women (HR for interquartile range [IQR], 3% vs 0% = 1.30, 1.19–1.42) than for men (HR for IQR = 1.13, 1.06–1.21) (*P* for interaction = .01) in the adjusted model over a median of 9.3 years (**Fig. 3**).[55]

SUMMARY AND RESEARCH AGENDA

In conclusion, the available evidence suggests that women are not spared from the potential cardiovascular consequences of OSA, but the results are not consistent, and the aforementioned underrepresentation of women in this field prevents any definitive comparisons or conclusions. There is an urgent need for additional basic, translational, and clinical research addressing this important research area. Particular attention should be devoted to exploring whether OSA and its components (mainly intermittent hypoxia) have distinct effects on men and women. It would be also interesting to explore the potential benefits of estrogens and hormone reposition in mitigating the cardiovascular effects of OSA in women. Larger longitudinal and interventional studies are needed in order to identify all the clinical variables, biomarkers, and intermediary pathways that may play a role in the OSA-cardiovascular association and to determine if OSA management should differ according to sex and age.

CLINICS CARE POINTS

- Cardiovascular disease is the leading cause of death in women, accounting for 35% of female deaths worldwide in 2019. Sleep apnea is a prevalent condition among individuals with hypertension, heart failure, coronary artery disease, atrial fibrillation, and stroke, yet it remains underdiagnosed and undertreated in clinical practice.
- Many studies investigating the detection and treatment of cardiovascular diseases underrepresent the female population, which limits the ability to measure the safety and efficacy of therapies for women and identify specific sex differences. Given the relationship between OSA, the development of cardiovascular risk factors, it is necessary to address the specificities and impact of sleep apnea and cardiovascular diseases in females.
- In summary, we acknowledge the shortcomings in the current literature regarding OSA in women and its association with cardiovascular problems. It is crucial to invest in more comprehensive and robust studies to fill these gaps and better understand the effects of sleep apnea in women, aiming for more personalized approaches to diagnosis and treatment.

REFERENCES

1. Drager LF, McEvoy RD, Barbe F, et al. INCOSACT initiative (international collaboration of sleep apnea cardiovascular trialists). Sleep apnea and cardiovascular disease: lessons from recent trials and need for team science. Circulation 2017;136(19):1840–50.
2. Heinzer R, Vat S, Marques-Vidal P, et al. Prevalence of sleep-disordered breathing in the general population: the HypnoLaus study. Lancet Respir Med 2015;3(4):310–8.
3. Redline S, Kump K, Tishler PV, et al. Gender differences in sleep disordered breathing in a community-based sample. Am J Respir Crit Care Med 1994;149(3 Pt 1):722–6.
4. Bixler EO, Vgontzas AN, Lin HM, et al. Prevalence of sleep-disordered breathing in women: effects of gender. Am J Respir Crit Care Med 2001;163(3 Pt 1):608–13.
5. Daitch V, Turjeman A, Poran I, et al. Underrepresentation of women in randomized controlled trials: a systematic review and meta-analysis. Trials 2022;23(1):1038.
6. Wenger NK, Arnold A, Bairey Merz CN, et al. Hypertension across a woman's life cycle. J Am Coll Cardiol 2018;71(16):1797–813.
7. Schenck-Gustafsson K. Risk factors for cardiovascular disease in women. Maturitas 2009;63(3):186–90.
8. Tsao CW, Aday AW, Almarzooq ZI, et al. Heart disease and stroke statistics-2022 update: a report from the American heart association. Circulation 2022;145(8):e153–639.
9. Levy D, Larson MG, Vasan RS, et al. The progression from hypertension to congestive heart failure. JAMA 1996;275(20):1557–62.
10. Celermajer DS, Sorensen KE, Spiegelhalter DJ, et al. Aging is associated with endothelial dysfunction in healthy men years before the age-related decline in women. J Am Coll Cardiol 1994;24(2):471–6.
11. Hay M. Sex, the brain and hypertension: brain oestrogen receptors and high blood pressure risk factors. Clin Sci (Lond) 2016;130(1):9–18.
12. Garovic VD, August P. Preeclampsia and the future risk of hypertension: the pregnant evidence. Curr Hypertens Rep 2013;15(2):114–21.
13. Patel AR, Patel AR, Singh S, et al. The association of obstructive sleep apnea and hypertension. Cureus 2019;11(6):e4858.
14. Drager LF, Santos RB, Silva WA, et al. OSA, short sleep duration, and their interactions with sleepiness and cardiometabolic risk factors in adults: the ELSA-Brasil study. Chest 2019;155(6):1190–8.
15. Peppard PE, Young T, Palta M, et al. Prospective study of the association between sleep-disordered breathing and hypertension. N Engl J Med 2000;342(19):1378–84.
16. Marin JM, Agusti A, Villar I, et al. Association between treated and untreated obstructive sleep apnea and risk of hypertension. JAMA 2012;307(20):2169–76.
17. Drager LF, Bortolotto LA, Figueiredo AC, et al. Obstructive sleep apnea, hypertension, and their interaction on arterial stiffness and heart remodeling. Chest 2007;131(5):1379–86.
18. Drager LF, Bortolotto LA, Krieger EM, et al. Additive effects of obstructive sleep apnea and hypertension on early markers of carotid atherosclerosis. Hypertension 2009;53(1):64–9.
19. Hedner J, Bengtsson-Boström K, Peker Y, et al. Hypertension prevalence in obstructive sleep apnoea and sex: a population-based case-control study. Eur Respir J 2006;27(3):564–70.

20. Jenner R, Fatureto-Borges F, Costa-Hong V, et al. Association of obstructive sleep apnea with arterial stiffness and nondipping blood pressure in patients with hypertension. J Clin Hypertens 2017;19(9):910–8.
21. Pedrosa RP, Barros IML, Drager LF, et al. OSA is common and independently associated with hypertension and increased arterial stiffness in consecutive perimenopausal women. Chest 2014;146(1):66–72.
22. Cano-Pumarega I, Barbé F, Esteban A, et al. Sleep apnea and hypertension: are there sex differences? The vitoria sleep cohort. Chest 2017;152(4):742–50.
23. Freitas LS, Drager LF. Gender and cardiovascular impact of obstructive sleep apnea: work in progress. J Thorac Dis 2017;9(10):3579–82.
24. Fatureto-Borges F, Lorenzi-Filho G, Drager LF. Effectiveness of continuous positive airway pressure in lowering blood pressure in patients with obstructive sleep apnea: a critical review of the literature. Integr Blood Press Control 2016;9:43–7.
25. Montesi SB, Edwards BA, Malhotra A, et al. The effect of continuous positive airway pressure treatment on blood pressure: a systematic review and meta-analysis of randomized controlled trials. J Clin Sleep Med 2012;8(5):587–96.
26. Fava C, Dorigoni S, Dalle Vedove F, et al. Effect of CPAP on blood pressure in patients with OSA/hypopnea a systematic review and meta-analysis. Chest 2014;145(4):762–71.
27. Pengo MF, Soranna D, Giontella A, et al. Obstructive sleep apnoea treatment and blood pressure: which phenotypes predict a response? A systematic review and meta-analysis. Eur Respir J 2020;55(5):1901945.
28. Campos-Rodriguez F, Gonzalez-Martinez M, Sanchez-Armengol A, et al. Effect of continuous positive airway pressure on blood pressure and metabolic profile in women with sleep apnoea. Eur Respir J 2017;50(2):1700257.
29. Huffman MD, Berry JD, Ning H, et al. Lifetime risk for heart failure among white and black Americans: cardiovascular lifetime risk pooling project. J Am Coll Cardiol 2013;61(14):1510–7.
30. Bozkurt B, Khalaf S. Heart failure in women. Methodist Debakey Cardiovasc J 2017;13(4):216–23.
31. Mozaffarian D, Benjamin EJ, Go AS, et al, Writing Group Members. Heart disease and stroke statistics-2016 update: a report from the American heart association. Circulation 2016;133(4):e38–360.
32. Chami HA, Devereux RB, Gottdiener JS, et al. Left ventricular morphology and systolic function in sleep-disordered breathing: the Sleep Heart Health Study. Circulation 2008;117(20):2599–607.
33. Lévy P, Naughton MT, Tamisier R, et al. Sleep apnoea and heart failure. Eur Respir J 2022;59(5):2101640.
34. Roca GQ, Redline S, Claggett B, et al. Sex-specific association of sleep apnea severity with subclinical myocardial injury, ventricular hypertrophy, and heart failure risk in a community-dwelling cohort: the atherosclerosis risk in communities-sleep heart health study. Circulation 2015;132(14):1329–37.
35. Javaheri S, Sharma RK, Wang R, et al. Association between obstructive sleep apnea and left ventricular structure by age and gender: the multi-ethnic study of atherosclerosis. Sleep 2016;39(3):523–9.
36. Ljunggren M, Byberg L, Theorell-Haglöw J, et al. Increased risk of heart failure in women with symptoms of sleep-disordered breathing. Sleep Med 2016;17:32–7.
37. Lebek S, Hegner P, Tafelmeier M, et al. Female patients with sleep-disordered breathing display more frequently heart failure with preserved ejection fraction. Front Med 2021;8:675987.
38. Gottlieb DJ, Yenokyan G, Newman AB, et al. Prospective study of obstructive sleep apnea and incident coronary heart disease and heart failure: the sleep heart health study. Circulation 2010;122(4):352–60.
39. Bernal O, Moro C. [Cardiac arrhythmias in women]. Rev Esp Cardiol 2006;59(6):609–18.
40. Curtis AB, Narasimha D. Arrhythmias in women. Clin Cardiol 2012;35(3):166–71.
41. Linde C. Women and arrhythmias. Pacing Clin Electrophysiol 2000;23(10 Pt 1):1550–60.
42. Moreira DAR, Habib RG. Arritmias Cardiadas na Mulher. Rev Soc Cardiol Estado de São Paulo 2009;19(4):503–10.
43. Yarnoz MJ, Curtis AB. More reasons why men and women are not the same (gender differences in electrophysiology and arrhythmias). Am J Cardiol 2008;101(9):1291–6.
44. Volgman AS, Bairey Merz CN, Benjamin EJ, et al. Sex and race/ethnicity differences in atrial fibrillation. J Am Coll Cardiol 2019;74(22):2812–5.
45. May AM, Van Wagoner DR, Mehra R. OSA and cardiac arrhythmogenesis: mechanistic insights. Chest 2017;151(1):225–41.
46. Mou L, Norby FL, Chen LY, et al. Lifetime risk of atrial fibrillation by race and socioeconomic status: ARIC study (atherosclerosis risk in communities). Circ Arrhythm Electrophysiol 2018;11(7):e006350.
47. Emdin CA, Wong CX, Hsiao AJ, et al. Atrial fibrillation as risk factor for cardiovascular disease and death in women compared with men: systematic review and meta-analysis of cohort studies. BMJ 2016;532:h7013.
48. Mehra R, Chung MK, Olshansky B, et al. Sleep-disordered breathing and cardiac arrhythmias in adults: mechanistic insights and clinical implications: a scientific statement from the American heart association. Circulation 2022;146(9):e119–36.
49. Geovanini GR, Lorenzi-Filho G. Cardiac rhythm disorders in obstructive sleep apnea. J Thorac Dis 2018;10(Suppl 34):S4221–30.

50. Linz D, Nattel S, Kalman JM, et al. Sleep apnea and atrial fibrillation. Card Electrophysiol Clin 2021;13(1): 87–94.
51. Mokhlesi B, Ham SA, Gozal D. The effect of sex and age on the comorbidity burden of OSA: an observational analysis from a large nationwide US health claims database. Eur Respir J 2016;47(4): 1162–9.
52. Medeiros AKL, Coutinho RQ, Barros IML, et al. Obstructive sleep apnea is independently associated with subclinical coronary atherosclerosis among middle-aged women. Sleep Breath 2017; 21(1):77–83.
53. Weinreich G, Wessendorf TE, Erdmann T, et al. Association of obstructive sleep apnoea with subclinical coronary atherosclerosis. Atherosclerosis 2013; 231(2):191–7.
54. Campos-Rodriguez F, Martinez-Garcia MA, de la Cruz-Moron I, et al. Cardiovascular mortality in women with obstructive sleep apnea with or without continuous positive airway pressure treatment: a cohort study. Ann Intern Med 2012;156(2):115–22.
55. Kendzerska T, Leung RS, Atzema CL, et al. Cardiovascular consequences of obstructive sleep apnea in women: a historical cohort study. Sleep Med 2020;68:71–9.

The Impact of Maternity and Working Demands in Women's Sleep Pattern

Lisie P. Romanzini, MSc, Isabela A. Ishikura, MSc, Gabriel Natan Pires, PhD, Sergio Tufik, MD, PhD, Monica L. Andersen, PhD*

KEYWORDS

• Sleep • Maternity • Motherhood • Work • Pregnancy • Postpartum • Woman

KEY POINTS

- Motherhood affects women's level of sleep satisfaction.
- Poor sleep quality and sleep restriction are highly prevalent during pregnancy and postpartum.
- High professional demands seem related to stress factors and recurrent sleep complaints.

INTRODUCTION

In the last decades changes occurred in female behavior related to their different roles in society, with more freedom to follow their professional and domestic goals. Along with social, economic, cultural, and professional achievements, the conflict between building a solid professional career and taking care of the children arises.[1] Maternal and professional responsibilities bring a set of demands that begin to interfere significantly in women sleep, changing the quality, quantity, and sleep satisfaction level.[2,3]

Many studies reveal an association between mothers' sleep restrictions and the activities related to taking care of infants during the night.[4] What is observed are parents, in particular those who have young children, that have shown lower total time of sleeping and poor quality of sleep when compared with adults without children.[5]

Although fathers and mothers have changes in their sleep, there are signs that maternal sleep is more fragmented,[6] including long periods of time awake after sleep onset, in addition to showing a nonrestorative sleep. Changes in fathers' sleep satisfaction and duration after a child's birth are less frequent than that observed in mothers. This event is related to the fact that mothers, including working women, have more responsibilities in raising the child and dedicate more time to this task.[7]

Considering the professional perspective, it is observed that work overload and stress situations related to sleep complaints,[8–10] and the more the demand, the more the sleeping problems.[2] Mothers that work more time away from home tend to have more necessity of sleeping earlier, maybe because of professional requirements of the next workday. In addition, mothers tend to present a parenting less positive during the child's bedtime.[11]

Professional and domestic requirements faced by mothers after maternity interfere drastically in sleep routine and quality of life. Thus, it becomes essential that professionals from the heath field address issues related to sleep during their appointments, with the aim to improve the well-being of those women.

GOALS

The goal of this study was to gather some relevant findings from literature regarding the way that responsibilities related to maternity and the demands of work impact women's sleep, examining the possible risks and protection factors. We seek to

Departamento de Psicobiologia, Universidade Federal de São Paulo (UNIFESP/EPM), São Paulo, Brazil
* Corresponding author. Universidade Federal de São Paulo, Napoleão de Barros, 925 Vila Clementino, 04024-002, São Paulo/SP, Brazil.
E-mail address: ml.andersen12@gmail.com

Sleep Med Clin 18 (2023) 481–487
https://doi.org/10.1016/j.jsmc.2023.06.009

join the results in a narrative revision for a discussion of how sleep is interfered with by maternity and professional activities.

SLEEP IN WOMEN

Recently, society has been acting incorrectly when the subject is associated with sleep. The idea that sleep is lost time has been constantly and unfortunately incorporated into current lifestyle, although it is known that having an adequate night of sleep is essential for healthy bodily functioning and to be physiologically balanced.

To achieve a good quality of life, it is important to have adequate nights of sleeping, because they impact positively on the immunologic system, memory consolidation, and humor stability.[12] Research findings about the effects of sleep restrictions on human physiologic functioning and neurobehavior recommends a total sleep time from 7 to 8 hours per night for adults.[13,14]

In recent years there has been a drop in the number of people that maintained a weekly sleep routine of 8 hours, from around 38% of respondents in 2001 to 26% in 2005[15] One British study has found similar average sleep duration (7 hours) with 18% of respondents complaining of insufficient sleep.[16]

Although the general population is experiencing problems related to sleep, there is a difference between men and women. In addition to gender differences, there are other issues, such as regular menstrual cycles, women taking oral contraceptives, pregnant and lactating women, and women entering menopause. Each of these time-points is associated with a hormonal situation, and it is important to point out that there are clinically significant differences in the sleep of women in these stages of life.[17]

The hormonal changes that occur in the menstrual cycle, pregnancy, and menopause make understanding sleep in women an important topic to be analyzed separately. Over the years, the risk of sleep disorders increases and requires different management in women. Poor sleep quality, sleep deprivation, obstructive sleep apnea, restless legs syndrome, and insomnia may be caused by hormonal changes.[18]

During the first trimester of pregnancy there is a marked increase in gonadal steroid hormones, generating physical discomfort associated with the growing fetus during the second and third trimesters. The dizzying drop in hormones after childbirth and the baby's irregular feeding and sleeping schedules are pertinent reasons for sleep disturbances.[17]

If we consider sleep parameters during a woman's reproductive life, the findings are controversial, ranging from modifications in sleep characteristics throughout the menstrual cycle to the absence of significant alterations in sleep patterns.[17,19–23]This statement contrasts with the period after menopause, in which studies indicated drastic changes in sleep patterns, with daytime effects.[24–26]

Studies using polysomnography to assess women's sleep during the menstrual cycle are scarce, mainly because of some factors inherent in women's lives, and the difficulty in obtaining polysomnographic data throughout the menstrual cycle. In addition, the examination is expensive, requires the presence of qualified professionals specialized in sleep, and enough space to meet the demand of women throughout the menstrual cycle. Hormone tests are also recommended to confirm menstrual cycle phase during sleep recording. Hence, a study of the sleep pattern in women in the reproductive phase becomes difficult and expensive.

Because of these numerous factors inherent to the female gender, studies have found that sleep complaints are greater in women when compared with men.[27]

SLEEP DURING MATERNITY

The birth of a child changes the life of a couple, especially the mother, who generally assumes most of the responsibilities and care activities. Motherhood is a new stage of life that tends to generate stress because of the adaptation required, with greater intensity in the first 3 months of the baby's life, when the needs tend to be exacerbated. Among the main situations that cause stress during the baby's first year of life are maternal fatigue, sleep restriction, and daily commitment to meet the needs of the newborn.[28] Although pregnancy, childbirth, and the postpartum period can be a rewarding and exciting experience for a woman, they are also fraught with considerable sleep disruption.[17]

The postpartum period, which is associated with considerable sleep disruption, begins with childbirth and ends for most women approximately 6 to 12 months later when the baby sleeps through the night.[29] After childbirth, there is a rapid decrease in placental-derived hormones, which is primarily responsible for the short duration of "postnatal melancholy" experienced by most women (75%–80%) from 3 to 5 days after birth. Hormonal changes can also have a profound effect on sleep.[17] It is important to highlight that 10% to 15% of new mothers develop postpartum depression.[30]

Women have more sleep disturbances and greater fatigue postpartum compared with late pregnancy.[31] Drowsiness is frequent during pregnancy, but it is in the postpartum period that sleep satisfaction decreases markedly, with insomnia symptoms being highly prevalent and sleep duration decreasing significantly,[32,33] with primiparous mothers more heavily affected than those going through their second or third child.[13]

When evaluating the number of hours of sleep of many mothers in the first 4 months of the baby's life, it was observed that the total sleep time was 3 hours per night. This sleep deprivation resulted in marital problems, because the mothers revealed that they preferred sleeping to having sex with their husbands.[33] Some factors may be involved in the worsening of maternal sleep, including the baby's crying, frequent breastfeeding, physical pain related to childbirth, and the anguish linked to maternal demands.[28]

The feeding method can affect the sleep of mothers with young children, although this subject has not been much addressed in the literature and the existing studies are divergent in their findings. Mainly, studies pointed that breastfeeding impairs women's sleep, because newborns who are breastfed wake up more often during the night, staying awake longer and with less consolidated sleep.[34,35] Other studies showed that such an act does not significantly impact sleep; and there are still those who claim to have a positive association between sleep and breastfeeding.[31,36–38] In a study of actigraphy in the United States, women who exclusively breastfed had an average of 30 minutes more nightly sleep than women who used formula at night, but they did not significantly differ in terms of sleep fragmentation.[36]

A study involving mothers who were evaluated during the fourth postpartum week found that those who breastfed had more awakenings and tended to sleep fewer hours during the night than women who did not breastfeed.[39] However, another study revealed that lactation was associated with significant increases in slow wave sleep in women who breastfed (182 minutes) when compared with women who bottle fed (63 minutes).[40] Irregular bedtime and/or sleeping very late were also factors associated with a worsening of parental quality with babies at bedtime, compared with mothers with more regular and consistent sleep patterns.[41]

Problems related to sleep in the gestational period and after childbirth tend to decrease after 3 months of the baby's life, because of regularity in wakefulness and sleep patterns, making mothers' sleep more continuous.[42] A cohort study carried out in Germany with 2541 women, in the period from 2008 to 2015, found that sleep only returns to being similar to that before the birth of the child after 6 years of the child's life.[33]

Women recognize their daily difficulties and report that they would like more information and advice on how to care for their babies.[43] Thus, it becomes relevant to understand these difficulties in this period that is so important for women and to seek ways to alleviate greater concerns.

Demands of Work and Maternity Affecting Mothers' Sleep

Adults spend one-third of their lives sleeping, another one-third working, with the rest of their time filled with family and domestic experiences and responsibilities. The growth and consolidation of women's participation in the labor market, together with the hectic routine of life, have been transforming family roles in recent years, especially those played by the mother.[28]

To solve domestic, maternal, and professional demands, women often find themselves in a stressful situation. Stress associated with childcare can affect parents' sleep and, consequently, daily productivity.[44] Stress factors generated by work can also interfere with the individual's interaction with his or her partner and children, creating difficulties that influence sleep.[8–10] The greater the professional demand, the greater the sleep problems.[2]

When analyzing the interface between quality of sleep and negative experiences at home and at work, different sleep patterns were observed in parents of children younger than 6 years old, mostly younger than 2 years old.[11,31,41,45] The literature is scarce regarding the various stress domains that can interfere with sleep considering the professional scenario combined with the maternity period.[10] This fact demonstrates the need to develop studies involving the sleep of women with children and who work away from home.

The support network is one of the possible ways for women to reconcile family life with professional life. The various forms of care given to children that are alternatives for mothers include schools, day care centers, nannies, neighbors, and grandparents, among others.[28] The option for each choice of care depends on the family context. The combination of work and parenthood, however, is additionally influenced by the availability and affordability of childcare, the affordability of flexible working arrangements, and gender roles within families with respect to the division of paid work and care responsibilities after parenthood.[28,46]

Regarding breastfeeding and careers, the United States has one of the highest percentages of working mothers with young babies and little workplace support for breastfeeding mothers, such as lactation programs or maternity leave.

Employers who support breastfeeding through policies benefit from reduced maternity leave and absenteeism, higher productivity, and lower health care costs.[47]

All these responsibilities of meeting a new reality as a working woman need to favor the family economically and psychologically the new mothers. It is necessary to consider the expectations and interests, which, in turn, can generate anxiety and stress, which are clearly active factors in the quality of sleep.[28] Women with higher stress take longer to fall asleep and report more sleep problems.[11]

With all the demand that motherhood requires, together with the professional demand, mothers become an audience at greater risk for the development of sleep problems, from sleep deprivation to insomnia. Sleep complaints can have drastic daytime consequences, facilitating the onset of depression, attention deficits, and changes in memory and focus, among others.[13,14,48] Clearly, all these consequences significantly harm the professional, social, and marital life of these women.

Prevention and Risk

Having regular bedtimes and good sleep hygiene are essential factors for mothers to reduce sleep-related problems and possible psychological disorders.[41] Daytime naps when the baby falls asleep is also an effective strategy to help compensate for sleep deprivation or fragmentation that occurs during the night.[6] Sleep-related problems, such as sleep deprivation, assessed using actigraphy, were associated with less positive parenting; that is, improving mothers' sleep helps to improve the mother-baby relationship.[41]

For these reasons, social support becomes fundamental for the performance of the maternal task, reducing risks and increasing prevention of future problems, for women and children.

DISCUSSION

The literature on sleep suggests that motherhood and work used objective measures of actigraphy in their methodology, between 7 and 10 days, and/or subjective measures, such as questionnaires or self-reports to assess the participants' sleep.

Articles about motherhood and sleep present a diverse amount in terms of sample size, from 70 to 2500 participants, with the age range of women being 19 to 50 years old, with an approximate average of 30 years old. Most of them are living with their partner (85% or more), with at least 30% being primiparous mothers, ranging in age from 0 to 6 years. The work variable was present in 49% to 72% of employed mothers, but many studies did not present this information in their analysis.

In general, motherhood results in a decrease in total sleep time, an increase in awakenings, and a decrease in satisfaction with sleep after the baby is born, especially in primiparous mothers. The findings found in relation to women were that sleep satisfaction and duration decrease with childbirth and reach a maximum peak in the first 3 months of the baby's life. Up to 6 months, there was a greater impairment in the mother's sleep.[33,41] Another variable was the increase in awake time after sleep onset,[31] thus, mothers started to have more awakenings and a longer time awake after the onset of sleep after childbirth.

Specifically in relation to the number of children, after the birth of the baby, mothers slept less, on average 41 minutes after the first child, 39 minutes after the second child, and 44 minutes after the third.[33] In this sense, one can understand that the arrival of the first child generates greater negative effects on the mothers' total sleep time. These effects are smaller when considering the second child, with a worsening with the third child, probably because of the increased demands.

According to studies, there is a considerable disruption of sleep that begins with childbirth and ends for most women when the baby reaches its first year of life.[17] During the first 2 years of the child, the mother experiences a decrease in total sleep time and recovers over the months. This could be evidenced in a study that found that at 32 weeks of gestation women slept 7 hours and 16 minutes, reducing to 6 hours and 31 minutes at 8 weeks postpartum and 6 hours and 52 minutes 2 years after the baby's birth.[29] This fact demonstrates how sleep is affected with the arrival of the newborn and, little by little, with the regularity of the child's sleep to monophasic, it is possible to notice an improvement in maternal sleep. Another factor addressed is that mothers who sleep late and who change their bedtime have higher levels of stress and worse parenting quality when putting the child to sleep.[11,41] The consistency in bedtime and going to bed early are favorable factors for achieving a better quality of sleep.

When dealing with the professional demands in which women are involved, it was possible to verify that mothers try to divide themselves into career and motherhood, often overloading themselves and affecting their quality of sleep. Aspects related to work and marital issues can lead to stress and sleep disturbances.[11] No associations were found between working hours and sleep problems in the maternity ward.[11,29,31,41]

Fatigue ratings were generally higher postpartum than during pregnancy, with nocturnal fatigue increasing more than daytime fatigue. Women who worked in the last month of pregnancy slept less at night, less during the day, and an average of 67 minutes less total sleep when compared with women who did not work. Women who worked in the last month of pregnancy also reported significantly higher levels of morning and evening fatigue.[31]

The differences in sleep and fatigue observed in beginner and experienced mothers reflect the new challenges in the maternal role in the group of primigravidae. They suggested that the process of integrating and acquiring competence in maternal behaviors, along with sleep deprivation, may put new mothers at greater risk for postpartum depression. The results of this study highlight the need for social support so that mothers can adequately deal with the complexity of situations involving baby care and motherhood in general. The participation of family members, friends, and professionals seems to contribute enormously, not only in the immediate resolution of possible needs in the care of the baby, but also in providing the mother with the peace of mind she needs to take care of her first child in all dimensions of physical and psychological care.[10,11,31]

Sleep research during pregnancy and the postpartum period is limited because of different data collection strategies, small and often nonrepresentative sample sizes, poorly controlled studies, and data pooled in ways that may obscure individual participant variation.

SUMMARY

The alertness of sleep complaints in working mothers has become more prevalent. The literature points out that having children, especially small ones, significantly interferes with women's sleep, reducing the quality and duration of sleep. These changes in sleep can lead to physical and/or psychological health problems. Studies addressing the influence of work on mothers are scarce, and more research is warranted to confirm how much this condition affects mothers' sleep. Sleep hygiene as an important intervention to improve mothers' sleep has been widely discussed, because sleeping at usual times and not late improves sleep quality. A support network is also essential for women to succeed in their demands, whether they are maternal, professional, or leisure, because it reduces fatigue and satisfies their need for sleep, benefiting their quality of life.

CLINICS CARE POINTS

- The level of satisfaction with sleep decreases with the birth of the first child.
- Women with children have less sleep time compared with women without children.
- The first 3 months after the newborn's birth is the period when sleep suffers the greatest change.
- Primiparous women have less sleep time compared with mothers with two or more children.
- Taking care of domestic and professional demands increases fatigue and stress in mothers.
- Breastfeeding may or may not interfere with sleep.
- It is important that health professionals advise patients to maintain sleep hygiene.
- Having a support network is essential for women not to develop sleep or stress problems.
- Treating sleep complaints is beneficial in improving women's quality of life.

FUNDING

Our studies are supported by the Associação Fundo de Incentivo à Pesquisaa (AFIP). M.L.A. is a recipient of a Conselho Nacional de Desenvolvimento Científico e Técnologico (CNPq) fellowship. No funding or sponsorship was received for the publication of this review. This research did not receive any specific grant from funding agencies in the public, commercial, or not-for-profit sectors.

DISCLOSURE

The authors have nothing to disclose.

REFERENCES

1. Silva MA, Pereira MMO, Antunes LGR, et al. Conciliando maternidade e carreira profissional: percepções de professoras do Ensino Superior. Revista Vianna Sapiens 2019;10(2):190–216.
2. Åkerstedt T, Garefelt J, Richter A, et al. Work and sleep: a prospective study of psychosocial work factors, physical work factors, and work scheduling. Sleep 2015;38(7):1129–36.
3. Rechtschaffen A, Bergmann BM. Sleep deprivation in the rat: an update of the 1989 paper. Sleep 2002;25(1):18–24.
4. Insana SP, Garfield CF, Montgomery-Downs HE. A mixed-method examination of maternal and

paternal nocturnal caregiving. J Pediatr Health Care 2014;28(4):313–21.
5. Hagen EW, Mirer AG, Palta M, et al. The sleep-time cost of parenting: sleep duration and sleepiness among employed parents in the Wisconsin Sleep Cohort Study. Am J Epidemiol 2013;177(5):394–401.
6. Insana SP, Montgomery-Downs HE. Sleep and sleepiness among first-time postpartum parents: a field- and laboratory-based multimethod assessment. Dev Psychobiol 2013;55(4):361–72.
7. Mencarini L, Sironi M. Happiness, housework and gender inequality in Europe. Eur Sociol Rev 2012; 28(2):203–19.
8. Walsh JK, Coulouvrat C, Hajak G, et al. Nighttime insomnia symptoms and perceived health in the America insomnia survey (AIS). Sleep 2011;34(8): 997–1011.
9. Ohayon MM, Bader G. Prevalence and correlates of insomnia in the Swedish population aged 19-75 years. Sleep Med 2010;11(10):980–6.
10. Burgard SA, Ailshire JA. Putting work to bed: stressful experiences on the job and sleep quality. J Health Soc Behav 2009;50(4):476–92.
11. McQuillan ME, Bates JE, Staples AD, et al. Maternal stress, sleep, and parenting. J Fam Psychol 2019; 33(3):349–59.
12. Oginska H, Pokorski J. Fatigue and mood correlates of sleep length in three age-social groups: school children, students, and employees. Chronobiol Int 2006;23(6):1317–28.
13. Belenky G, Wesensten NJ, Thorne DR, et al. Patterns of performance degradation and restoration during sleep restriction and subsequent recovery: a sleep dose-response study. J Sleep Res 2003;12(1):1–12.
14. Van Dongen HP, Maislin G, Mullington JM, et al. The cumulative cost of additional wakefulness: dose-response effects on neurobehavioral functions and sleep physiology from chronic sleep restriction and total sleep deprivation. Sleep 2003;26(2):117–26.
15. Hirshkowitz M, Whiton K, Albert SM, et al. National Sleep Foundation's sleep time duration recommendations: methodology and results summary. Sleep Health 2015;1(1):40–3.
16. Groeger JA, Zijlstra FRH, Dijk DJ. Sleep quantity, sleep difficulties and their perceived consequences in a representative sample of some 2000 British adults. J Sleep Res 2004;13(4):359–71.
17. Moline ML, Broch L, Zak R. Sleep in women across the life cycle from adulthood through menopause. Med Clin 2004;88(3):705–36.
18. Pengo MF, Won CH, Bourjeily G. Sleep in women across the life span. Chest 2018;154(1):196–206.
19. Baker FC, Driver HS. Circadian rhythms, sleep, and the menstrual cycle. Sleep Med 2007;8(6):613–22.
20. Baker FC, Sassoon SA, Kahan T, et al. Perceived poor sleep quality in the absence of polysomnographic sleep disturbance in women with severe premenstrual syndrome. J Sleep Res 2012;21(5): 535–45.
21. Lee KA, Shaver JF, Giblin EC, et al. Sleep patterns related to menstrual cycle phase and premenstrual affective symptoms. Sleep 1990;13(5):403–9.
22. Parry BL, Mendelson WB, Duncan WC, et al. Longitudinal sleep EEG, temperature, and activity measurements across the menstrual cycle in patients with premenstrual depression and in age-matched controls. Psychiatry Res 1989;30(3):285–303.
23. Sharkey KM, Crawford SL, Kim S, et al. Objective sleep interruption and reproductive hormone dynamics in the menstrual cycle. Sleep Med 2014; 15(6):688–93.
24. Dugral E, Ordu G. Differences in polysomnography parameters of women in the post and transitional phases of menopause. Cureus 2021;13(12): e20570.
25. Hachul H, Frange C, Bezerra AG, et al. The effect of menopause on objective sleep parameters: data from an epidemiologic study in São Paulo, Brazil. Maturitas 2015;80(2):170–8.
26. Young T, Rabago D, Zgierska A, et al. Objective and subjective sleep quality in premenopausal, perimenopausal, and postmenopausal women in the Wisconsin Sleep Cohort study. Sleep 2003;26(6):667–72.
27. Krishnan V, Collop NA, Williams L. Gender differences in sleep disorders. Curr Opin Pulm Med 2006;12(6):383–9.
28. Rapoport AP, Piccinini CA. Motherhood and stressful situations in the baby's first year of life. Psico-UFS 2011;16(2):215–25.
29. Teti DM, Shimizu M, Crosby B, et al. Sleep arrangements, parent-infant sleep during the first year, and family functioning. Dev Psychol 2016;52(8): 1169–81.
30. Coble PA, Reynolds CF, Kupfer DJ, et al. Childbearing in women with and without a history of affective disorder. II. Electroencephalographic sleep. Compr Psyhiatry 1994;35(3):215–24.
31. Gay CL, Lee KA, Lee SY. Sleep patterns and fatigue in new mothers and fathers. Biol Res Nurs 2004;5(4): 311–8.
32. Ohayon MM, Carskadon MA, Guilleminault C, et al. Meta-analysis of quantitative sleep parameters from childhood to old age in healthy individuals: developing normative sleep values across the human lifespan. Sleep 2004;27(7):1255–73.
33. Richter D, Krämer MD, Tang NKY, et al. Long-term effects of pregnancy and childbirth on sleep satisfaction and duration of first-time and experienced mothers and fathers. Sleep 2019;42(4). https://doi.org/10.1093/sleep/zsz015.
34. Ramamurthy MB, Sekartini R, Ruangdaraganon N, et al. Effect of current breastfeeding on sleep patterns in infants from Asia-Pacific region. J Paediatr Child Health 2012;48(8):669–74.

35. Mindell JA, du Mond C, Tanenbaum JB, et al. Long-term relationship between breastfeeding and sleep. Child Health Care 2012;41(3):190–203.
36. Doan T, Gardiner A, Gay CL, et al. Breast-feeding increases sleep duration of new parents. J Perinat Neonatal Nurs 2007;21(3):200–6.
37. Montgomery-Downs HE, Clawges HM, Santy EE. Infant feeding methods and maternal sleep and daytime functioning. Pediatrics 2010;126(6). https://doi.org/10.1542/peds.2010-1269.
38. Smith JP, Forrester RI. Association between breastfeeding and new mothers' sleep: a unique Australian time use study. Int Breastfeed J 2021;16(1). https://doi.org/10.1186/s13006-020-00347-z.
39. Quillin SI. Infant and mother sleep patterns during 4th postpartum week. Issues Compr Pediatr Nurs 1997;20(2):115–23.
40. Blynton DM, Sullivan CE, Edwards N. Lactation is associated with an increase in slow-wave sleep in women. J Sleep Res 2002;11(4):297–303.
41. Bai L, Whitesell CJ, Teti DM. Maternal sleep patterns and parenting quality during infants' first 6 months. J Fam Psychol 2020;34(3):291–300.
42. Shinkoda H, Matsumoto K, Park YM. Changes in sleep-wake cycle during the period from late pregnancy to puerperium identified through the wrist actigraph and sleep logs. Psychiatr Clin Neurosci 1999;53(2):133–5.
43. Thompson JF, Roberts CL, Currie M, et al. Prevalence and persistence of health problems after childbirth: associations with parity and method of birth. Birth 2002;29(2):83–94.
44. Meltzer LJ, Meltzer LJ, Mindell J a, et al. Sleep and sleep disorders in children and adolescents. Psychiatr Clin North Am 2006;29(4):1059–76.
45. Kalogeropoulos C, Burdayron R, Laganière C, et al. Sleep patterns and intraindividual sleep variability in mothers and fathers at 6 months postpartum: a population-based, cross-sectional study. BMJ Open 2022;12(8):e060558.
46. Kuo PX, Volling BL, Gonzalez R. Gender role beliefs, work-family conflict, and father involvement after the birth of a second child. Psychol Men Masc 2018; 19(2):243–56.
47. Rollins NC, Bhandari N, Hajeebhoy N, et al. Why invest, and what it will take to improve breastfeeding practices? Lancet 2016;387:491–505.
48. Banks S, Dinges DF. Behavioral and physiological consequences of sleep restriction. J Clin Sleep Med 2007;3(5):519–28.

COVID-19
A Challenge to the Safety of Assisted Reproduction

Marise Samama, MD, PhD[a,b,1,*], Frida Entezami, MD, MSc[c,2], Daniela S. Rosa, PhD[d,3], Amanda Sartor[b,e], Rita C.C.P. Piscopo, MD[b,4], Monica L. Andersen, PhD[e,5], Joao Sabino Cunha-Filho, MD, PhD[f,6], Zsuzsanna I.K. Jarmy-Di-Bella, MD, PhD[a,7]

KEYWORDS

• Pandemic • COVID-19 • Ovarian stimulation • Human IVF • Cytokine storm • Assisted reproductive technology • Sleep • Immune system

KEY POINTS

- Mitigating the risk of COVID-19 and preventing the cytokine storm is crucial during assisted reproductive technology (ART) treatment.
- The impact of SARS-CoV-2 on asymptomatic and pre-symptomatic infertile patients poses challenges in ART protocols, particularly in managing hormonal, immunologic, and prothrombotic risks associated with controlled ovarian stimulation (COS), ART surgery, and IVF laboratory procedures.
- High levels of estradiol should be avoided or reduced as the primary strategy to prevent complications, including the potential cytokine storm in COVID-19 cases, highlighting the need for careful monitoring.
- Consideration should be given to the potential effects of viral infection on ovulation process efficacy and the risks it poses to IVF cycle outcomes and early fetal development.
- Safety procedures must be followed at fertility clinics to minimize contamination risks for health care providers and patients, encompassing hormone treatment, surgical procedures, and gamete/embryo processing and storage in the laboratory, especially as COVID-19 becomes an endemic disease.

BACKGROUND

The COVID-19 pandemic unleashed by SARS-CoV-2 has infected more than 630 million people worldwide and caused more than 6.5 million deaths. Despite the discovery of new therapies and licensing of several vaccines against COVID-19[1] the contagion returns wave after wave mainly caused by the emergence of the variants of concern (VOCs). Disease transmission occurs from symptomatic, pre-symptomatic, and asymptomatic (75%)

[a] Department of Gynecology, Federal University of São Paulo, São Paulo, Brazil; [b] GERA Institute of Reproductive Medicine, São Paulo, Brazil; [c] American Hospital of Paris, IVF Unit, Neuilly-Sur-Seine, France; [d] Department of Microbiology, Immunology and Parasitology, Federal University of São Paulo, São Paulo, Brazil; [e] Department of Psychobiology, Federal University of São Paulo, São Paulo, Brazil; [f] Faculdade de Medicina, Universidade Federal do Rio Grande do Sul, Porto Alegre, Brazil
[1] Rua Teodoro Sampaio 352/117, São Paulo-SP, 05406-000, Brazil.
[2] 55, Bd du Château, 92200 Neuilly sur Seine
[3] Rua Botucatu 862, 4Andar, São Paulo-SP, 04023-062, Brazil
[4] Rua Brasilia 133, Araras-SP, 13600-710, Brazil
[5] Rua Botucatu 862, 1Andar, São Paulo-SP, 04724-000, Brazil
[6] Rua Nilo Peçanha 2821/905, Porto Alegre-RS, Brazil
[7] Av. Brig. Faria Lima 2927/14, São Paulo-SP, 01452-010, Brazil
* Corresponding author. Rua Teodoro Sampaio 352/117, São Paulo-SP 05406-000, Brazil.
E-mail address: marisesamama@yahoo.com.br

Sleep Med Clin 18 (2023) 489–497
https://doi.org/10.1016/j.jsmc.2023.06.012
1556-407X/23/

carriers.[2] SARS-CoV-2 infects host cells through the spike protein binding to the angiotensin-converting enzyme (ACE)2 cellular receptor, and internalization occurs mainly by type II transmembrane serine protease (TMPRSS2).[3] In severe cases, higher levels of D-dimer, lactate dehydrogenase, C-reactive protein, ferritin and increased neutrophil counts were reported. Moreover, lower $CD4^+$ and $CD8^+$ T lymphocytes, and reduced numbers of cytotoxic natural killer (NK) cells have been associated with a rise in proinflammatory cytokines leading to a cytokine storm, that could be the major cause of Acute Respiratory Distress Syndrome (ARDS) and multiple-organ failure.[2]

As a public health issue affecting 15% of couples worldwide, infertility treatments were affected and postponed during pandemic. Now it seems to be an endemic disease as COVID-19 is not likely to be eradicated, treatment centers and fertility care resumed in a new COVID-19 environment. To mitigate the risk of virus spread, fertility treatments programs need to monitor local conditions and mutant strains that vary in contagion and severity. According to the ASRM (American Society for Reproductive Medicine), a prudent strategy is to encourage vaccination and booster shots in all patients who are considering pregnancy and employees, self-diagnostic tests before treatment and masking.[4]

Infertility treatments result in thousands of controlled ovarian stimulation (COS) cycles annually. COS with gonadotrophins is the corner stone of fertility treatments for assisted reproductive technology (ART). The immunologic and prothrombotic profiles of COS indicated striking similarities with the mechanisms of COVID-19 that can lead to a cytokine storm. The similar profiles found in both conditions and the oocyte retrieval procedure may increase the risk of triggering COVID-19 in asymptomatic SARS-CoV-2 carriers.

Since the beginning of the global pandemic, sleep disorders, sleep deprivation and poor sleep quality have been related to negative COVID-19 outcomes.[5–7] Some studies have speculated that sleep disturbances, particularly sleep deprivation and obstructive sleep apnea (OSA), might decrease the efficacy of immunization against COVID-19,[8–10] although it has not been properly investigated yet. This assumption is based on previous studies that demonstrated that sleep deprivation and short sleep duration decrease immune response after vaccination for H1N1, influenza, and hepatitis A,[11–15] although a study found no impaired antibody response to influenza vaccination among OSA individuals.[16] Collectively, it can be stated that sleep is an important feature that impacts both the imunological profile and psychological aspects related to ART.

Given the high number of asymptomatic patients and the uncertainties from conception during COVID-19 infection,[17] the hypothesis proposed herein recommends more cautious strategies for ovarian stimulation in ART to prevent complications. The aim of the review is to produce a comprehensive overview of the potential risks associated with fertility treatments during the COVID-19 period, with a focus on assisted reproduction, and to suggest risk mitigation strategies.

SEARCH METHODS

In order to collect comprehensive data from the literature on the subject of COVID-19 in relation to fertility, a search of the PubMed database was conducted using the keywords "coronavirus," "COVID-19," "SARS-CoV-2" and "pregnancy," "fertility," "urogenital system," "vertical transmission," "assisted human reproduction," "controlled ovarian stimulation," "oocyte retrieval," "in vitro fertilization," "hormones," "surgical procedures," "embryos," "oocytes," "sperm," "semen," "ovary," "testis," "ACE-2 receptor," "immunology," "cytokine storm," and "coagulation," from January 2020 to July 2022.

CLINICAL CHALLENGE

COVID-19 and Pregnancy

A systematic review on SARS-CoV-2-positive pregnant women showed a high level of prematurity (42%), mainly caesarean section deliveries (92%)[18] and fetal distress.[19,20] A few studies showed evidence of perinatal contamination of the newborn. Zeng and colleagues (2020)[21] tested 33 newborns from COVID-19 mothers, 3 of which proved to be infected.

Li and colleagues (2020)[22] revealed in their study that the SARS-CoV-2 receptor was widely spread in specific cell types of the maternal-fetal interface and fetal organs. The high expression of *ACE2* receptor in the syncytiotrophoblast suggests that the placenta has the potential to be infected by SARS-CoV-2, and might cause placental dysfunction and pregnancy complications. Stanley and colleagues (2020)[23] reported that the BeWo choriocarcinoma cell line displays the co-expression of all proteins that are relevant for SARS-CoV-2 binding and entry into the host cell (ACE-2, TMPRSS2, Basigin, and Cathepsin L). A case of miscarriage during the second trimester of pregnancy in a woman with COVID-19 appeared related to placental infection with SARS-CoV-2, and was supported by virologic findings in the placenta.[24,25] The first proven case of transplacental transmission of SARS-CoV-2 from a pregnant woman affected by COVID-19 during late pregnancy to her offspring was reported.[25] A systematic review suggests that vertical transmission from mother to child could be exceptionally possible at the time of delivery or breastfeeding. Another reported recently that pregnant women with COVID-19 are more likely to be hospitalized, and are at increased risk for intensive care unit (ICU) admission and mechanical ventilation.[26] It is recommended that pregnant women should be aware of their potential risk for severe illness, and measures to prevent infection with SARS-CoV-2 should be emphasized.

COVID-19 and the Urogenital System

A search for ACE2 mRNA in the Human Protein Atlas database conducted by Chen Y. et al. (2020)[27] showed expression of the transcript in different parts of the urogenital system: kidneys, testis, epididymis, ductus deferens, seminal vesicle, ovary, vagina, uterus, and the placenta. The presence of *ACE2* mRNA does not prove viral interaction or invasion in those tissues, but considering that the levels of expression were higher than those found in the lung, the most affected organ in COVID-19, this data might point to other viral targets and other modes of viral transmission that warrant investigation, such as co-expression of *TMPRSS2* or a novel route for entry using CD147 (Basigin)[28] or Cathepsin L.[29] Recently, Boudry and colleagues analyzed 16 women infected with SARS-CoV-2 who underwent ART, and viral RNA was undetectable in the follicular fluid, cumulus cells, and endometrium.[30]Contrary to other authors, Li and colleagues (2020)[31] reported the presence of SARS-CoV-2 in the semen of 16% of patients in the acute and recovery phases of COVID-19. Donders and colleagues (2022) observed in their study that SARS-CoV-2 is non-infectious in a week or more after this infection (mean of 53 days), however, seminal quality after SARS-COV-2 infection may be suboptimal. The estimated recovery time is 3 months.[32] However, there is no robust information about sexual transmission.[23]

Some studies show that SARS-CoV-2 infection can result in poor-quality oocytes and embryos due to the oxidative stress caused by the infection, and thus alter female fertility. In another cited study, a lower mean number of euploid embryos per patient was also observed.[33] The transmission risks, the risks (directly or indirectly) to fertility, and the long-term risks to men and women's reproductive health require further clarification.

Possible Risks Related to COVID-19 in the Fertility Context

In vitro fertilization (IVF) treatment involves several stages before reaching its final objective, which is pregnancy. These include: COS, anesthesia, the surgical procedure for egg retrieval, manipulation of the biological material in the IVF laboratory, and embryo transfer and/or cryostorage of gametes and embryos. The risks related to COVID-19 should be considered for every stage.

The immunologic and prothrombotic profiles of patients with COVID-19 and their relation to the hormonal, immunologic, and prothrombotic risks of COS in ART, anesthesia, and the surgical procedure for egg retrieval are considered later in discussion. Indeed, alongside strategies to be used in ovarian stimulation and oocyte retrieval to prevent complications that could increase the risk of disease in asymptomatic SARS-CoV-2 infected patients, or even in non-infected ones.

Risks in controlled ovarian stimulation

Hormonal and immunologic risks The ovary is a major site of interaction between the immune and endocrine systems. Estradiol (E2), the predominant estrogen, plays an important role in the immune response. Estrogens attract $CD8^+$ T cells in the growing follicles and stimulate their proliferation and differentiation.[34] In COS, E2 can increase up to ten-fold when compared to non-stimulated cycles. Additionally, the total number of blood leukocytes increases with the rise of E2, mainly due to neutrophils and monocytes.[35] In patients infected with SARS-CoV-2, the severity of disease correlates with an increase in neutrophils and monocytes and a decrease in $CD8^+$ and $CD4^+$ T cell counts in peripheral blood.[2] Thus, the rise in neutrophils and monocytes observed with high levels of estradiol in COS could contribute to the severity of COVID-19. Moreover, if $CD8^+$ T cells are reduced during SARS-CoV-2 infection, successful ovarian stimulation could be compromised, resulting in a dose escalation of gonadotrophins, and subsequently in an increase of E2.

The ovarian renin–angiotensin system, including angiotensinogen, ACE, angiotensin II, and the Ang II receptors, was reported to be involved in ovarian physiology as a regulator of follicular development, steroidogenesis, ovulation, and oocyte maturation. In animal models, sex hormones modulate the expression of *ACE2,* which has also been described in ovarian granulosa cells where its expression increases with the luteinizing hormone (LH) surge. Angiotensin-(1–7) is an intermediate of gonadotrophin-induced oocyte maturation in the preovulatory follicle, promoting meiotic oocyte resumption. LH increases both Ang-(1–7) and ACE2 in preovulatory follicles and upregulates the ACE2–Ang-(1–7)–Mas axis.[36] In patients with

COVID-19, ACE2 is activated and down-regulated by the spike protein of SARS-CoV-2, which reduces angiotensin-(1–7) production[37] and could, therefore, affect oocyte maturation, luteal angiogenesis, endometrial regular changes, and embryo development.[37] Furthermore, the androgen receptor (AR) regulates the transcription of *TMPRSS2*. Genetic variants of AR have been associated with polycystic ovary syndrome (PCOS) and may be linked with host susceptibility for SARS-CoV-2[38] (**Fig. 1**).

Prothrombotic risks Controlled ovarian stimulation promotes supra physiologic levels of estradiol and vascular endothelial growth factor (VEGF),[39] elevated coagulation factors (eg, Von Willebrand factor, factors VIII and V, fibrinogen), and activated protein C resistance, while reducing antithrombin, and protein C and S activity. Levels of several markers of fibrinolysis such as tissue plasminogen activator (tPA) and plasminogen activator inhibitor type I (PAI-1) decline. All these changes suggest the possible development of a "prothrombotic" state. This state in the coagulation and fibrinolysis systems favors the development of ovarian hyper stimulation syndrome (OHSS)[40] and is associated with thrombophilic disorders, including inherited disorders. The risk of venous thrombosis from OHSS is the same as during pregnancy, which can be ten times the risk of non-pregnant women at reproductive age.[41,42] In Wuhan, in February 2020, Tang and colleagues[43] retrospectively analyzed 183 patients with COVID-19 and observed that the non-survivors revealed significantly higher D-dimer and fibrin degradation product (FDP) levels, longer prothrombin time and activated partial thromboplastin time (aPTT) compared to survivors on admission. Considering the increased levels of E2, coagulation, and immune disorders in ovarian stimulation for IVF, COVID-19 can potentially be facilitated or worsened during the incubation period in asymptomatic patients.

Risks of ovarian hyperstimulation syndrome Ovarian hyper stimulation syndrome is the most serious iatrogenic complication of the controlled ovarian stimulation cycles used in ART. Its prevalence is between 20% and 33% in milder forms[44] and 1% to 5% in moderate and severe forms.[45] It has a high incidence in patients with PCOS. An increased risk of developing OHSS is observed in patients with high antral follicle count (AFC) and previous OHSS occurrence. The pathophysiology is driven by high levels of E2, LH and human chorionic gonadotropin (hCG),[46] which induce high levels of VEGF that promote hyperpermeability of ovarian blood vessels, and the shift of fluid from the intravascular to the third space.[47] The syndrome generally includes ovarian enlargement, ascites, hemoconcentration, and hypercoagulability. Proinflammatory cytokines and the renin-angiotensin system are also involved in the pathogenesis of OHSS symptoms. Some patients will need culdocentesis, prophylactic anticoagulation, anti-inflammatory treatment, and dopamine-receptor agonist administration, such as cabergoline, to reduce VEGF production.[44] In a study with 126 patients at risk of OHSS, early administration of cabergoline was shown to be safe, and potentially a more effective approach for prophylaxis against OHSS. Cabergoline was administered (0.5 mg/d) for 8 days when the size of the leading follicle reached 15 mm.[48]

In patients with COVID-19, data demonstrated higher levels of VEGF when compared to healthy controls.[49] VEGF might have a detrimental role by increasing vascular permeability, inducing pulmonary edema and ultimately ARDS. There is evidence indicating that VEGF and other proinflammatory mediators, especially IL-6, IL-1, and TNFα are present in follicular fluid, ascitic fluid and in the blood of women after stimulation.[50] These mediators participate in the development of OHSS and are known to play an important role in the pathogenesis of ARDS and severe COVID-19.

COS for IVF treatments increases the risk of a thromboembolic event by 10-fold or more, and OHSS by 100-fold compared to the risk in pregnant women not submitted to fertility treatments, increasing almost all inflammatory and thromboembolic markers.[51] If increased levels of estradiol can promote immunologic, prothrombotic status and increased VEGF, and LH and hCG also increase VEGF, then hormonal assisted reproductive technology and pregnancy can contribute to a higher risk of developing more severe forms of COVID-19 by facilitating the development of the cytokine storm. Procedures that induce such an inflammatory milieu might be detrimental for the patient and must be considered in ART.

Risks during oocyte retrieval

Risks related to anesthesia and surgical procedures SARS-CoV-2 is contagious in asymptomatic, presymptomatic, and symptomatic patients, making it highly difficult to control its spread,[52] which takes place mainly via respiratory droplets, aerosols, and contaminated surfaces.[53] Health care professionals are among the most vulnerable populations, especially when they perform procedures such as tracheal intubation and mechanical ventilation, and because of the use of orofacial masks

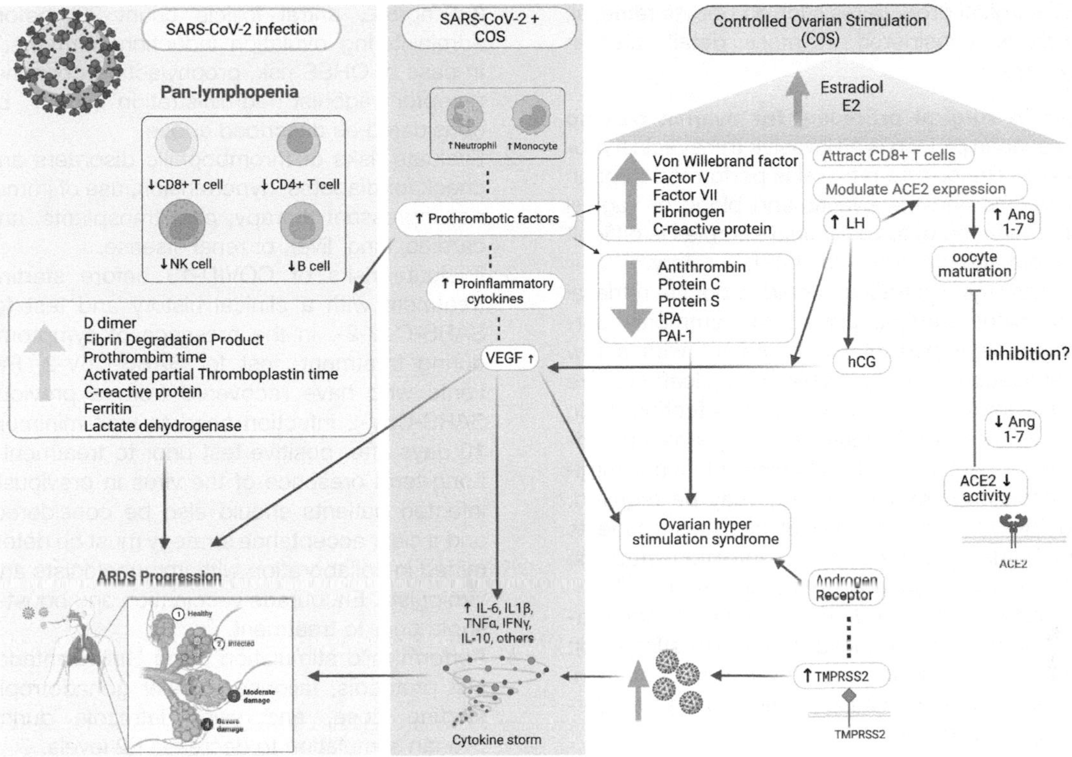

Fig. 1. Immunologic and prothrombotic aspects of COVID-19 and controlled ovarian stimulation (COS).COS and COVID-19 commonly have an increased number of neutrophils, monocytes, prothrombotic factors, and proinflammatory cytokines that can lead to increased VEGF production and cytokine storm. SARS-CoV-2 binds to ACE2, reducing its activity, and the number of $CD8^+$, $CD4^+$ T cell, and NK cells. SARS-CoV-2 could exploit interferon-driven (IFN α and γ) upregulation of *ACE2* to enhance infection by exploitation of the host cytokine response to infection. Moreover, higher levels of D-dimer, lactate dehydrogenase, C-reactive protein, and ferritin are observed. Severe disease is characterized by increased levels of proinflammatory cytokines and VEGF that leads to cytokine storm and ARDS. COS promotes high levels of E2, elevates prothrombotic factors such as Von Willebrand factor, factors VIII and V, fibrinogen, and C-reactive protein, while reducing antithrombin, proteins C and S activities, tPA and PAI-1. E2 attracts $CD8^+$ T cells in growing follicles. The peak of E2 increases LH and modulates *ACE2* expression, increasing angiotensin (Ang1-7) and promoting oocyte maturation. High levels of E2, LH and hCG can induce high levels of VEGF, which associated with increased numbers of neutrophils, monocytes, prothrombotic factors, and proinflammatory cytokines, leads to OHSS. COS and COVID-19 together can promote a cytokine storm leading to ARDS. In gray: SARS-CoV-2 spike protein downregulates ACE2 that, in turn decrease angiotensin (Ang 1–7) production that may affect oocyte maturation. In light blue: alternate pathway that correlates COS and COVID-19: the androgen receptor regulates the transcription of *TMPRSS2*, which is required for SARS-CoV-2 infectivity. The androgen receptor is upregulated in PCOS, and could be associated with host susceptibility, contributing to OHSS and the cytokine storm.

during general anesthesia for surgery that could generate aerosols and respiratory droplets. The generated aerosols may remain in the environment for hours.[53,54] In the case of laparoscopic surgery, the equipment used such as ultrasonic knives or other electronic equipment may produce smoke, causing a high concentration of particles that could bind to viruses and remain in the room, bringing a higher risk to the medical team. An effective method for smoke evacuation is required.[55,56] Surgery and invasive procedures, thus, pose a high risk to health professionals, and also to patients, who are susceptible to contagion in the hospital environment, particularly as low levels of immunity are associated with the post-surgery period. A study in Wuhan demonstrated that all 34 patients submitted to surgery at the beginning of the pandemic were asymptomatic, but, on average, presented pneumonia associated with COVID-19 3 days after the procedure. Of these patients, 44% needed ICU hospitalization, of whom 20% died. The study suggests that performing surgery may induce an early systemic inflammatory response and be responsible for the acceleration or worsening of the disease.[57] This must be taken into account in respect of

ART surgical procedures such as oocyte retrieval, which is considered in more detail later in discussion.

Risks in surgical procedure for ovarian pick up The ovarian pick up is an invasive transvaginal procedure. The oocyte retrieval is performed through the vagina and the ovaries and blood or vaginal contamination of follicular fluid samples is difficult to avoid and can reach the IVF laboratory.[58]

Transvaginal ultrasound-guided oocyte retrieval is a minor surgical procedure commonly performed as a part of IVF treatment with a low complication rate; possible complications are intraabdominal bleeding[56] and infection.[57] In case of hemoperitoneum, hemodynamically unstable or persistent intrabdominal infection, surgical assistance by laparoscopy may be required, and this may put the patient at risk. In patients with hematoma, bleeding, or infection after the OPU, antibiotic coverage is recommended.[56]

Transvaginal procedures, and even the transvaginal ultrasounds required for ovarian stimulation monitoring, could increase the risk of contagion. by potentially transmitting the virus to the staff during the procedures.

Risks for embryo development The impact on embryo development remains an open question.[58] Orvieto and colleagues reported a decrease in the proportion of top-quality embryos for IVF cycles conducted within 90 days after SARS-COV-2 infection, when compared with cycles performed before infection for the same couples.[59]

Assisted Reproductive Technology Treatments

Considering the hormonal, immunologic, and prothrombotic risks of controlled ovarian stimulation, anesthesia, and surgical procedures related to COVID-19, treatment must be carefully tailored for each patient to eliminate risks during the endemic period. Gonadotrophin Releasing Hormone (GnRH) antagonist protocols (triggering ovulation with GnRH agonists) should be used instead of hCG, given the effects of hCG described above.

Some protocols using minimal stimulation, such as the use of aromatase inhibitors (letrozole)[60] to prevent high levels of estradiol and decrease the effect on thromboembolic markers was largely used during pandemic, and must be considered in ART. The main strategies are detailed later in discussion.

Strategies Before and During Ovarian Stimulation During the Endemic COVID-19 Period

1. Identify patients at a high risk for OHSS (PCOS profile, age<30y, Anti-Müllerian hormone > 3.4 ng/mL, antral follicle count>20) before administering ovulation induction hormone.[44] In case of OHSS risk, prophylactic dopamine-receptor agonist administration could be considered as described above.
2. Evaluate risks of thrombophilic disorders and check for diabetes, hypertension, use of immunosuppressant therapy, past transplants, and cardiac, lung, liver, or renal disease.
3. Evaluate risks of COVID-19 before starting treatment with a clinical history and test for SARS-CoV-2-. In the presence of symptoms during treatment, test for SARS-CoV-2. Patients who have recovered from a previous SARS-CoV-2 infection need to wait minimum 10 days after positive test prior to treatment.[4] Long-term presence of the virus in previously infected patients should also be considered, and a clear acceptance strategy must be determined in collaboration with immunologists and virologists. Encourage vaccination and booster shots prior to treatment.
4. Perform mild stimulation using GnRH antagonist protocols, tailoring a lower gonadotropin starting dose, and using letrozole during ovarian stimulation to decrease E2 levels.
5. use the GnRH agonist for final follicular maturation instead of using hCG must be considered depending on severity of local conditions and mutant strains of varying contagion
6. Adopt the freeze-all oocytes and/or embryos strategy if at high risk according to local conditions or for patients with active SARS-COV-2 infection after oocyte retrieval
7. Cancel the cycle if testing positive and proceed to oocyte retrieval and embryo transfer only after giving the patient risk information and obtaining their consent and checking if no clinical history of infection and testing positive

SUMMARY

There is a need to mitigate the risk of developing COVID-19 during ART treatment, and to prevent the cytokine storm that could lead to a severe form of the disease.

The possible impact of SARS-CoV-2 on asymptomatic and pre-symptomatic infertile patients presents a challenge to the performance of ART protocols while avoiding the possible hormonal, immunologic, and prothrombotic risks related to COS, ART surgery, and IVF laboratory procedures. Up to 33% of patients receiving COS develop mild forms of OHSS, and 1% to 5% more severe forms. COS elevates estradiol, prothrombotic factors, proinflammatory cytokines, and VEGF. The avoidance or reduction of high levels of estradiol should, therefore, be the main strategy to prevent complications, such as a potential cytokine storm in the case of COVID-19. In addition, the possibility that the efficacy of the ovulation process could be affected by the viral infection needs to be considered. The impact of acute infection on IVF cycle outcomes and early fetal development remains a potential risk for cycle and embryo transfer cancellation.[61]

Reported data on pregnancy has shown some evidence for vertical transmission, a higher incidence of prematurity and cesarean delivery, and an increased risk to develop severe COVID-19.

Now that it seems to be an endemic disease, all fertility clinics should continue to use safety procedures to lower contamination risks, both for health care providers and patients, at every step of the process, from hormone treatment to surgical procedures. This should extend to gamete and embryo processing, and storage in the laboratory.[58]

AUTHOR CONTRIBUTIONS

M Samama, F Entezami, M L. Andersen, and ZIKJDB designed the study. M Samama, F Entezami, D S. Rosa, AS, RCCP collected the data. M Samama, F Entezami, A Sartor, D S. Rosa analyzed the data. M Samama wrote the article with F Entezami, D S. Rosa, MLA, and A Sartor contribution. M Samama designed the figure with F Entezami and D S. Rosa contribution. All the authors revised the article. M Samama, corresponding author, had full access to all the data in the study and had final responsibility for the decision to submit for publication.

CLINICS CARE POINTS

- Screen patients for potential sleep disorders, such as obstructive sleep apnea, and consider appropriate diagnostic testing or referral to a sleep specialist if indicated.
- Apply strategies to optimize sleep hygiene and promote healthy sleep habits. Encourage patients to maintain a consistent sleep schedule, create a conducive sleep environment, and practice relaxation techniques before bedtime.
- Implement strict monitoring protocols for pregnant women with SARS-CoV-2 infection to identify and manage prematurity and fetal distress promptly. Consider individualized care plans and interventions to optimize maternal and fetal well-being.
- Enhance prenatal screening programs to detect placental dysfunction and pregnancy complications in COVID-19-positive pregnant women. Implement regular ultrasound monitoring and laboratory assessments to identify potential issues early on.
- Establish specialized care pathways for pregnant women with COVID-19 who require hospitalization. Ensure access to intensive care resources and mechanical ventilation when needed, while prioritizing the safety and well-being of both mother and fetus.

DECLARATIONS OF INTEREST

All other authors report no conflicts of interest.

DISCLOSURE

The authors have nothing to disclose.

ACKNOWLEDGMENTS

MLA, ZIKJDB, and DSR are recipients of CNPq fellowships. Our studies are supported by Associação Fundo de Incentivo à Pesquisa, Brazil (AFIP).

REFERENCES

1. Andrews N, Tessier E, Stowe J, et al. Duration of Protection against mild and severe disease by COVID-19 vaccines. N Engl J Med 2022;386(4):340–50.
2. Tay MZ, Poh CM, Rénia L, et al. The trinity of COVID-19: immunity, inflammation and intervention. Nat Rev Immunol 2020;(6):363–74.
3. Ziegler CGK, Allon SJ, Nyquist SK, et al. SARS-CoV-2 receptor ACE2 is an interferon-stimulated Gene in human airway epithelial cells and is detected in specific cell subsets across tissues. Cell 2020;181(5):1016–35.e19.
4. American Society for Reproductive Medicine. Patient Management and Clinical Recommendations During The Coronavirus (COVID-19) Pandemic. 2020 Available in: https://www.asrm.org/news-and-publications/COVID-19/statements/patient-management-and-clinical-recommendations-during-the-coronavirus-COVID-19-pandemic/. Accessed in 21 July 10, 2022.
5. Li P, Zheng X, Ulsa MC, et al. Poor sleep behavior burden and risk of COVID-19 mortality and hospitalization. Sleep 2021;44(8):zsab138.
6. Tufik S, Gozal D, Ishikura IA, et al. Does obstructive sleep apnea lead to increased risk of COVID-19 infection and severity? J Clin Sleep Med 2020;16(8):1425–6.
7. Tufik S. Obstructive sleep apnea as a comorbidity to COVID-19. Sleep Sci 2020;(3):181–2.
8. Zhu J, Zhang M, Sanford LD, Tang X. Advice for COVID-19 vaccination: get some sleep. Sleep Breath 2021;25(4):2287–8.

9. Rayatdoost E, Rahmanian M, Sanie MS, et al. Sufficient Sleep, Time of Vaccination, and Vaccine Efficacy: A Systematic Review of the Current Evidence and a Proposal for COVID-19 Vaccination. Yale J Biol Med 2022;95(2):221–35.
10. Xue P, Merikanto I, Chung F, et al. Persistent short nighttime sleep duration is associated with a greater post-COVID risk in fully mRNA-vaccinated individuals. Transl Psychiatry 2023;13(1):32.
11. Benedict C, Brytting M, Markström A, et al. Acute sleep deprivation has no lasting effects on the human antibody titer response following a novel influenza A H1N1 virus vaccination. BMC Immunol 2012;13:1.
12. Lange T, Perras B, Fehm HL, et al. Sleep enhances the human antibody response to hepatitis A vaccination. Psychosom Med 2003;65(5):831–5.
13. Spiegel K, Sheridan JF, Van Cauter E. Effect of sleep deprivation on response to immunization. JAMA 2002;288(12):1471–2.
14. Prather AA, Pressman SD, Miller GE, et al. Temporal links between self-reported sleep and antibody responses to the influenza vaccine. Int J Behav Med 2021;28(1):151–8.
15. Prather AA, Hall M, Fury JM, et al. Sleep and antibody response to hepatitis B vaccination. Sleep 2012;35(8):1063–9.
16. Dopp JM, Wiegert NA, Moran JJ, et al. Humoral immune responses to influenza vaccination in patients with obstructive sleep apnea. Pharmacotherapy 2007;11:1483–9.
17. Carvalho BR, Adami KS, Gonçalves-Ferri WA, et al. COVID-19: uncertainties from conception to birth. Rev Bras Ginecol Obstet 2021;43(1): 54–60.
18. Zaigham M, Andersson O. Maternal and perinatal outcomes with COVID-19: a systematic review of 108 pregnancies. Acta Obstet Gynecol Scand 2020;7:823–9.
19. Chen H, Guo J, Wang C, et al. Clinical characteristics and intrauterine vertical transmission potential of COVID-19 infection in nine pregnant women: a retrospective review of medical records. Lancet 2020;395(10226):809–15.
20. Chen L, Li Q, Zheng D, et al. Clinical characteristics of pregnant women with covid-19 in wuhan, China. N Engl J Med 2020;382(25):e100.
21. Zeng L, Xia S, Yuan W, et al. Neonatal early-onset infection with SARS-CoV-2 in 33 neonates born to mothers with COVID-19 in wuhan, China. JAMA Pediatr 2020;174(7):722–5.
22. Li M, Chen L, Zhang J, et al. The SARS-CoV-2 receptor ACE2 expression of maternal-fetal interface and fetal organs by single-cell transcriptome study. PLoS One 2020;15(4):e0230295.
23. Stanley KE, Thomas E, Leaver M, et al. Coronavirus disease-19 and fertility: viral host entry protein expression in male and female reproductive tissues. Fertil Steril 2020;114(1):33–43.
24. Baud D, Greub G, Favre G, et al. Second-trimester miscarriage in a pregnant woman with SARS-CoV-2 infection. JAMA 2020;323(21):2198–200.
25. Vivanti AJ, Vauloup-Fellous C, Prevot S, et al. Transplacental transmission of SARS-CoV-2 infection. Nat Commun 2020;11(1):3572.
26. Ramirez Ubillus GC, Sedano Gelvet EE, Neira Montoya CR. Gestational complications associated with SARS-CoV-2 infection in pregnant women during 2020-2021: systematic review of longitudinal studies. J Perinat Med 2022;51(3):291–9.
27. Chen Y, Guo Y, Pan Y, et al. Structure analysis of the receptor binding of 2019-nCoV. Biochem Biophys Res Commun 2020;525(1):135–40.
28. Wang K, Chen W, Zhang Z, et al. CD147-spike protein is a novel route for SARS-CoV-2 infection to host cells. Sig Transduct Target Ther 2020;5(1):283.
29. Ou X, Liu Y, Lei X, et al. Characterization of spike glycoprotein of SARS-CoV-2 on virus entry and its immune cross-reactivity with SARS-CoV. Nat Commun 2020;11(1):1620.
30. Boudry L, Essahib W, Mateizel I, et al. Undetectable viral RNA in follicular fluid, cumulus cells, and endometrial tissue samples in SARS-CoV-2-positive women. Fertil Steril 2022;117(4):771–80.
31. Li D, Jin M, Bao P, et al. Clinical characteristics and results of semen tests among men with coronavirus disease 2019. JAMA Netw Open 2020;3(5): e208292.
32. Donders GGG, Bosmans E, Reumers J, et al. Sperm quality and absence of SARS-CoV-2 RNA in semen after COVID-19 infection: a prospective, observational study and validation of the SpermCOVID test. Fertil Steril 2022;117(2):287–96.
33. Carp-Veliscu A, Mehedintu C, Frincu F, et al. The effects of SARS-CoV-2 infection on female fertility: a review of the literature. Int J Environ Res Public Health 2022;19(2):984.
34. Vinatier D, Dufour P, Tordjeman-Rizzi N, et al. Immunological aspects of ovarian function: role of the cytokines. Eur J Obstet Gynecol Reprod Biol 1995; 63(2):155–68.
35. Habib P, Dreymueller D, Rösing B, et al. Estrogen serum concentration affects blood immune cell composition and polarization in human females under controlled ovarian stimulation. J Steroid Biochem Mol Biol 2018;178:340–7.
36. Palumbo A, Ávila J, Naftolin F. The ovarian renin-angiotensin system (ovras): a major factor in ovarian function and disease. Reprod Sci 2016;23(12): 1644–55.
37. Jing Y, Run-Qian L, Hao-Ran W, et al. Potential influence of COVID-19/ACE2 on the female reproductive system. Mol Hum Reprod 2020;26(6):367–73.

38. Wambier CG, Goren A, Vaño-Galván S, et al. Androgen sensitivity gateway to COVID-19 disease severity. Drug Dev Res 2020;81(7):771–6.
39. Malamitsi-Puchner A, Sarandakou A, Tziotis J, et al. Circulating angiogenic factors during periovulation and the luteal phase of normal menstrual cycles. Fertil Steril 2004;81(5):1322–7.
40. Chan WS. The 'ART' of thrombosis: a review of arterial and venous thrombosis in assisted reproductive technology. Curr Opin Obstet Gynecol 2009;21(3): 207–18.
41. Kierkegaard A. Incidence and diagnosis of deep vein thrombosis associated with pregnancy. Acta Obstet Gynecol Scand 1983;62(3):239–43.
42. Andersen BS, Steffensen FH, Sørensen HT, et al. The cumulative incidence of venous thromboembolism during pregnancy and puerperium–an 11 year Danish population-based study of 63,300 pregnancies. Acta Obstet Gynecol Scand 1998;77(2):170–3.
43. Tang N, Li D, Wang X, et al. Abnormal coagulation parameters are associated with poor prognosis in patients with novel coronavirus pneumonia. J Thromb Haemost 2020;18(4):844–7.
44. Nelson SM. Prevention and management of ovarian hyperstimulation syndrome. Thromb Res 2017; 151(Suppl 1):S61–4.
45. Practice Committee of the American Society for Reproductive Medicine. Electronic address: ASRM@asrm.org; Practice Committee of the American Society for Reproductive Medicine. Prevention and treatment of moderate and severe ovarian hyperstimulation syndrome: a guideline. Fertil Steril 2016;(7):1634–47.
46. Neulen J, Yan Z, Raczek S, et al. Human chorionic gonadotropin-dependent expression of vascular endothelial growth factor/vascular permeability factor in human granulosa cells: importance in ovarian hyperstimulation syndrome. J Clin Endocrinol Metab 1995;80(6):1967–71.
47. Mourad S, Brown J, Farquhar C. Interventions for the prevention of OHSS in ART cycles: an overview of Cochrane reviews. Cochrane Database Syst Rev 2017;1(1):CD012103.
48. Gaafar S, El-Gezary D, El Maghraby HA. Early onset of cabergoline therapy for prophylaxis from ovarian hyperstimulation syndrome (OHSS): a potentially safer and more effective protocol. Reprod Biol 2019;19(2):145–8.
49. Huang C, Wang Y, Li X, et al. Clinical features of patients infected with 2019 novel coronavirus in Wuhan, China. Lancet 2020;395(10223):497–506.
50. Chen CD, Wu MY, Chen HF, et al. Prognostic importance of serial cytokine changes in ascites and pleural effusion in women with severe ovarian hyperstimulation syndrome. Fertil Steril 1999;72(2): 286–92.
51. Sennström M, Rova K, Hellgren M, et al. Thromboembolism and in vitro fertilization - a systematic review. Acta Obstet Gynecol Scand 2017;96(9): 1045–52.
52. Li R, Pei S, Chen B, et al. Substantial undocumented infection facilitates the rapid dissemination of novel coronavirus (SARS-CoV-2). Science 2020;368(6490): 489–93.
53. Peng PWH, Ho PL, Hota SS. Outbreak of a new coronavirus: what anaesthetists should know. Br J Anaesth 2020;124(5):497–501.
54. Chen R, Zhang Y, Huang L, et al. Safety and efficacy of different anesthetic regimens for parturients with COVID-19 undergoing Cesarean delivery: a case series of 17 patients. Can J Anaesth 2020;67(6): 655–63.
55. Mintz Y, Arezzo A, Boni L, et al. We read in detail the comments regarding our article "A low cost, safe, and effective method for smoke evacuation in laparoscopic surgery for suspected coronavirus Patients"! and would like to reply. Ann Surg 2021, 274(6):e776–7.
56. Zheng MH, Boni L, Fingerhut A. Minimally invasive surgery and the novel coronavirus outbreak: lessons learned in China and Italy. Ann Surg 2020;272(1): e5–6.
57. Lei S, Jiang F, Su W, et al. Clinical characteristics and outcomes of patients undergoing surgeries during the incubation period of COVID-19 infection. EClinicalMedicine 2020;1:100331.
58. Entezami F, Samama M, Dejucq-Rainsford N, et al. SARS-CoV-2 and human reproduction: an open question. EClinicalMedicine 2020;25:100473.
59. Orvieto R, Segev-Zahav A, Aizer A. Does COVID-19 infection influence patients' performance during IVF-ET cycle?: an observational study. Gynecol Endocrinol 2021;37(10):895–7.
60. Haas J, Casper RF. In vitro fertilization treatments with the use of clomiphene citrate or letrozole. Fertil Steril 2017;108(4):568–71.
61. Clain E, Johnson J, Roeca C. Triggered with COVID: what are my chances. Doc? Fertil Steril. 2022; 117(4):781–2.

The Integration of the Maternal Care with Sleep During the Postpartum Period

Luciana Benedetto, PhD[a,*], Florencia Peña, BS[a], Mayda Rivas, PhD[a], Annabel Ferreira, PhD[b], Pablo Torterolo, PhD[a]

KEYWORDS

• NREM • Maternal behavior • Milk ejection • Sleep deprivation • Nursing

KEY POINTS

- All mammalian mothers have sleep disturbances at some point during the postpartum period.
- Sleep fragmentation is the most common sleep disturbance.
- Mother rats are capable to sleep and nurse at the same time.
- The mother integrates the maternal care of the offspring to her routine before sleep.
- Sleep is not necessary for milk ejection in rats.

SLEEP AS A MOTIVATED BEHAVIOR

Motivated behaviors can be divided into an appetitive and a consummatory phase,[1,2] and among the different motivational concepts, it has been posited that motivated behaviors may serve to return some of the physiologic variables to the homeostatic levels.[3] Like the need to ingest food and water, the need for sleep satisfies some elementary need that has not yet been fully clarified. "Sleep is as essential as food and water: the physiologic and psychological pressure to sleep is so great that it can overwhelm all other needs."[4] From this point of view, sleep could be considered a motivated behavior, where animals do not only sleep at some point due to sleep pressure, but they actively seek for sleep, preparing themselves and the environment to achieve this goal in optimal conditions. In this sense, in many species, before the animal goes to sleep, it exhibits certain behaviors that promote sleep onset, such as nest building, look for a safe and warm environment.[5] In fact, humans perform several routines before sleep.[6–8] The search for the appropriate conditions for sleep initiation could be identified as the appetitive phase, as it not only precedes sleep but also promotes it,[5] whereas sleep itself would be the consummatory phase.

The mammalian sleep is organized in two stages: non-rapid eye movement (NREM; also called slow wave sleep [SWS]) sleep and rapid eye movement (REM) sleep,[9] each stage having its own function.[10] Also, sleep deprivation leads to the alteration of innumerable physiologic variables in such a way that if sleep deprivation is perpetuated, it could determine the animal's own death.[11–20] In this way, the motivation to sleep would come from internal stimuli,[5] generated by imbalances in the body. This physiologic imbalance during the deprivation of a motivated behavior determines an amplification of this behavior, usually observed in the post-deprivation period. In this regard, after a sleep deprivation period, there is an increase in sleep duration and depth, a phenomenon known as sleep rebound.[21] These characteristics make sleep meet the features of motivated behavior and show the essentiality of this behavioral state for survival.

[a] Departamento de Fisiología, Facultad de Medicina, Universidad de la República, Montevideo, Uruguay; [b] Sección de Fisiología y Nutrición, Facultad de Ciencias, Universidad de la República, Montevideo, Uruguay
* Corresponding author. Departamento de Fisiología, Facultad de Medicina, Universidad de la República, General Flores 2125, Montevideo 11800, Uruguay.
E-mail address: lbenedet@fmed.edu.uy

Sleep Med Clin 18 (2023) 499–509
https://doi.org/10.1016/j.jsmc.2023.06.013

In addition to the well-documented sleep propensity and circadian rhythm in the onset of sleep, a variety of external and internal needs can also regulate its initiation.[22] In the context of motherhood, the needs of the pups that require active maternal care might influence the sleep of the mother.

MATERNAL BEHAVIOR AS A MOTIVATED BEHAVIOR

Any behavior directed to the offspring that increases the probability of its survival can be defined as maternal behavior, being one of the most rewarding motivated behaviors in nature.[2,23] Pups are a natural potent reward,[24–27] which has been deeply studied in laboratory animals. In rats, it has been described that the mothers significantly reduce the cocaine self-administration in chronically cocaine exposed animals,[28] overcome potentially dangerous obstacles to get access to their pups,[29] and prefer an environment associated with their pups over one associated with food, despite of being food-deprived.[27] The fact that pups are a powerful reinforcing stimulus has also been documented in operant conditioning paradigms, in which mothers learn to press a lever to gain access to pups.[26] Unlike other motivated behaviors, maternal behavior has no satiety.[26] All these features make maternal behavior to be considered as a highly motivated behavior.[30]

Maternal behavior can be divided into active behaviors (or appetitive phase) and passive behaviors (consummatory phase).[1,2] In rats, the active maternal repertoire includes the retrieval of the pups into the nest, the grooming of the pups (both corporal and anogenital licking), and the rearrangements of the pups in the nest (mouthing),[23] whereas passive maternal behavior includes mainly nursing.

Despite the diversity of maternal behavior in different species, nursing is the most generalizable behavior that defines us as mammals.[2] Nursing behavior transcends milk ejection and nutrition. In fact, it includes huddling that provides shelter and reduces the probability that predators harm the pups. Also grants the adequate temperature of the offspring, critical in some altricial mammals that are unable to control their own temperature during the first days after birth.[2,23,31] Indeed, if non-lactating rats are repeatedly exposed to newborn pups, they develop maternal behaviors, being capable to adopt nursing postures.[32,33]

ARE SLEEP AND MATERNAL BEHAVIOR COMPATIBLE BEHAVIORS?

From a behavioral point of view, sleep can be defined as a rapidly reversible state, where response and interaction with the environment and awareness of it are reduced. Thus, sleep constitutes a period of great fragility for the individual, and in the case of a mother, it also represents a moment of vulnerability for her offspring.

Non-lactating rats spend approximately half of the entire day sleeping. However, the first days after giving birth, mother rats spend most of their day (above 80% of the time) in contact with the pups.[34] Thus, the mother either sleeps and takes care of the pups at the same time or she is sleep deprived. Hence, work from our laboratory shows that mother rats are capable to sleep and nurse at the same time (**Figs. 1** and **2**). In fact, in the earliest postpartum stage, the mother rat sleeps more than 80% of the time whereas she is nursing in low kyphosis, the most typical nursing position[35] (see **Fig. 2**). Mothers barely leave the nest to eat, drink, or perform self-grooming, and in general, they do not sleep outside the nest. In addition, another nursing position, the supine posture (see **Fig. 1**), is associated with higher percentages of

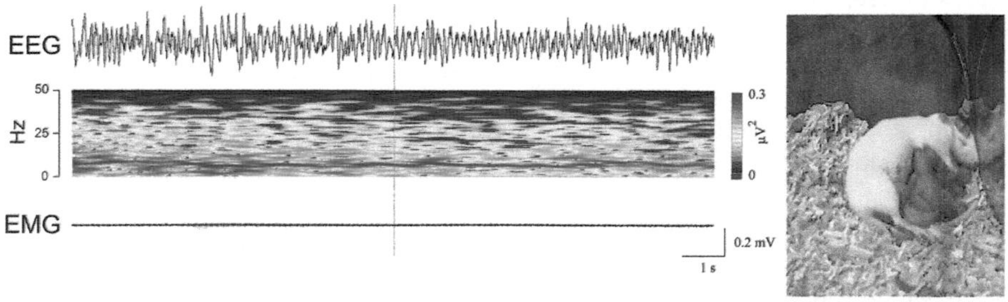

Fig. 1. Mother rat sleeping during a nursing posture. Figure shows the raw electroencephalogram (EEG), its correspondent spectrogram below, and the electromyogram (EMG). It can be observed that the mother is transitioning from NREM to REM sleep during supine nursing posture. The vertical line indicates the moment when the photo was taken. (*Adapted from* ref[35]; this animal was not included in the data analysis of the mentioned article.)

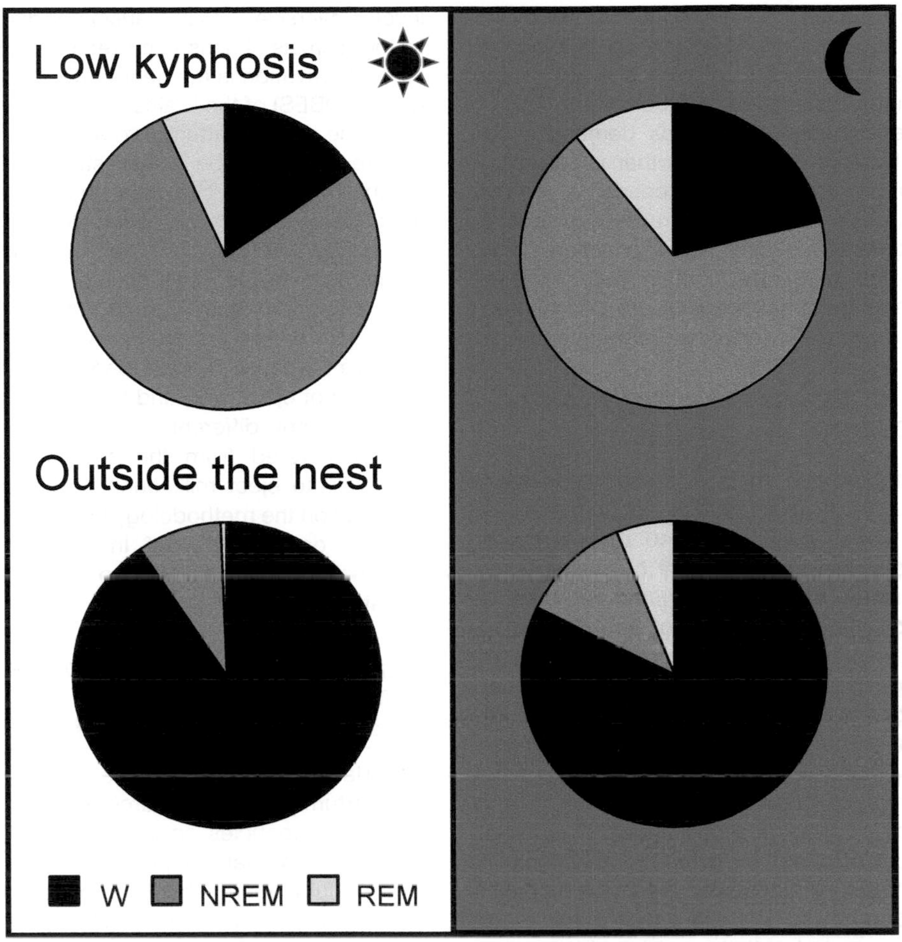

Fig. 2. Graphic charts showing the percentage of wakefulness (W), NREM, and REM sleep during different maternal behaviors. Data represent the mean percentage of each behavioral state in low kyphosis (the most common nursing posture) and outside the nest, in the light (left column) and dark (right column) phases during the first postpartum week. (*Adapted from* ref.[35])

REM sleep compared with other positions. As postpartum progresses to the second postpartum week, the sleeping time decreases during certain nursing positions, such as high kyphosis, possibly because the pups are more mobile compared with the first postpartum days. In contrast, other positions, such as low kyphosis, have similar percentages of sleeping time during the first and second postpartum weeks (for details see ref[35]). As the pups grow older, the mother also spends more time away from the nest and begins to sleep more time outside the nest compared with the early stages, compensating, in part, for the time they are awake during nursing at this stage.[35]

Thus, the mother can sleep and nurse at the same time. In this sense, sleep and nursing share common features that enable a joint occurrence: the animal should remain calm, find a comfortable or unique posture,[9,36] an adequate temperature (either of the environment or the nest[36,37]) and need a reduction in the external stimuli.[38,39] In fact, the sucking of the offspring encourages the mother to remain in the nest and adopt nursing postures, typically inhibiting all active behaviors.[23,36] Therefore, we hypothesized that the sensory stimulation from the suckling offspring promotes the conditions that facilitate both behaviors. Thus, nursing is not only compatible with sleep but would promote each other.

Regarding the preparatory phase of sleep and nursing, the appetitive phase of sleep includes seeking of a safe place without disturbing stimuli,[38,39] building a nest and self-grooming.[5,22] In the same sense, the mothers must also retrieve the pups to the nest and lick them before they can lay together in the nest and nurse them.[23] Thus, the mother would have to care for the pups' needs and integrity before sleep. We proposed that the appetite phase of sleep and maternal behavior overlaps and takes place at the same time, ensuring the display of the consummatory phases of both behaviors.

However, whenever the pups demand active maternal behavior while the mother is asleep, or if the pups' stimulation exceeds a certain threshold, sleep would be interrupted, generating sleep fragmentation or sleep deprivation. Thus, when the appetitive and consummatory phases of sleep and maternal behavior are desynchronized, these two behaviors would compete.

IS SLEEP NECESSARY FOR NURSING AND MILK EJECTION?

In most studied mammals, suckling is necessary and enough for milk ejection occurrence.[40,41] However, it has been described that in mother rats, the suckling stimulus must be preceded by a SWS episode to eject milk. If mother rats are prevented from sleep by means of gentle handling (GH), milk ejection would not occur.[42–44] Although, in other species such as rabbit[40] and pig,[41] sleep would not be necessary for milk letdown. In addition, although in humans there is no need to sleep for milk ejection, a non-stressful state favors the maintenance of breast milk production.[45,46] In this regard, Poulain and colleagues[41] proposed that sleep would not be a requirement for milk ejection in rats. Instead, sleep would be a parallel event induced by suckling. In a recent article, the authors demonstrated that sleep is not necessary for milk ejection in rats, but rather the methodology used to prevent sleep determines if milk letdown occurs or not.[47]

Sleep deprivation is a stressful situation itself.[48–50] However, most common practices to prevent sleep in laboratory environments, usually involve aversive stimuli, causing additional stress to the animals. A less used technique to achieve sleep deprivation is the deep brain electrical stimulation (DBES) of the brainstem reticular formation when the animals attempt to sleep.[51,52] This procedure seems to be a less stressful procedure for the mother rat.[53] In this regard, mother rats are capable of eject milk when sleep is prevented by using DBES in the peduncle-pontine tegmentum. In fact, milk ejections events do not vary compared with control rats (**Fig. 3**), and pups gain weight as much as controls (**Fig. 4**). However, when GH was used to sleep deprive, rats did not eject milk, and the weight gain of the pups did not differentiate from the pups that were separated from the mother.[47] Thus, the capability to eject milk during sleep deprivation depends on the methodology implemented, rather than the deprivation itself. In summary, as other mammals, the rat is able to eject milk during wakefulness.[40,41]

SLEEP DURING MOTHERHOOD IN RATS, HUMANS, AND DOLPHINS

General Sleep Characteristics in Rats

Reports of sleep architecture in rats during the postpartum period are scarce. Although there are some discrepancies among authors, there is an agreement in that an increment in the waking time occurs during the light phase of the first days after giving birth, together with a sleep fragmentation.[54–56]

A first report by Rocha and Hoshino shows that between postpartum days 2 (PPD2) and PPD20 , mother rats remain more time awake, display more awakening episodes, and less REM sleep compared with virgin females and male rats when recorded for 7 hours during the light phase.[56]

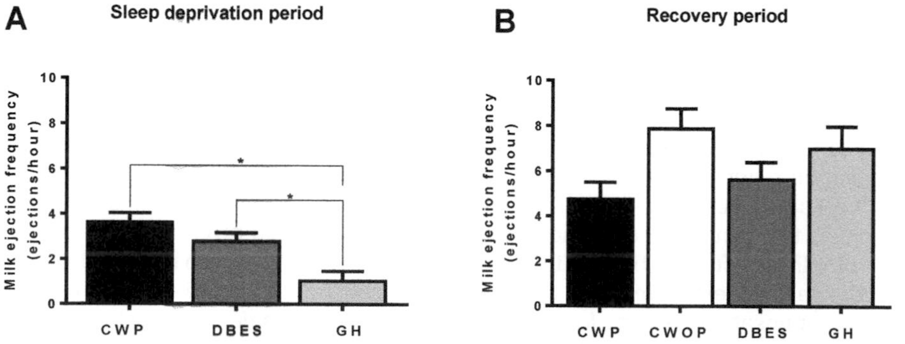

Fig. 3. Impact of sleep deprivation on milk ejection. The graphs show milk ejection frequency during a 3-hour-period of sleep deprivation (*A*) and the following recovery period (*B*). Sleep deprivation was achieved by gentle handling (GH) and deep brain stimulation (DBES). Two control groups (with and without pups [CWP and CWOP, respectively]) are also shown. Data are presented as mean ± standard error ($n = 8$). Statistical analysis was performed using a one-way ANOVA followed by the Tukey test was used. Asterisks (*) symbols indicate significant differences ($P < .05$). CWP, control with pups; CWOP, control without pups. (*Adapted from* ref.[47])

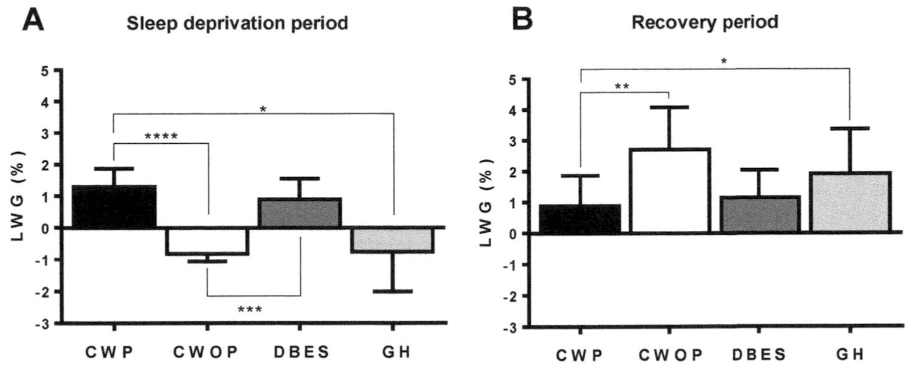

Fig. 4. Impact of sleep deprivation on the litter weight gain (LWG). Variations in the percentage of LWG after a 3-hour-period of sleep deprivation (*A*) and the following recovery period (*B*). Sleep deprivation was achieved by gentle handling (GH) and deep brain stimulation (DBES). Two control groups (with and without pups [CWP and CWOP, respectively]) are also shown. Data are presented as mean ± standard error ($n = 8$). Statistical analysis was performed using a one-way ANOVA followed by the Tukey test was used. Asterisks (*) symbols denote significant differences between groups (*$P < .05$; **$P < .01$; ***$P < .001$; ****$P < .0001$). (*Adapted from* ref.[47])

An elegant report from Sivadas and colleagues provides detailed data about sleep across pregnancy, postpartum, and postweaning periods.[54] Their main findings were a reduction in light NREM sleep and an increment in active wakefulness during the light phase, almost during the entire postpartum, until weaning. In addition, they found a reduction in the bout duration of light NREM sleep also during the light period in all postpartum days. During the dark phase of middle and late postpartum days, an increase in the frequency of wakefulness and light NREM sleep was observed, which could be interpreted as sleep fragmentation.[54] In this sense, we have observed that the mother rat experiences more sleep fragmentation while nursing their pups compared with when she sleeps outside the nest, both in the light and dark periods in the first and second postpartum weeks (**Table 1**). However, sleep depth did not differ between these two behaviors (for details see ref[35]). Related to REM sleep, Sivadas and colleagues observed a specific increase on postpartum day (PPD)2 and PPD10 during the dark period.[54] Although Rocha and Hoshino show a decrease in REM sleep, this decrement was observed during the light phase and the analysis was based on an average between PPD2 and PPD20 [56].

More recently, Toth and colleagues also found an increase in the time of wakefulness during the postpartum period, mainly on PPD2 during the light phase.[55] This increment in wakefulness seems to be at the expense of a reduction in NREM and REM sleep. However, during the dark phase, the time in wakefulness decreased compared with the diestrous phase of female rats.

Sleep in Human Mothers

General characteristics

The early stages of the postpartum period in human mothers consistently lead to sleep alterations.[57,58] All reports in postpartum women show sleep fragmentation. Regarding sleep deprivation, some studies report partial sleep deprivation,[59] whereas

Table 1
Sleep fragmentation during non-rapid eye movement sleep in the first postpartum week (PPW) and second PPW during the light and dark phases

Brief Awakenings (*Episodes/h of NREM*)	First PPW/Light	First PPW/Dark	Second PPW/Light	Second PPW/Dark
Nursing	15.4 ± 2.2[a]	15.6 ± 3.5[a]	20.4 ± 1.9[a,b]	18.2 ± 3.5[a]
Outside of the nest	2.1 ± 1.3	2.1 ± 0.7	7.5 ± 2.0	3.0 ± 1.2

Data are presented as mean ± standard error and analyzed using a dependent *t*-test.
[a] Significant differences (P < .05) compared with outside the nest in the same phase.
[b] Significant difference compared with nursing during first PPW/light.
Adapted from ref[35].

others do not.[45,60] In nondepressed mothers, total sleep time is 7.8 hours at 8 weeks after giving birth,[61] 7.2 both between 4 and 10 weeks[60] and between 2 and 16 weeks.[62]

Most pronounced sleep disruptions are mainly found during the first weeks after giving birth,[59,63] continuing at 6 months.[64] However, the mother will still have sleep disruption until the baby manages to sleep through the night.[65]

Sleep is influenced by a complex interplay between psychosocial, physiologic, and environmental factors.[66] During the postpartum period, several factors would influence maternal sleep, including the age of the mother, parity, culture, and social environment.[65] Regarding the social environment, various findings show that the sleeping arrangements in the family context modify the quality of mothers' sleep; for example, the place where the child sleeps as well as the collaboration of another adult determines the mother's sleep.[66,67] However, the main sleep disturbances during the early stages of motherhood are caused by the frequency of feeding of the baby at night and the polycyclic sleep pattern of the newborn.[68] Thus, to understand when the mother returns to a "healthy" sleep pattern, we have to acknowledge the development of sleep during childhood.

Humans are born with a polycyclic sleep pattern and an undeveloped circadian rhythm.[69,70] Sleep consolidation (process often named "sleeping through the night"),[71,72] is the main sleep change during the first years of life, beginning at 2 to 3 months old with an important consolidation by the age of 6 months after birth.[73,74] Although at 12 months most babies have a more consolidated sleep[74] and are able to go back to sleep on their own for approximately half of their nocturnal awakenings,[75–77] not all children make it at that age.[71] In addition, different sleep disturbances may emerge, such as bedtime resistance and frequent nocturnal awakenings[78,79] which, although these alterations are reduced as the child grows, in many of them persist for a long time.[80,81] Sleep problems affect approximately more than 20% of preschool and school children,[80,81] which can vary according to the sample (20%–30% of children aged 1–3 years,[82–84] around 10% of children 4–5 years of age,[81,85] 25%–50% in preschool age children[86]), with the most frequent disturbances being due to frequent awakenings and the inability of children to go back to sleep without the help of an adult. These problems are associated with several consequences in children,[87] but they are also related to poor maternal health, and affecting the capability of the mother to sleep the entire night without interruptions.[88]

Consequences of sleep disturbances in human mothers

Regardless of how natural the sleep alterations during the postpartum period are, their consequences are similar to that found in different sleep pathologies.[57] Although sleep disturbances during the postpartum period are not considered a pathological condition,[68] several studies found an association of sleep fragmentation (or disruption) with daytime fatigue, from the first days up to 3 months after giving birth.[89–91] Also, using the psychomotor vigilance test, Insana and colleagues found that the neurobehavioral performance is decreased in first-time mothers compared with their partners and control women.[92] In addition, poor sleep quality increases mood disturbances at 36 months postpartum.[93] In the same direction, in mothers with poorer objective sleep continuity, both the ability to understand the signals of their infants[94] and their patience about the baby are reduced.[95] Furthermore, many articles report an association between depression and poor sleep due to maternity.[96,97] However, as sleep disturbances may be caused by depression itself, this association has been argued.[98] Interestingly, sleep disturbances during the early postpartum period may have a negative impact on human milk production.[99]

Natural mechanisms of mothers to cope with sleep disturbances and take appropriate care of the newborn

The most common advice to women with newborn babies is "taking a nap while the baby sleeps," to compensate for the lack of restorative nighttime sleep. Indeed, naps, but not nocturnal sleep, have been associated with better mother–infant interaction.[100] However, the opportunity of napping will be determined by several factors, such as the return to work and the care of other children at home, and so forth.[57] In addition, approximately half of the women do not nap, and the ones they do, they nap for about 30 minutes a day.[101] Another study show that less than 50% of the women napped at the third postpartum week, and only 25% to 35% of women took naps by the 11th week.[62] In addition, sleep is more restorative when sleep pressure and the circadian rhythm go together. Thus, maternal napping could help, to some extent, to cope with the deleterious consequences of sleep disturbances during nighttime,[57] but few mothers put it into practice.

Interestingly, mothers who breastfeed their babies have a significant increment in deep NREM sleep, and their light NREM sleep is reduced compared with control women and mothers that bottle-feed their babies, despite that both mothers experience sleep fragmentation.[45] Doan and colleagues also found a positive relationship between breastfeeding and sleep.[102] A possible explanation for these findings could be the highly elevated circulating levels of prolactin in lactating women, hormone that not only promotes milk synthesis but also promotes sleep.[45,103] All this could suggest that sleep in breastfeeding mothers is more efficient or more restorative. In this way, the human mother could partially adapt her sleep physiology to this new stage. Thus, the introduction of bottle feeding in many cultures would reduce the capability of the mother to deal with her sleep disturbances.

Above all, we hypothesized that the main mechanism that the mother has to cope with the lack of a full restorative sleep and still take care of her offspring is the highly rewarding value the newborn has for most mothers, which transcends her own physiology.

Sleep in Aquatic Mammals in the Postpartum Period

A peculiarity of the sleep of some aquatic mammals, in particular dolphins, is that they are able to sleep with one hemisphere of the brain and remain awake with the other, which allows them to continue swimming.[10] This behavior is invariably associated with the closure of the contralateral eye to the hemisphere with slow waves (the sleeping hemisphere), being able to remain with the other eye open, possibly to monitor the environment and thus avoiding predation or maintaining visual contact with members of its family group.[104] Unlike the terrestrial habitat, there are few safe places to sleep or rest in the ocean.[10] Thus, these animals are exceptional, being able to be asleep and stay alert at the same time.[105] These animals rest by remaining motionless both on the surface of the water and on the bottom, and most frequently they rest swimming.

In the case of mother dolphins, they and their calves remain practically without sleeping for the first few days after giving birth. The behavioral sleep pattern is different from that of a non-maternal adult and it is clearly diminished during the first and second months after giving birth in the mother and her calf; then, they gradually return to the normal daily sleep rhythms of a non-maternal adult. In these mothers, the behavior of resting on the surface disappears, and they remain with both eyes open during the postpartum period, without subsequently having an apparent rebound of this behavior. Possibly, this is an adaptive mechanism to the environment due to the lack of a safe place or nest for the newborn to avoid predation at the early stages of their development. Thus, the period when the mother sleeps represents a highly fragile moment for the newborn dolphin, apparently making sleep incompatible with the care of the calf.[105]

SUMMARY

Sleep during the postpartum period has been studied in very few species. In general, the main sleep disturbances during motherhood are determined by the constant care of the pups, the sleeping pattern and the feeding frequency of the progeny, and the characteristics of the environment. Similar to what has been described for human mothers, the type of environment, the social behavior, and the ability or possibility of creating a safe space for their offspring, will determine how the mother will sleep in other species. Although it has not been studied the general characteristics of sleep in the mother rabbit, as they nurse approximately once or twice a day,[106,107] it could be speculated that they probably would not have any sleep disturbances. Animals that raise their offspring in groups such as meerkats[108] might have the opportunity to sleep more. However, in the human or the rat, as the mother spends almost the entire day taking care of their pups during the early stages of the postpartum period, sleep disturbances are unavoidable. Although each species has developed different mechanisms to cope with whatever sleep disruption the mother might have, the lack of sleep continuity or sleep fragmentation that emerges during this stage will still have physiologic consequences.

CLINICS CARE POINTS

- Sleep disruptions are most commonly experienced in the initial weeks following childbirth persisting up to 6 months.
- Mothers often experience sleep disruptions until their babies are able to sleep through the night.
- Most sleep disturbances during the early stages of motherhood are caused by the frequency of feeding of the baby at night and the polycyclic sleep pattern of the newborn.
- The consequences of sleep disruptions during the postpartum period are similar to those observed in various sleep disorders.
- Poor sleep quality increases mood disturbances.
- Mothers who experience poorer objective sleep continuity often have reduced the ability to understand their infants' signals and exhibit lower levels of patience toward their babies.

DISCLOSURE

The authors declare that they have no known competing financial interests or personal relationships that could have appeared to influence the work reported in this article.

FUNDING

Partially financed by PEDECIBA.

REFERENCES

1. Vanderwolf CH. The role of the cerebral cortex and ascending activating systems in the control of behavior. In: Satinoff E, Teitelbaum P, editors. Handbook of behavioral Neurobiology: motivation. 1985. p. 67–104.
2. Stern JM. Maternal behavior: sensory, hormonal and neural determinants. In: Brush FR, Levine S, editors. Psychoendocrinology. New York: Academic Press; 1989. p. 103–226. chap 3.
3. Berridge KC. Motivation concepts in behavioral neuroscience. Physiology & behavior 2004;81(2): 179–209.
4. Aldrich M. Sleep Medicine. New York: Oxford University Press, Inc.; 1999.
5. Sotelo MI, Tyan J, Markunas C, et al. Lateral hypothalamic neuronal ensembles regulate pre-sleep nest-building behavior. Curr Biol 2022;32(4):806–822 e7.
6. Ellis C, Lemmens G, Parkes D. Pre-sleep behaviour in normal subjects. Journal of Sleep Research 1995;4(4):199–201.
7. Anderson JR. Sleep-related behavioural adaptations in free-ranging anthropoid primates. Sleep Med Rev 2000;4(4):355–73.
8. Philippens N, Janssen E, Kremers S, et al. Determinants of natural adult sleep: an umbrella review. PLoS One 2022;17(11):e0277323.
9. Siegel JM. Do all animals sleep? Review. Trends Neurosci 2008;31(4):208–13.
10. Siegel JM. Clues to the functions of mammalian sleep. Nature 2005;437(7063):1264–71.
11. Everson CA. Sustained sleep deprivation impairs host defense. American journal of physiology 1993;265(5 Pt 2):R1148–54.
12. Everson CA. Functional consequences of sustained sleep deprivation in the rat. Behav Brain Res 1995;69(1–2):43–54.
13. Everson CA, Bergmann BM, Rechtschaffen A. Sleep deprivation in the rat: III. Total sleep deprivation. Sleep 1989;12(1):13–21.
14. Everson CA, Laatsch CD, Hogg N. Antioxidant defense responses to sleep loss and sleep recovery. Am J Physiol Regul Integr Comp Physiol 2005; 288(2):R374–83.
15. Everson CA, Reed HL. Pituitary and peripheral thyroid hormone responses to thyrotropin-releasing hormone during sustained sleep deprivation in freely moving rats. Endocrinology 1995;136(4): 1426–34.
16. Everson CA, Szabo A. Repeated exposure to severely limited sleep results in distinctive and persistent physiological imbalances in rats. PLoS One 2011;6(8):e22987.
17. Brussaard AB, Herbison AE. Long-term plasticity of postsynaptic GABAA-receptor function in the adult brain: insights from the oxytocin neurone. Trends in Neurosciences 2000;23(5):190–5.
18. Spiegel K, Leproult R, Van Cauter E. [Impact of sleep debt on physiological rhythms]. Rev Neurol (Paris) 2003;159(11 Suppl):6S11, 20. Impact d'une dette de sommeil sur les rythmes physiologiques.
19. Wei R, Duan X, Guo L. Effects of sleep deprivation on coronary heart disease. Korean J Physiol Pharmacol 2022;26(5):297–305.
20. Rechtschaffen A, Gilliland MA, Bergmann BM, et al. Physiological correlates of prolonged sleep deprivation in rats. Science 1983;221(4606):182–4.
21. Borbély A. Sleep Homeostasis and models of sleep regulation. In: Kryger MH, Roth T, Dement WC, editors. Principles and practice of sleep Medicine. 5th edition. St. Louis, MO: Elsevier; 2011. p. 431–44. chap 37.
22. Sotelo MI, Tyan J, Dzera J, et al. Sleep and motivated behaviors, from physiology to pathology. Current Opinion in Physiology 2020;15:159–66.
23. Stern JM. Somatosensation and materna care in Norway rats. In: Rosenblatt JS, Snowdon CT, editors. Advances in the study of behavior, Parental care: Evolution, mechanisms, and adaptive significance. San Diego, CA: Academic Press; 1996. p. 243–94.
24. Wansaw MP, Pereira M, Morrell JI. Characterization of maternal motivation in the lactating rat: contrasts between early and late postpartum responses. Horm Behav 2008;54(2):294–301.
25. Wilsoncroft WE. Babies by bar-press: maternal behavior in the rat. Behav ResMeth& Instru 1969; 1(6):229–30.
26. Lee A, Clancy S, Fleming AS. Mother rats bar-press for pups: effects of lesions of the mpoa and limbic sites on maternal behavior and operant responding for pup-reinforcement. Behavioural Brain Research 1999;100(1–2):15–31.
27. Fleming AS, Korsmit M, Deller M. Rat pups are potent reinforcers to the maternal animal: effects of experience, parity, hormones, and dopamine function. Psychobiology 1994;22(1):44–53.
28. Hecht GS, Spear NE, Spear LP. Changes in progressive ratio responding for intravenous cocaine throughout the reproductive process in female rats. Developmental psychobiology 1999;35(2): 136–45.

29. Fahrbach SE, Pfaff DW. Hormonal and neural mechanisms underlying maternal behavior in the rat. In: Pfaff DW, editor. The physiological mechanisms of motivation. New York: Springer-Verlag; 1982. p. 253–85.
30. Pereira M, Morrell JI. The medial preoptic area is necessary for motivated choice of pup- over cocaine-associated environments by early postpartum rats. Neuroscience 2010;167(2):216–31.
31. Stern JM, Johnson SK. Ventral somatosensory determinants of nursing behavior in Norway rats. I. Effects of variations in the quality and quantity of pup stimuli. Physiology & Behavior 1990;47(5): 993–1011.
32. Stolzenberg DS, Champagne FA. Hormonal and non-hormonal bases of maternal behavior: the role of experience and epigenetic mechanisms. Horm Behav 2016;77:204–10.
33. Ferreira A, Agrati D, Uriarte N, et al. The rat as a model for studying maternal behavior. In: Arriaga-ramírez SEC-MaJCP. In: Behavioral animal Models. Kerala, India: Research Signpost; 2012.
34. Grota LJ, Ader R. Behavior of lactating rats in a dual-chambered maternity cage. Horm Behav 1974;5(4):275–82.
35. Benedetto L, Rivas M, Pereira M, et al. A descriptive analysis of sleep and wakefulness states during maternal behaviors in postpartum rats. Arch Ital Biol 2017;155(3):99–109.
36. Stern JM, Lonstein JS. Neural mediation of nursing and related maternal behaviors. Prog Brain Res 2001;133:263–78.
37. Haskell EH, Palca JW, Walker JM, et al. The effects of high and low ambient temperatures on human sleep stages. Electroencephalogr Clin Neurophysiol 1981;51(5):494–501.
38. Neckelmann D, Ursin R. Sleep stages and EEG power spectrum in relation to acoustical stimulus arousal threshold in the rat. Sleep 1993;16(5): 467–77.
39. Stern JM, Azzara AV. Thermal control of mother-young contact revisited: hyperthermic rats nurse normally. Physiology & Behavior 2002;77(1):11–8.
40. Neve HA, Paisley AC, Summerlee AJ. Arousal a prerequisite for suckling in the conscious rabbit? Physiology & Behavior 1982;28(2):213–7.
41. Poulain DA, Rodriguez F, Ellendorff F. Sleep is not a prerequisite for the milk ejection reflex in the pig. Exp Brain Res 1981;43(1):107–10.
42. Lincoln DW, Hentzen K, Hin T, et al. Sleep: a prerequisite for reflex milk ejection in the rat. Exp Brain Res 1980;38(2):151–62.
43. Sutherland RC, Juss TS, Wakerley JB. Prolonged electrical stimulation of the nipples evokes intermittent milk ejection in the anaesthetised lactating rat. Exp Brain Res 1987;66(1):29–34.
44. Voloschin LM, Tramezzani JH. Milk ejection reflex linked to slow wave sleep in nursing rats. Endocrinology 1979;105(5):1202–7.
45. Blyton DM, Sullivan CE, Edwards N. Lactation is associated with an increase in slow-wave sleep in women. Journal of sleep research 2002;11(4): 297–303.
46. Nishihara K, Horiuchi S, Eto H, et al. Delta and theta power spectra of night sleep EEG are higher in breast-feeding mothers than in non-pregnant women. Neurosci Lett 2004;368(2):216–20.
47. Peña F, Rivas M, Serantes D, et al. Is sleep critical for lactation in rat? Physiology & behavior 2022; 258:114011.
48. Pires GN, Bezerra AG, Tufik S, et al. Effects of experimental sleep deprivation on anxiety-like behavior in animal research: systematic review and meta-analysis. Neuroscience and biobehavioral reviews 2016;68:575–89.
49. Meerlo P, Koehl M, van der Borght K, et al. Sleep restriction alters the hypothalamic-pituitary-adrenal response to stress. Journal of neuroendocrinology 2002;14(5):397–402.
50. Mirescu C, Peters JD, Noiman L, et al. Sleep deprivation inhibits adult neurogenesis in the hippocampus by elevating glucocorticoids. Proceedings of the National Academy of Sciences of the United States of America 2006;103(50):19170–5.
51. Mallick BN, Chhina GS, Sundaram KR, et al. Activity of preoptic neurons during synchronization and desynchronization. Experimental Neurology 1983; 81(3):586–97.
52. Moruzzi G, Magoun HW. Brain stem reticular formation and activation of the EEG. Electroencephalogr Clin Neurophysiol 1949;1(4):455–73.
53. Oonk M, Krueger JM, Davis CJ. Voluntary sleep loss in rats. Sleep 2016;39(7):1467–79.
54. Sivadas N, Radhakrishnan A, Aswathy BS, et al. Dynamic changes in sleep pattern during postpartum in normal pregnancy in rat model. Behavioural brain research 2016;320:264–74.
55. Toth A, Petho M, Keseru D, et al. Complete sleep and local field potential analysis regarding estrus cycle, pregnancy, postpartum and post-weaning periods and homeostatic sleep regulation in female rats. Sci Rep 2020;10(1):8546.
56. Rocha L, Hoshino K. Some aspects of the sleep of lactating rat dams. Sleep Science (Sao Paulo, Brazil) 2009;2(2):88–91.
57. Stremler R, Sharkey K, Wolfson A. Postpartum Period and early motherhood. In: Kryger MH, Roth T, Dement WC, editors. Principles and practice of sleep Medicine. Philadelphia, PA: Elsevier; 2017. p. 1547–52. chap 158.
58. Lee KA. Alterations in sleep during pregnancy and postpartum: a review of 30 years of research. Sleep medicine reviews 1998;2(4):231–42.

59. Nishihara K, Horiuchi S. Changes in sleep patterns of young women from late pregnancy to postpartum: relationships to their infants' movements. Percept Mot Skills 1998;87(3 Pt 1):1043–56.
60. Thomas KA, Burr RL. Melatonin level and pattern in postpartum versus nonpregnant nulliparous women. J Obstet Gynecol Neonatal Nurs 2006; 35(5):608–15.
61. Dorheim SK, Bondevik GT, Eberhard-Gran M, et al. Subjective and objective sleep among depressed and non-depressed postnatal women. Acta Psychiatr Scand 2009;119(2):128–36.
62. Montgomery-Downs HE, Insana SP, Clegg-Kraynok MM, et al. Normative longitudinal maternal sleep: the first 4 postpartum months. Am J Obstet Gynecol 2010;203(5):465 e1–e7.
63. Signal TL, Gander PH, Sangalli MR, et al. Sleep duration and quality in healthy nulliparous and multiparous women across pregnancy and postpartum. Aust N Z J Obstet Gynaecol 2007;47(1): 16–22.
64. Wu J, Einerson B, Shaw JM, et al. Association between sleep quality and physical activity in postpartum women. Sleep Health 2019;5(6):598–605.
65. Stremler R, Wolfson A. The postpartum period. In: Kryger MH, Roth T, Dement WC, editors. Principles and practice of sleep Medicine. 5th edition. Canada: Elsevier; 2011. p. 1587–91. chap 139.
66. Volkovich E, Bar-Kalifa E, Meiri G, et al. Mother-infant sleep patterns and parental functioning of room-sharing and solitary-sleeping families: a longitudinal study from 3 to 18 months. Sleep 2018; 41(2). https://doi.org/10.1093/sleep/zsx207.
67. Mosko S, Richard C, McKenna J. Maternal sleep and arousals during bedsharing with infants. Sleep 1997;20(2):142–50.
68. Hunter LP, Rychnovsky JD, Yount SM. A selective review of maternal sleep characteristics in the postpartum period. J Obstet Gynecol Neonatal Nurs 2009;38(1):60–8.
69. Rudzik AEF, Ball HL. Biologically normal sleep in the mother-infant dyad. Am J Hum Biol 2021; 33(5):e23589.
70. Rivkees SA. Developing circadian rhythmicity in infants. Pediatr Endocrinol Rev 2003;1(1):38–45.
71. Pennestri MH, Laganiere C, Bouvette-Turcot AA, et al. Uninterrupted infant sleep, development, and maternal mood. Pediatrics 2018;142(6). https://doi.org/10.1542/peds.2017-4330.
72. Kalogeropoulos C, Burdayron R, Laganiere C, et al. Sleep patterns and intraindividual sleep variability in mothers and fathers at 6 months postpartum: a population-based, cross-sectional study. BMJ Open 2022;12(8):e060558.
73. Mindell JA, Leichman ES, Composto J, et al. Development of infant and toddler sleep patterns: real-world data from a mobile application. Journal of sleep research 2016;25(5):508–16.
74. Henderson JM, France KG, Blampied NM. The consolidation of infants' nocturnal sleep across the first year of life. Sleep Med Rev 2011;15(4): 211–20.
75. Burnham MM, Goodlin-Jones BL, Gaylor EE, et al. Nighttime sleep-wake patterns and self-soothing from birth to one year of age: a longitudinal intervention study. J Child Psychol Psychiatry 2002; 43(6):713–25.
76. Quin N, Tikotzky L, Stafford L, et al. Preventing postpartum insomnia by targeting maternal versus infant sleep: a protocol for a randomized controlled trial (the Study for Mother-Infant Sleep "SMILE"). Sleep Adv 2022;3(1):zpab020.
77. Tikotzky L, Bar-Shachar Y, Volkovich E, et al. A longitudinal study of the links between maternal and infant nocturnal wakefulness. Sleep Health 2022;8(1):31–8.
78. Field T. Infant sleep problems and interventions: a review. Infant Behav Dev 2017;47:40–53.
79. Kuhn BR, Elliott AJ. Treatment efficacy in behavioral pediatric sleep medicine. J Psychosom Res 2003;54(6):587–97.
80. Archbold KH, Pituch KJ, Panahi P, et al. Symptoms of sleep disturbances among children at two general pediatric clinics. Journal of Pediatrics 2002; 140(1):97–102.
81. Owens JA, Spirito A, McGuinn M, et al. Sleep habits and sleep disturbance in elementary school-aged children. J Dev Behav Pediatr 2000; 21(1):27–36.
82. Richman N, Stevenson JE, Graham PJ. Prevalence of behaviour problems in 3-year-old children: an epidemiological study in a London borough. J Child Psychol Psychiatry 1975;16(4): 277–87.
83. Richman N. A community survey of characteristics of one- to two- year-olds with sleep disruptions. J Am Acad Child Psychiatry 1981;20(2):281–91.
84. Ramchandani P, Wiggs L, Webb V, et al. A systematic review of treatments for settling problems and night waking in young children. BMJ 2000;320(7229):209–13.
85. Bax MC. Sleep disturbance in the young child. British medical journal 1980;280(6224):1177–9.
86. Anders TF, Eiben LA. Pediatric sleep disorders: a review of the past 10 years. J Am Acad Child Adolesc Psychiatry 1997;36(1):9–20.
87. Fallone G, Owens JA, Deane J. Sleepiness in children and adolescents: clinical implications. Sleep Med Rev 2002;6(4):287–306.
88. Boergers J, Hart C, Owens JA, et al. Child sleep disorders: associations with parental sleep duration and daytime sleepiness. J Fam Psychol 2007;21(1):88–94.

89. Lee KA, Zaffke ME. Longitudinal changes in fatigue and energy during pregnancy and the postpartum period. J Obstet Gynecol Neonatal Nurs. Mar-Apr 1999;28(2):183–91.
90. Rychnovsky J, Hunter LP. The relationship between sleep characteristics and fatigue in healthy postpartum women. Wom Health Issues 2009;19(1): 38–44.
91. Gay CL, Lee KA, Lee SY. Sleep patterns and fatigue in new mothers and fathers. Biol Res Nurs 2004;5(4):311–8.
92. Insana SP, Williams KB, Montgomery-Downs HE. Sleep disturbance and neurobehavioral performance among postpartum women. Sleep 2013; 36(1):73–81.
93. Wang G, Deng Y, Jiang Y, et al. Trajectories of sleep quality from late pregnancy to 36 months postpartum and association with maternal mood disturbances: a longitudinal and prospective cohort study. Sleep 2018;41(12). https://doi.org/10.1093/sleep/zsy179.
94. King LS, Rangel E, Simpson N, et al. Mothers' postpartum sleep disturbance is associated with the ability to sustain sensitivity toward infants. *Sleep medicine*. Jan 2020;65:74–83.
95. Ran-Peled D, Bar-Shachar Y, Horwitz A, et al. Objective and subjective sleep and caregiving feelings in mothers of infants: a longitudinal daily diary study. Sleep 2022;45(7). https://doi.org/10.1093/sleep/zsac090.
96. Huang CM, Carter PA, Guo JL. A comparison of sleep and daytime sleepiness in depressed and non-depressed mothers during the early postpartum period. J Nurs Res 2004;12(4):287–96.
97. Goyal D, Gay C, Lee K. Fragmented maternal sleep is more strongly correlated with depressive symptoms than infant temperament at three months postpartum. Arch Womens Ment Health 2009;12(4):229–37.
98. Ross LE, Murray BJ, Steiner M. Sleep and perinatal mood disorders: a critical review. J Psychiatry Neurosci 2005;30(4):247–56.
99. Carrega J, Lee SY, Clark P, et al. Impact of the quality of postpartum sleep and its health determinants on human milk volume. MCN Am J Matern Child Nurs Sep/2020;45(5):289–95.
100. Ronzio CR, Huntley E, Monaghan M. Postpartum mothers' napping and improved cognitive growth fostering of infants: results from a pilot study. Behav Sleep Med 2013;11(2):120–32.
101. Cottrell L, Karraker KH. Correlates of nap taking in mothers of young infants. Journal of sleep research 2002;11(3):209–12.
102. Doan T, Gardiner A, Gay CL, et al. Breast-feeding increases sleep duration of new parents. J Perinat Neonatal Nurs 2007;21(3):200–6.
103. Frieboes RM, Murck H, Stalla GK, et al. Enhanced slow wave sleep in patients with prolactinoma. The Journal of clinical endocrinology and metabolism 1998;83(8):2706–10.
104. Lilly J. Animals in aquatic environments: adaptations of mammals to the ocean. In: Dill D, editor. Handbook of physiology — environment. Washington, DC: American Physiology Society; 1964. p. 741–7.
105. Lyamin O, Pryaslova J, Kosenko P, et al. Behavioral aspects of sleep in bottlenose dolphin mothers and their calves. Physiology & behavior 2007;92(4): 725–33.
106. Zarrow MX, Denenberg VH, Anderson CO. Rabbit: frequency of suckling in the pup. Science 1965; 150(3705):1835–6.
107. Gonzalez-Mariscal G, Caba M, Martinez-Gomez M, et al. The rabbit as a model system in the study of mammalian maternal behavior and sibling interactions. Hormones and behavior 2016;77:30–41.
108. Clutton-Brock TH, Brotherton PN, O'Riain MJ, et al. Individual contributions to babysitting in a cooperative mongoose, Suricata suricatta. Proc Biol Sci 2000;267(1440):301–5.

Insomnia as a Risk Factor for Substance Use Disorders in Women

Laís F. Berro, PhD

KEYWORDS

• Insomnia • Substance use disorders • Women • Sleep • Addiction

KEY POINTS

- Insomnia is a highly prevalent sleep disorder, and its diagnostic criteria have changed in recent years to include a more specific set of nighttime and associated daytime symptoms.
- Insomnia and insufficient sleep predict and put individuals at a higher risk for substance use and associated psychosocial problems.
- Women show a higher prevalence of insomnia compared with men and also show a greater vulnerability to the effects of drugs of abuse.
- Insomnia shares several risk factors with substance use disorders, and women are disproportionally affected by many of those factors.
- Higher rates of insomnia among women may be a risk factor for substance use disorders.

INTRODUCTION

In recent years, the scientific field has taken huge steps toward better understanding sex and gender differences in a variety of health conditions. After decades of male-centric research, studies finally started demonstrating how women are differentially—and often, more severely—affected than men by many disorders. Even before the focus on sex as a biological variable, the field of psychiatry already suggested that women are more likely to be affected by some psychiatric disorders than men. However, the definition of "woman" has changed over the years to incorporate more up-to-date science on sex versus gender differences. This vocabulary has allowed us to better understand the differences between biology and environmental determinants, such as social roles and cultural factors, in psychiatric disorders. It is now commonly accepted that sex refers to biological determinants of male and female based on a person's reproductive organs determined by genetics, whereas gender is a person's self-identification as man or woman.[1]

The distinction between sex and gender is extremely important in psychiatry, especially for disorders that can be heavily influenced by environmental factors and personal experiences. Of note, gender differences have been shown for both insomnia and substance use disorders, with women more likely to have insomnia and showing increased susceptibility to the effects of drugs than men, despite social factors deterring drug use among women. Importantly, a growing body of evidence suggests that insufficient sleep predicts and puts individuals at a higher risk for substance use and associated psychosocial problems. However, the role of insomnia in substance use disorders among women remains poorly understood. The present article discusses gender differences in insomnia and in substance use disorders and reviews evidence suggesting

Department of Psychiatry and Human Behavior, University of Mississippi Medical Center, 2500 North State Street, Jackson, MS 39216, USA
E-mail address: lberro@umc.edu

Sleep Med Clin 18 (2023) 511–520
https://doi.org/10.1016/j.jsmc.2023.06.010
1556-407X/23/

that an increased prevalence of insomnia may be a risk factor for substance use disorders in women.

INSOMNIA: DIAGNOSIS AND PATHOPHYSIOLOGY

Every human has experienced what is commonly referred to as "insomnia," or being unable to fall or stay asleep at night, at least once in their lifetime. Globalization, busy lifestyles, and the advent of the "24/7 society" have contributed to a generation of insomniacs, with society going as far as to glamorize lack of sleep and associate sleeping with lack of productivity. Because of the growing prevalence of sleep and insomnia complaints in the general population, the medical field has seen a major change in the diagnostic criteria for insomnia in recent years. The 10th edition of the *International Classification of Diseases* (*ICD-10*), which went into effect in 1993[2] and was last updated in 2019, defined "nonorganic insomnia" as changes in sleep quantity and/or quality that persist for a "considerable period of time." The most recent version of this manual, the *ICD-11*,[3] which is now in effect as of January 2022, brings a much more detailed definition of this sleep disorder, with 2 subclassifications: short-term and chronic insomnia. Short-term insomnia is defined as difficulty initiating or maintaining sleep despite adequate opportunity for sleep, leading to sleep dissatisfaction and daytime impairment (eg, excessive daytime sleepiness, cognitive impairment), of less than 3 months' duration. Chronic insomnia, on the other hand, is defined when the sleep disturbance and associated daytime symptoms occur several times per week for at least 3 months. This new definition and subclassification not only brings to light the different ways in which insomnia can be experienced by an individual but also emphasizes the daytime consequences of this disorder, now a determinant symptom in its diagnosis. Based on its medical definition, insomnia is one of the most prevalent sleep disorders in the world, affecting 10% to 30% of the population, with a total estimated cost of $92.5 to $107.5 billion annually for the United States alone.[4–8]

The pathophysiology of insomnia has been studied extensively in humans. Available evidence indicates increased activity of the hypothalamic-pituitary-adrenal axis and of the autonomic nervous system in insomnia, as well as circadian process misalignment (changes in melatonin secretion) and dysfunction of the homoeostatic process (changes in extracellular adenosine levels[9]). Specific sleep- and electroencephalography (EEG)-related changes also have been reported in patients with insomnia, with reduced amounts of both slow-wave and rapid eye movement sleep[10] and increased EEG β power during non–rapid eye movement sleep in patients with insomnia.[9] The sleep of many patients with insomnia is also characterized by an increased frequency of brief events, such as shifts in sleep stages, brief periods of awakening, and microarousals,[11] indicating that changes in sleep-wake regulation at the neurochemical levels might also be affected in insomnia. Particularly, reduced GABA release and increased orexin activation at night have been proposed as neurobiological mechanisms underlying insomnia.[9,12]

Several studies also have investigated the negative consequences of chronic insomnia, including decreased quality of life, increased likelihood of accidents, decreased work productivity, and physical health consequences, such as diabetes and cardiovascular disease.[6,13] It is well known that sleep plays an integral role in health, and insufficient sleep—associated with insomnia or not—can have a negative impact on virtually every system in the body, with broad-ranging clinical and public health consequences. Importantly, although it is not as largely studied, a growing body of evidence indicates that lack of sleep predicts substance use and associated psychosocial problems and puts individuals at a higher risk for substance use disorders.

INSOMNIA AS A RISK FACTOR FOR SUBSTANCE USE DISORDERS

Substance use disorders represent an important—and growing—public health concern. The 2022 World Drug Report estimates that more than 350 million people worldwide use illicit drugs, with nearly 35 million people meeting diagnostic criteria for substance use disorders.[14] As defined by the *Diagnostic and Statistical Manual of Mental Disorders* (Fifth Edition) (*DSM-5*), substance use disorder is a chronic, relapsing disorder characterized by a set of symptoms that determine the recurrent use of alcohol and/or drugs leading to significant health and life consequences. Symptoms include tolerance to the drug effects, abstinence syndrome, increased drug use over time, persistent and unsuccessful attempts to discontinue or reduce drug use, spending increasing amounts of time to obtain the drug and/or recover from drug effects, reduced social and work-related activities in order to seek and/or use drugs, and continued drug use despite significant negative consequences associated with its use.[15] According to the World Health Organization, more than 180 thousand deaths were directly associated with substance use disorders in 2019.[16] Although drug use is high worldwide, with general increased rates of cannabis, amphetamines, opioids, and cocaine use in recent years, the type of drug most commonly used and available varies between different regions and countries.[14]

Many factors can contribute to initiation of and increased drug use, including adverse life experiences, psychiatric disorders, and socioeconomic and genetic factors.[17,18] However, one commonly neglected contributor to drug use and abuse is insufficient sleep. Several aspects of substance use and sleep impairment have prompted researchers to investigate relationships between these 2 factors.[19] For example, individuals using drugs often show a pattern of nocturnal drug taking owing to professional, academic, and/or social demands. Conversely, individuals with substance use disorders who present sleep problems are more likely to relapse during treatment.[20] Finally, and completing what likely is a vicious cycle, sleep impairment is frequent in individuals with substance use disorders, who are 5 to 10 times more likely to present with sleep problems than the general population.[21] In fact, most drugs of abuse impair sleep in all phases of addiction.[22–27] Given this striking and seemingly bidirectional interaction, it has become clear that neurobiological mechanisms seem to link sleep impairment and stimulant abuse, although the specific mechanisms are yet to be elucidated. In accordance with studies showing altered dopaminergic neuroplasticity following sleep deprivation,[28,29] the mesolimbic dopaminergic system has been proposed as the main pathway mediating drug-induced sleep impairment.[30]

In addition to the nocturnal pattern of drug use, the fact that sleep impairment predisposes relapse and that drug use and abuse can affect sleep quality, recent studies also suggest that poor sleep predicts substance use and associated psychosocial problems and puts individuals at a higher risk for substance use disorders. Initial evidence for this relationship was demonstrated in preclinical studies showing that sleep loss can potentiate many behaviors associated with the abuse-related effects of drugs of abuse. Studies in rodents show that sleep deprivation can potentiate the rewarding and locomotor stimulant effects of drugs,[31–34] as well as drug intake[35,36] and drug-seeking behavior.[37,38]

Clinically, most of the evidence linking insufficient sleep and a substance use disorder emerged from prospective clinical studies in children and adolescents investigating associations between sleep patterns at baseline and subsequent substance use. Childhood sleep problems during ages 3 to 5 years have been associated with early onset use of alcohol, cannabis, illicit drugs, and cigarettes.[39] Wong and colleagues[40] also studied a relationship between insufficient sleep and substance use in the National Longitudinal Study of Adolescent Health and showed that sleep difficulties and hours of sleep were significant predictors of substance-related problems in adolescents. Corroborating these findings, Pieters and colleagues[41] showed that sleep problems seem to be important predictors of substance use in adolescence. Specifically, inconsistent sleep-wake patterns and greater daytime sleepiness mediate increased lifetime use of all substances in adolescents.[42] Of note, difficulty sleeping during childhood predicts sleep problems during adolescence, which then increases the risk for drug-related problems in young adulthood.[43] In this latter study, the number of illicit drugs used and several alcohol-related problems in young adulthood was associated with increased childhood tiredness.[43]

A direct relationship between insomnia and risk for substance use also has been shown in both adolescents and adults.[44] Roane and Taylor[45] showed that adolescents with insomnia at baseline were more likely to use alcohol, cannabis, and other drugs during a 6- to 7-year follow up. An association between insomnia symptoms and problematic drug use also has been reported among university students.[46] In adults, an insomnia diagnosis has been associated with increased risk for next-year alcohol use,[47] as well as increased risk of illicit substance use disorder and nicotine dependence.[48] Insomnia also moderates drug-related problems in adults, including increased aggression associated with cocaine use[49] and alcohol-related consequences, such as public embarrassment, drinking on nights they had planned not to drink, and passing out from drinking.[50]

Together, these studies indicate that insufficient sleep is a major predictor of future substance use and related problems, with a direct association between insomnia and increased risk for drug use. Importantly, gender differences may play a major role in the relationship between insomnia and drug use. Although investigating gender differences in insomnia and substance use disorders may seem straightforward, many biological, psychological, cultural, and social factors can differentially contribute to the emergence of sleep problems and to drug use in women compared with men.

SEX DIFFERENCES IN INSOMNIA AND SUBSTANCE USE DISORDERS

Several potential risk factors have been identified in chronic insomnia, including gender and genetic factors,[51–53] and it is well established that insomnia complaints are most prevalent in women.[54,55] Gender differences in insomnia have been reported as early as in adolescence,[56] with a peak in insomnia symptoms among girls ages 11 to 12 years—likely associated with puberty.[57] In fact, a study by Johnson and colleagues[58] showed that this increased risk for insomnia in adolescent girls is only observed after onset of menstruation, when girls show a 2.75-fold increased risk for insomnia. In adults, epidemiologic studies show that as many as 48.6% of women present insomnia symptoms,[55] in addition to a higher prevalence of objective (polysomnography-based) insomnia in women compared with men.[8] According to Castro and colleagues,[8] an epidemiologic sleep study showed that 71.4% of participants who met *DSM-IV* criteria for insomnia diagnosis were women. A meta-analysis also confirmed a female predisposition for insomnia, showing that women are 1.5 times more likely to have insomnia than men.[59] In addition to gender, population-based studies show family history as a predisposing factor to insomnia,[60] indicating a potential role for genetic factors in the genesis and heritability of this sleep disorder. Several twin studies strongly suggest that genetic factors influence insomnia and account for approximately one-third of the variance in insomnia complaints,[61–63] with one study on 7500 male and female twins showing that women have a higher genetic risk of developing insomnia than men.[64]

Although it is very clearly established that being a woman increases the risk for developing insomnia, this association is not as clear when it comes to substance use disorders. Generally, men are more likely to use most drugs than women.[14] However, gender differences in drug use vary by region, by country, and by drug, which is likely associated with whether women have the opportunity to use drugs owing to accessibility, social factors preventing women from using drugs, and potential cultural barriers to drug use among women.[14] Nevertheless, women consistently outnumber men in both medical and nonmedical use of a specific class of drugs: sedatives and tranquilizers, such as benzodiazepines and benzodiazepine-type drugs.[14] The most recent World Drug Report showed an increase in the use of sedatives and tranquilizers in recent years, particularly among women.[14] Benzodiazepines and related drugs are commonly used for the treatment of anxiety and sleep disorders, being one of the most largely prescribed treatments for insomnia.[65] Therefore, the increased prevalence of insomnia, as well as anxiety disorders,[66] among women likely contributes to an increased prevalence of sedative/tranquilizer use in recent years. Women also show a high prevalence of nonmedical use of other pharmaceutical drugs, particularly opioids, surpassing men in some regions.[14] The misuse of prescription opioids is often associated with self-medication for pain, which is also highly prevalent among women,[67] and can contribute to—and be affected by—insomnia.[68]

Despite the fact that gender differences in rates of drug use are not consistent across drug classes, significant gender differences have been reported in drug use patterns and in the progression from drug use to substance use disorders. Of major importance, women show a faster progression from drug use to abuse. Studies show a more rapid progression to treatment admission for women who are dependent on opioids, cannabis, and alcohol, with women reporting more severe psychiatric and medical complications related to drug use than men.[69] Studies also show that women are less sensitive to the effects of some drugs,[70] which could contribute to higher drug intake, and develop drug-related brain damage more rapidly than men.[71] Westermeyer and Boedicker[72] reported that despite women using drugs for a shorter period of time compared with men, women and men had similar dependence rates, indicating that women may develop dependence faster. The interval between first-time drug use and treatment-seeking also seems to be shorter in women than men.[73]

Women with substance use disorders also have more difficulty quitting drug use and are more likely to relapse compared with men. Studies have shown that women are more likely than men to engage in heavy alcohol drinking to deal with unpleasant emotions.[74] Considering that preoccupation/anticipation is one of the final stages of substance use disorders, leading to relapse, this coping mechanism, combined with increased craving among women,[75] might put women at a higher risk for relapse.[76] Enhanced craving and relapse risk in women also have been reported for opioids, psychostimulants, and nicotine.[76] Nevertheless, despite higher relapse rates, women are generally underrepresented when it comes to treatment of substance use disorders.[14] Studies suggest that several factors contribute to decreased treatment seeking among women, including fear of legal repercussions, such as losing child custody, in addition to social and cultural factors, such as increased stigma and heavier household responsibilities placed on women.[14,77] Consequently, women with substance use disorders are more likely to be living with HIV and hepatitis C[78] and show higher mortalities compared with men.[79]

Several factors can contribute to increased vulnerability to insomnia and substance use disorders in women. Importantly, many of these risk factors are common between the 2 disorders. Specifically, regarding sex differences, studies have shown a role for sex hormones in insomnia and substance use disorders. Female sex hormones, including luteinizing hormone and progesterone, can alter circadian rhythms and disrupt sleep.[80] On the other hand, higher endogenous estrogen levels are associated with better sleep in women,[81] although the effects of estrogen on sleep may depend on the menstrual cycle phase.[80] In fact, insomnia is highly prevalent among women undergoing menopause,[82,83] when ovarian hormone production decreases, and hormone therapy with estrogen improves sleep in postmenopausal women.[84] Estrogen also has been shown to contribute to the increased vulnerability to substance use disorders in women,[85] with greater subjective effects of drugs experienced during high-estrogen and low-progesterone levels.[86] It is important to note, however, that changes in reproductive hormones can only explain the biological role of sex in disease, but not gender differences. This is an important distinction considering that both insomnia and substance use disorders can be influenced by psychological, environmental, and social factors, which emphasize that sex differences alone cannot explain the increased vulnerability to these disorders in women and their relationship.

Psychological risk factors common to both insomnia and substance use disorders include anxiety, depression, and stress.[48,87–90] Insomnia is highly comorbid with other psychiatric disorders, with studies showing that individuals with 2 psychiatric disorders are 2.2 to 3.2 times more likely to have sleep problems, a rate that increases to 4.6 to 6.3 times for individuals with 3 or more psychiatric disorders.[91] In fact, psychiatric comorbidities seem to mediate the interaction between insomnia and substance use disorders. In patients with comorbid anxiety and substance use disorders, anxiety sensitivity was associated with symptoms of insomnia.[92] Anxiety symptoms seem to mediate insomnia induced by emotional dysregulation in patients with alcohol use disorder.[93] A social anxiety disorder diagnosis has been associated with an increased likelihood of both alcohol use disorder and insomnia diagnosis, with insomnia contributing to the interaction between anxiety and alcohol use disorder.[94] Sleep also has been shown as a significant mediator between psychiatric symptoms (anxiety and depression) and drug use in epidemiologic studies.[95] Of note, anxiety and depression are more prevalent in women,[66,96] and women are also more vulnerable to the effects of stress than men.[97] Therefore, an increased prevalence of psychiatric risk factors for both insomnia and substance use disorders would place women at a higher risk for the development of these disorders.

Importantly, socioeconomic factors also contribute to both insomnia and substance use disorders. Studies show that a low socioeconomic status is a strong predictor of short sleep duration, with insomnia being more frequent among those with lower income and lower educational levels.[98,99] Low income and education and exposure to poverty during childhood also are risk factors for the development of substance use disorders.[100,101] Of note, a study by Abreu and colleagues[102] showed that lower family income, insomnia symptoms, and long working hours were associated with an increased likelihood of substance use among truck drivers. Therefore, socioeconomic factors may mediate the relationship between insomnia and drug use, although further research is needed to investigate this relationship. Regarding gender differences, it is well known that women generally show lower education attainment and lower income regardless of education compared with men,[103] which could contribute to gender differences in insomnia and substance use disorders. Importantly, black women are disproportionally affected by the influence of socioeconomic factors in sleep[104,105] and drug use.[106]

Importantly, biological, psychiatric, and socioeconomic risk factors may interact to mediate the relationship between insomnia and substance use disorders. In a recent study, Marees and colleagues[107] showed that high alcohol consumption quantity was genetically associated with low socioeconomic status and high risk of substance use disorders and other psychiatric disorders, including insomnia. A convergent model also showed that sleep quality, psychiatric symptoms (anxiety and depression), and socioeconomic factors interacted to mediate risk for tobacco consumption in an epidemiologic sleep study.[95] Although no studies to date have investigated gender differences specifically in these interactions, it seems clear that the relationship between insomnia and substance use disorders is multifactorial and involves factors that generally pose women at a higher risk for the development of substance use disorders.

DISCUSSION: INSOMNIA AS A RISK FACTOR FOR SUBSTANCE USE DISORDERS IN WOMEN

Over the last century, an increase in the number of women participating in the economy and working outside the home has been seen. With an increased presence of women in the labor force, women have had to adjust to managing a work-life balance to juggle their professional and personal lives. Oftentimes, women sacrifice their sleep to keep up with their many chores and responsibilities, which has led to a generation of women with insomnia. In fact, work characteristics and family responsibilities play a major role in the gender differences observed in insomnia, contributing to an increased prevalence of insomnia in women.[108–110]

Of note, this increase in the number of women reporting insufficient sleep has been accompanied by a narrowing in the gender gap in substance use disorders.[111] Importantly, an increase in the prevalence of substance use disorders among women also seems to be associated with the increased presence and importance of women in contemporary society. Lack of access to drugs, less opportunities for substance use, and negative attitudes toward the appropriateness of substance use represented the main barriers for drug use among women.[112–114] However, with a growth in the movement for gender equality, an increase in the prevalence of substance use disorders among women has also been seen.

This concomitant increase in the prevalence of insomnia and substance use disorders poses the possibility that insomnia may be a potential unique risk factor for substance use disorders among women. A causal relationship is difficult to determine, especially considering that both disorders have multiple contributing factors that also mediate each other. However, as reviewed in this article, several of the risk factors for insomnia are common to substance use disorders, with many affecting women disproportionally. Also, a growing body of evidence shows that insomnia and insufficient sleep predict and put individuals at a higher risk for substance use and associated psychosocial problems. Importantly, gender differences in insomnia emerge during adolescence,[56,57] emphasizing the importance of focusing on sleep promotion during prevention and early intervention strategies to reduce the impact of substance use.

SUMMARY

Gender differences exist for both insomnia and substance use disorders. Women show a higher prevalence of insomnia and increased susceptibility to the effects of drugs than men. Importantly, a growing body of evidence suggests that insufficient sleep predicts and puts individuals at a higher risk for substance use and associated psychosocial problems. The current literature suggests that an increased prevalence of insomnia may be a risk factor for substance use disorders in women. Many risk factors are common between insomnia and substance use disorders, including psychiatric disorders (anxiety, depression) and low socioeconomic status, and disproportionally affect women. Considering that gender differences in insomnia emerge as early as during adolescence, prevention and early intervention strategies to reduce the impact of substance use should focus on sleep promotion and education among teenagers and young adults.

CLINICS CARE POINTS

- Women show a higher prevalence of insomnia than men.
- Men show a higher prevalence of substance use disorders for most drugs of abuse compared with women; however, this gap is narrowing in recent years.
- Women may show a "telescoping" effect, presenting a faster progression from initial substance use to substance use disorder/dependence compared with men.
- Insufficient sleep and insomnia can predispose a patient to developing substance use disorders.
- Several risk factors are common between insomnia and substance use disorders, including psychiatric disorders (anxiety, depression) and low socioeconomic status.
- Those risk factors disproportionally affect women, posing them at a higher risk for insomnia and—consequently—substance use disorders.

DISCLOSURE

The author has nothing to disclose.

ACKNOWLEDGMENTS

Dr Berro is supported by the National Institutes of Health, United States (DA049886).

REFERENCES

1. Pinn VW. Sex and gender factors in medical studies: implications for health and clinical practice. JAMA 2003;289:397–400.
2. World Health Organization (WHO). The ICD-10 classification of mental and behavioural disorders. World Health Organization; 1993.

3. World Health Organization (WHO). International Classification of Diseases, Eleventh Revision (ICD-11), 2019/2021 Available at: https://icd.who.int/browse11. Accessed December 01, 2022.
4. Stoller MK. Economic effects of insomnia. Clin Ther 1994;16:873–97.
5. Ringdahl EN, Pereira SL, Delzell JE Jr. Treatment of primary insomnia. J Am Board Fam Pract 2004;17:212–9.
6. Roth T. Insomnia: definition, prevalence, etiology, and consequences. J Clin Sleep Med 2007;3(5 Suppl):S7–10.
7. Mack LJ, Rybarczyk BD. Behavioral treatment of insomnia: a proposal for a stepped-care approach to promote public health. Nat Sci Sleep 2011;3:87–99.
8. Castro LS, Poyares D, Leger D, et al. Objective prevalence of insomnia in the São Paulo, Brazil epidemiologic sleep study. Ann Neurol 2013;74:537–46.
9. Riemann D, Nissen C, Palagini L, et al. The neurobiology, investigation, and treatment of chronic insomnia. Lancet Neurol 2015;14:547–58.
10. Baglioni C, Regen W, Teghen A, et al. Sleep changes in the disorder of insomnia: a meta-analysis of polysomnographic studies. Sleep Med Rev 2014;18:195–213.
11. Feige B, Al-Shajlawi A, Nissen C, et al. Does REM sleep contribute to subjective wake time in primary insomnia? A comparison of polysomnographic and subjective sleep in 100 patients. J Sleep Res 2008; 17:180–90.
12. Krystal AD, Benca RM, Kilduff TS. Understanding the sleep-wake cycle: sleep, insomnia, and the orexin system. J Clin Psychiatry 2013;74(Suppl 1):3–20.
13. Jarrin DC, Alvaro PK, Bouchard MA, et al. Insomnia and hypertension: a systematic review. Sleep Med Rev 2018;41:3–38.
14. United Nations Office on Drugs and Crime (UNODC). World Drug Report 2022 (United Nations publication, 2022). Available at: https://www.unodc.org/unodc/en/data-and-analysis/world-drug-report-2022.html. Accessed December 01, 2022.
15. American Psychiatric Association. (2022). Diagnostic and statistical manual of mental disorders (5th ed., text rev.). https://doi.org/10.1176/appi.books.9780890425787. Accessed December 01, 2022.
16. Global Health Estimates. Deaths by cause, age, sex, by country and by region, 2000-2019. Geneva: World Health Organization; 2020.
17. Meyers JL, Dick DM. Genetic and environmental risk factors for adolescent-onset substance use disorders. Child Adolesc Psychiatr Clin N Am 2010;19:465–77.
18. Christensen H, Low LF, Anstey KJ. Prevalence, risk factors and treatment for substance abuse in older adults. Curr Opin Psychiatry 2006;19:587–92.
19. Berro LF, Howell LL, Tufik S, et al. Sleep and drug abuse. In: Preedy Victor R, editor. Neuropathology of drug addictions and substance misuse, 3. San Diego: Academic Press (Elsevier); 2016. p. 58–65.
20. Brooks AT, Kazmi N, Yang L, et al. Sleep-related cognitive/behavioral predictors of sleep quality and relapse in individuals with alcohol use disorder. Int J Behav Med 2021;28:73–82.
21. Mahfoud Y, Talih F, Streem D, et al. Sleep disorders in substance abusers: how common are they? Psychiatry (Edgmont) 2009;6:38–42.
22. Berro LF, Andersen ML, Tufik S, et al. Actigraphy-based sleep parameters during the reinstatement of methamphetamine self-administration in rhesus monkeys. Exp Clin Psychopharmacol 2016;24:142–6.
23. Berro LF, Andersen ML, Howell LL. Assessment of tolerance to the effects of methamphetamine on daytime and nighttime activity evaluated with actigraphy in rhesus monkeys. Psychopharmacology (Berl) 2017;234:2277–87.
24. Berro LF, Overton JS, Rowlett JK. Methamphetamine-induced sleep impairments and subsequent slow-wave and rapid eye movement sleep rebound in male rhesus monkeys. Front Neurosci 2022;16:866971.
25. Berro LF, Zamarripa CA, Talley JT, et al. Effects of methadone, buprenorphine, and naltrexone on actigraphy-based sleep-like parameters in male rhesus monkeys. Addict Behav 2022;135:107433.
26. Herrmann ES, Johnson PS, Bruner NR, et al. Morning administration of oral methamphetamine dose-dependently disrupts nighttime sleep in recreational stimulant users. Drug Alcohol Depend 2017;178:291–5.
27. Roehrs T, Sibai M, Roth T. Sleep and alertness disturbance and substance use disorders: a bi-directional relation. Pharmacol Biochem Behav 2021;203:173153.
28. Volkow ND, Tomasi D, Wang GJ, et al. Evidence that sleep deprivation downregulates dopamine D2R in ventral striatum in the human brain. J Neurosci 2012;32(19):6711–7.
29. Wiers CE, Shumay E, Cabrera E, et al. Reduced sleep duration mediates decreases in striatal D2/D3 receptor availability in cocaine abusers. Transl Psychiatry 2016;6:e752.
30. Vrajová M, Šlamberová R, Hoschl C, et al. Methamphetamine and sleep impairments: neurobehavioral correlates and molecular mechanisms. Sleep 2021;44:zsab001.
31. Berro LF, Hollais AW, Patti CL, et al. Sleep deprivation impairs the extinction of cocaine-induced environmental conditioning in mice. Pharmacol Biochem Behav 2014;124:13–8.
32. Berro LF, Tufik SB, Frussa-Filho R, et al. Sleep deprivation precipitates the development of

amphetamine-induced conditioned place preference in rats. Neurosci Lett 2018;671:29–32.
33. Saito LP, Fukushiro DF, Hollais AW, et al. Acute total sleep deprivation potentiates amphetamine-induced locomotor-stimulant effects and behavioral sensitization in mice. Pharmacol Biochem Behav 2014;117:7–16.
34. Berro LF, Santos R, Hollais AW, et al. Acute total sleep deprivation potentiates cocaine-induced hyperlocomotion in mice. Neurosci Lett 2014;579:130–3.
35. Puhl MD, Fang J, Grigson PS. Acute sleep deprivation increases the rate and efficiency of cocaine self-administration, but not the perceived value of cocaine reward in rats. Pharmacol Biochem Behav 2009;94:262–70.
36. García-García F, Priego-Fernández S, López-Muciño LA, et al. Increased alcohol consumption in sleep-restricted rats is mediated by delta FosB induction. Alcohol 2021;93:63–70.
37. Reeves-Darby JA, Berro LF, Rowlett JK, et al. Enhancement of cue-induced reinstatement of alcohol seeking by acute total sleep restriction in male Wistar rats. Pharmacol Biochem Behav 2021;205:173188.
38. Shahveisi K, Abdoli N, Farnia V, et al. REM sleep deprivation before extinction or reinstatement alters methamphetamine reward memory via D1-like dopamine receptors. Pharmacol Biochem Behav 2022;213:173319.
39. Wong MM, Brower KJ, Fitzgerald HE, et al. Sleep problems in early childhood and early onset of alcohol and other drug use in adolescence. Alcoholism: Clinical and Experimental Research 2004;28:578–87.
40. Wong MM, Robertson GC, Dyson RB. Prospective relationship between poor sleep and substance-related problems in a national sample of adolescents. Alcohol Clin Exp Res 2015;39:355–62.
41. Pieters S, Burk WJ, Van der Vorst H, et al. Prospective relationships between sleep problems and substance use, internalizing and externalizing problems. J Youth Adolesc 2015;44:379–88.
42. Nguyen-Louie TT, Brumback T, Worley MJ, et al. Effects of sleep on substance use in adolescents: a longitudinal perspective. Addict Biol 2018;23:750–60.
43. Wong MM, Brower KJ, Nigg JT, et al. Childhood sleep problems, response inhibition, and alcohol and drug outcomes in adolescence and young adulthood. Alcoholism: Clinical and Experimental Research 2010;34:1033–44.
44. Short NA, Austin AE, Naumann RB. Associations between insomnia symptoms and prescription opioid and benzodiazepine misuse in a nationally representative sample. Addict Behav 2023;137:107507.
45. Roane BM, Taylor DJ. Adolescent insomnia as a risk factor for early adult depression and substance abuse. Sleep: Journal of Sleep and Sleep Disorders Research 2008;31:1351–6.
46. Navarro-Martínez R, Chover-Sierra E, Colomer-Pérez N, et al. Sleep quality and its association with substance abuse among university students. Clin Neurol Neurosurg 2020;188:105591.
47. Weissman MM, Greenwald S, Nino-Murcia G, et al. The morbidity of insomnia uncomplicated by psychiatric disorders. General Hospital Psychiatry 1997;19:245–50.
48. Breslau N, Roth T, Rosenthal L, et al. Sleep disturbance and psychiatric disorders: a longitudinal epidemiological study of young adults. Biological Psychiatry 1996;39:411–8.
49. Sexton MB, Dawson S, Spencer RJ, et al. Relationships between insomnia and alcohol and cocaine use frequency with aggression among veterans engaged in substance use treatment. Sleep Med 2021;83:182–7.
50. Miller MB, DiBello AM, Carey KB, et al. Insomnia moderates the association between alcohol use and consequences among young adult veterans. Addict Behav 2017;75:59–63.
51. Klink ME, Quan SF, Kaltenborn WT, et al. Risk factors associated with complaints of insomnia in a general adult population. Influence of previous complaints of insomnia. Arch Intern Med 1992;152:1634–7.
52. Foley D, Ancoli-Israel S, Britz P, et al. Sleep disturbances and chronic disease in older adults: results of the 2003 National Sleep Foundation Sleep in America Survey. J Psychosom Res 2004;56:497–502.
53. Morin CM, LeBlanc M, Daley M, et al. Epidemiology of insomnia: prevalence, self-help treatments, consultations, and determinants of help-seeking behaviors. Sleep Med 2006;7:123–30.
54. Hilty D, Young JS, Bourgeois JA, et al. Algorithms for the assessment and management of insomnia in primary care. Patient Prefer Adherence 2009;3:9–20.
55. Lucena L, Polesel DN, Poyares D, et al. The association of insomnia and quality of life: Sao Paulo epidemiologic sleep study (EPISONO). Sleep Health 2020;6:629–35.
56. Blank M, Zhang J, Lamers F, et al. Health correlates of insomnia symptoms and comorbid mental disorders in a nationally representative sample of US adolescents. Sleep 2015;38:197–204.
57. Calhoun SL, Fernandez-Mendoza J, Vgontzas AN, et al. Prevalence of insomnia symptoms in a general population sample of young children and preadolescents: gender effects. Sleep Med 2014;15:91–5.
58. Johnson EO, Roth T, Schultz L, et al. Epidemiology of DSM-IV insomnia in adolescence: lifetime

prevalence, chronicity, and an emergent gender difference. Pediatrics 2006;117:e247–56.
59. Zhang B, Wing YK. Sex differences in insomnia: a meta-analysis. Sleep 2006;29:85–93.
60. Beaulieu-Bonneau S, LeBlanc M, Mérette C, et al. Family history of insomnia in a population-based sample. Sleep 2007;30:1739–45.
61. Heath AC, Kendler KS, Eaves LJ, et al. Evidence for genetic influences on sleep disturbance and sleep pattern in twins. Sleep 1990;13:318–35.
62. McCarren M, Goldberg J, Ramakrishnan V, et al. Insomnia in Vietnam era veteran twins: influence of genes and combat experience. Sleep 1994;17:456–61.
63. Watson NF, Goldberg J, Arguelles L, et al. Genetic and environmental influences on insomnia, daytime sleepiness, and obesity in twins. Sleep 2006;29:645–9.
64. Lind MJ, Aggen SH, Kirkpatrick RM, et al. A longitudinal twin study of insomnia symptoms in adults. Sleep 2015;38:1423–30.
65. Atkin T, Comai S, Gobbi G. Drugs for insomnia beyond benzodiazepines: Pharmacology, clinical applications, and discovery. Pharmacol Rev 2018;70:197–245.
66. Asher M, Asnaani A, Aderka IM. Gender differences in social anxiety disorder: a review. Clin Psychol Rev 2017;56:1–12.
67. Mogil JS, Bailey AL. Sex and gender differences in pain and analgesia. Prog Brain Res 2010;186:141–57.
68. Haack M, Simpson N, Sethna N, et al. Sleep deficiency and chronic pain: potential underlying mechanisms and clinical implications. Neuropsychopharmacology 2020;45:205–16.
69. Hernandez-Avila CA, Rounsaville BJ, Kranzler HR. Opioid-, cannabis- and alcohol-dependent women show more rapid progression to substance abuse treatment. Drug and Alcohol Dependence 2004;74:265–72.
70. Lynch WJ, Roth ME, Carroll ME. Biological basis of sex differences in drug abuse: preclinical and clinical studies. Psychopharmacology (Berl) 2002;164:121–37.
71. Mann K, Ackermann K, Croissant B, et al. Neuroimaging of gender differences in alcohol dependence: are women more vulnerable? Alcoholism: Clinical & Experimental Research 2005;29:896–901.
72. Westermeyer J, Boedicker AE. Course, severity, and treatment of substance abuse among women versus men. Am J Drug Alcohol Abuse 2000;26:523–35.
73. Brady KT, Randall CL. Gender differences in substance use disorders. Psychiatr Clin North Am 1999;22:241–52.
74. Lau-Barraco C, Skewes MC, Stasiewicz PR. Gender differences in high-risk situations for drinking: are they mediated by depressive symptoms? Addict Behav 2009;34:68–74.
75. Boykoff N, Schneekloth TD, Hall-Flavin D, et al. Gender differences in the relationship between depressive symptoms and cravings in alcoholism. Am J Addict 2010;19:352–6.
76. Riley AL, Hempel BJ, Clasen MM. Sex as a biological variable: drug use and abuse. Physiol Behav 2018;187:79–96.
77. United Nations Office on Drugs and Crime (UNODC). World drug Report 2021, booklet 2, global overview: drug demand, drug supply., 2021, 2. https://www.unodc.org/unodc/en/data-and-analysis/wdr2021.html
78. United Nations Programme on HIV/AIDS (UNAIDS). Women Who Inject Drugs More Likely to Be Living with HIV, Based on Data from Global AIDS Monitoring 2103–2017. 2019. https://www.unaids.org/en/resources/presscentre/featurestories/2019/june/20190611_women-who-inject-drugs
79. European Monitoring Centre for Drugs and Drug Addiction (EMCDDA). Mortality among drug users in Europe: new and old challenges for public health. Luxembourg: Publications Office of the European Union; 2015.
80. Nowakowski S, Meers J, Heimbach E. Sleep and women's health. Sleep Med Res 2013;4:1–22.
81. Morssinkhof MWL, van Wylick DW, Priester-Vink S, et al. Associations between sex hormones, sleep problems and depression: a systematic review. Neurosci Biobehav Rev 2020;118:669–80.
82. Hachul H, Castro LS, Bezerra AG, et al. Hot flashes, insomnia, and the reproductive stages: a cross-sectional observation of women from the EPISONO study. J Clin Sleep Med 2021;17:2257–67.
83. Hachul CH, Brandão LC, D 'Almeida V, et al. Sleep disturbances, oxidative stress and cardiovascular risk parameters in postmenopausal women complaining of insomnia. Climacteric 2006;9:312–9.
84. Rossouw JE, Anderson GL, Prentice RL, et al. Risks and benefits of estrogen plus progestogen in healthy postmenopausal women: principal results from the Women's Health Initiative randomized controlled trial. JAMA 2002;288:321–33.
85. Harp SJ, Martini M, Lynch WJ, et al. Sexual differentiation and substance use: a mini-review. Endocrinology 2020;161:bqaa129.
86. Justice AJ, de Wit H. Acute effects of d-amphetamine during the follicular and luteal phases of the menstrual cycle in women. Psychopharmacology (Berl) 1999;145:67–75.
87. Kotov R, Gamez W, Schmidt F, et al. Linking "big" personality traits to anxiety, depressive, and substance use disorders: a meta-analysis. Psychol Bull 2010;136:768–821.
88. Cox RC, Olatunji BO. A systematic review of sleep disturbance in anxiety and related disorders. Journal of Anxiety Disorders 2016;37:104–29.

89. Gao W, Ping S, Liu X. Gender differences in depression, anxiety, and stress among college students: a longitudinal study from China. J Affect Disord 2020;263:292–300.
90. Jansson-Frojmark M, Lindblom K. A bidirectional relationship between anxiety and depression, and insomnia? A prospective study in the general population. Journal of Psychosomatic Research 2008; 64:443–9.
91. Roth T, Jaeger S, Jin R, et al. Sleep problems, comorbid mental disorders, and role functioning in the national comorbidity survey replication. Biol Psychiatry 2006;60:1364–71.
92. Dixon LJ, Lee AA, Gratz KL, et al. Anxiety sensitivity and sleep disturbance: investigating associations among patients with co-occurring anxiety and substance use disorders. J Anxiety Disord 2018; 53:9–15.
93. Wołyńczyk-Gmaj D, Jakubczyk A, Trucco EM, et al. Emotional dysregulation, anxiety symptoms and insomnia in individuals with alcohol use disorder. Int J Environ Res Public Health 2022;19:2700.
94. Blumenthal H, Taylor DJ, Cloutier RM, et al. The links between social anxiety disorder, insomnia symptoms, and alcohol use disorders: findings from a large sample of adolescents in the United States. Behav Ther 2019;50:50–9.
95. Dokkedal-Silva V, Fernandes GL, Morelhão PK, et al. Sleep, psychiatric and socioeconomic factors associated with substance use in a large population sample: a cross-sectional study. Pharmacol Biochem Behav 2021;210:173274.
96. Piccinelli M, Wilkinson G. Gender differences in depression. Critical review. Br J Psychiatry 2000; 177:486–92.
97. Swaab DF, Bao AM. Sex differences in stress-related disorders: major depressive disorder, bipolar disorder, and posttraumatic stress disorder. Handb Clin Neurol 2020;175:335–58.
98. Bixler E. Sleep and society: an epidemiological perspective. Sleep Med 2009;10:S3–6.
99. Gellis LA, Lichstein KL, Scarinci IC, et al. Socioeconomic status and insomnia. J Abnorm Psychol 2005;114:111–8.
100. Patrick ME, Wightman P, Schoeni RF, et al. Socioeconomic status and substance use among young adults: a comparison across constructs and drugs. J Stud Alcohol Drugs 2012;73:772–82.
101. Manhica H, Straatmann VS, Lundin A, et al. Association between poverty exposure during childhood and adolescence, and drug use disorders and drug-related crimes later in life. Addiction 2021; 116:1747–56.
102. Abreu AMM, Costa RMFD, Jomar RT, et al. Factors associated with psychoactive substance use among professional truck drivers. Rev Bras Enferm 2022;75:e20210187.
103. Budig MJ, Lim M, Hodges MJ. Racial and gender pay disparities: the role of education. Soc Sci Res 2021;98:102580.
104. Amyx M, Xiong X, Xie Y, et al. Racial/ethnic differences in sleep disorders and reporting of trouble sleeping among women of childbearing age in the United States. Matern Child Health J 2017;21: 306–14.
105. Jackson CL, Ward JB, Johnson DA, et al. Concordance between self-reported and actigraphy-assessed sleep duration among African-American adults: findings from the Jackson Heart Sleep Study. Sleep 2020;43:zsz246.
106. McCabe SE, Morales M, Cranford JA, et al. Race/ethnicity and gender differences in drug use and abuse among college students. J Ethn Subst Abuse 2007;6:75–95.
107. Marees AT, Smit DJA, Ong JS, et al. Potential influence of socioeconomic status on genetic correlations between alcohol consumption measures and mental health. Psychol Med 2020;50:484–98.
108. Sekine M, Chandola T, Martikainen P, et al. Work and family characteristics as determinants of socioeconomic and sex inequalities in sleep: the Japanese Civil Servants Study. Sleep 2006;29:206–16.
109. Yoshioka E, Saijo Y, Kita T, et al. Gender differences in insomnia and the role of paid work and family responsibilities. Soc Psychiatry Psychiatr Epidemiol 2012;47:651–62.
110. Doi Y, Minowa M. Gender differences in excessive daytime sleepiness among Japanese workers. Soc Sci Med 2003;56:883–94.
111. McHugh RK, Votaw VR, Sugarman DE, et al. Sex and gender differences in substance use disorders. Clin Psychol Rev 2018;66:12–23.
112. Caris L, Wagner FA, Ríos-Bedoya CF, et al. Opportunities to use drugs and stages of drug involvement outside the United States: evidence from the Republic of Chile. Drug Alcohol Depend 2009;102:30–4.
113. Delva J, Van Etten ML, González GB, et al. First opportunities to try drugs and the transition to first drug use: evidence from a national school survey in Panama. Subst Use Misuse 1999;34:1451–67.
114. Van Etten ML, Anthony JC. Comparative epidemiology of initial drug opportunities and transitions to first use: marijuana, cocaine, hallucinogens and heroin. Drug Alcohol Depend 1999;54:117–25.

X-Chromosome Dependent Differences in the Neuronal Molecular Signatures and Their Implications in Sleep Patterns

Mariana Moysés-Oliveira, PhD[a], Bianca Pereira Favilla, MSc[b], Maria Isabel Melaragno PhD[b], Sergio Tufik, MD, PhD[a,c,*]

KEYWORDS

• X-chromosome • Gene regulation • Epigenetic • X inactivation • Sleep pattern • Sex differences

KEY POINTS

- Human sex dimorphisms are triggered by sex chromosomes composition during early developmental stages.
- Genes that scape X-chromosome inactivation in women correspond to a source of gene expression variability between males and females, which impact sex-related dimorphisms on brain transcriptional programs.
- The X-chromosome content is significantly enriched for genes associated to neurological conditions which are frequently related to sleep disorders.
- Males and females often do not manifest sleep patterns in the same way or respond identically to treatment, and the sex biased expression of X-linked genes are a putative underlying factor for these differences.

IMPORTANCE OF SEX CHROMOSOMES' EFFECT ON SLEEP

Human development, physiology, and disease manifest differently in males and females. Many human neurological traits, including brain anatomy, chemistry, and function, exhibit sex-biased characteristics.[1–4] Sleep and circadian patterns are included in those sex differences. Although women spend more time in bed and sleep longer, they report a poorer sleep quality than men.[5] The perception of a poorer sleep quality in women, when compared to men, is not endorsed by polysomnographic assessments, which indicate that women have less wakefulness after sleep onset, less light Stage 1 sleep, more slow-wave sleep, and more slow-wave activity.[5] Sex differences in circadian timing may also differentially impact the sleep quality of men and women.[6] Circadian timing in women is even earlier than the sex difference in sleep timing would predict. Women, therefore, may be sleeping at a later circadian time than men, which could contribute to the higher prevalence of insomnia, particularly sleep maintenance insomnia, in women.[7] Those differences between the sexes in incidence, prevalence, and severity of sleep disturbances might also be extended to response to treatment.[3] Therefore, ignoring that males and females exhibit divergencies in circadian patterns might complicate our understanding of and hinder our ability to prevent, treat, and cure sleep and rhythm disorders.

[a] Sleep Institute, Associação Fundo de Incentivo à Pesquisa, Rua Marselhea, 500, São Paulo, São Paulo, Brazil; [b] Genetics Division, Departamento de Morfologia e Genética, Universidade Federal de São Paulo, São Paulo, Brazil; [c] Departamento de Psicobiologia, Universidade Federal de São Paulo, São Paulo, Brazil
* Corresponding author.
E-mail address: Sergio.Tufik@afip.com.br

Sleep Med Clin 18 (2023) 521–531
https://doi.org/10.1016/j.jsmc.2023.06.014

The 2015 National Institutes of Health guidelines (NOT-OD-15–102) mandate researchers to consider sex in study designs and, in fact, physiological sex differences have been in focus for the last years in the field. The large majority of studies addressing sex differences in the nervous system are focused on exposure to gonadal hormones, which act on the neuronal circuitry across puberty and adulthood and permanently organize the neural substrate[8]. However, genetic factors and mechanisms that drive sex differences are still understudied and poorly understood.

Human sex differences are primarily orchestrated by developmental gene expression, and genes located in the sex chromosomes initiate sex-specific gene activity during early embryogenesis[9]. Even after birth, sex divergence in health and disease is partially driven by the inherent inequality of the sex chromosomes, such as the effects of the expression of Y-chromosome (chrY) genes, differences in dosage of X-chromosome (chrX) genes, and epigenetic effects[9]. As the average populational age becomes shifted towards the elder stages of life, sex hormones' impact tends to be attenuated, and the sex genotype consequences might be superficialized in clinical contexts, demonstrating the urgency of investigating the sex chromosome contribution to diseases on the development of future precision medicine approaches.

The chrX function and regulation have been historically excluded from general scientific efforts on many fronts. This comes from the fact that most *in vivo* and *in vitro* functional studies have been performed only on male experimental systems, many genetic sequence mapping approaches fail to consider sex chromosome composition biases the sex chromosomes and most Genome-Wide Association Studies (GWAS) have omitted sex chromosomes from their analyses.[10] There are many challenges in studying chromosomal sex as a biological variable. Because the sex chromosomes are intrinsically linked to gonadal development, and thereby hormonal differences, the dissection of the impact of the sex genotype (ie, XX vs. XY) on neurological phenotypes between female and male adult patients is generally hampered by sex hormonal bias.[8] Additionally, accounting for chromosomal sex demands ensuring adequate sample sizes for well-powered analyses of each sex. Genetic-focused studies in this field face even greater challenges, such as poor mapping quality in specific chromosomal sex regions, bias from homologous (ie, highly similar in sequence) regions between the chrX and chrY, and difficulty in dealing with sex dichotomy in bioinformatics pipelines.[11]

This review aims to discuss chrX-driven impacts on brain function and the extent to which those impacts are linked to sex differences in sleep and circadian patterns. Sex differences driven by chrX can promote sex-specific therapeutic responses, in which women are generally benefited.[12] The relevance of chrX-focused investigations is given by the growing need to provide individualized disease prevention and treatment as we advance into the precision medicine era, and the urge to include women patients in those medicine advancements.

SEX CHROMOSOMES GENOTYPE AND FUNCTIONAL IMBALANCES BETWEEN MALES AND FEMALES

The human sex chromosomes are substantially different in size, structure, content, and function (**Fig. 1**A). As a consequence of those differences, genes in the sex chromosomes, and the proteins they encode, propagate a cascade of signaling events within gene networks to drive sexual differentiation programs during development.[13] The best-documented example of this in mammals is the gene of the chrY sex-determining region, *SRY*. When *SRY* is expressed at the correct time and place, it causes the undifferentiated gonads to become testes. In turn, androgens produced by the male testes organize the brain to respond to male-typical steroid hormones.[13]

Despite all the stringing divergencies between human chrX and chrY, there are 2 homologous segments between both chromosomes: the pseudoautosomal regions (PAR).[14] Those regions, located at terminal euchromatic portions of the sex chromosomes, harbor genes that are present in 2 copies in males and females (**Fig. 1**B).[15] Another relevant chromosomal region in the chrX is the "X inactivation center" (see **Fig. 1**B). During the early development of a female individual with a normal karyotype, after recognizing that a single cell presents two chrX, the X inactivation center is initiated by the transcription of the non-coding *XIST* transcript, which is the central gene in triggering the chrX inactivation mechanism.[16] The chrX inactivation is the process in which one of the 2 copies of the chrX is inactivated in order to achieve dosage compensation of X-linked genes between males and females.[17] The non-coding *XIST* transcript is active exclusively in the chrX that is going to be subjected to inactivation (Xi), and it coats the X-chromatin in both directions from the X inactivation center. After the Xi *XIST* coating, repressive epigenetic marks are recruited and, as a result, most Xi genetic sequence is transcriptionally silenced.[16,18]

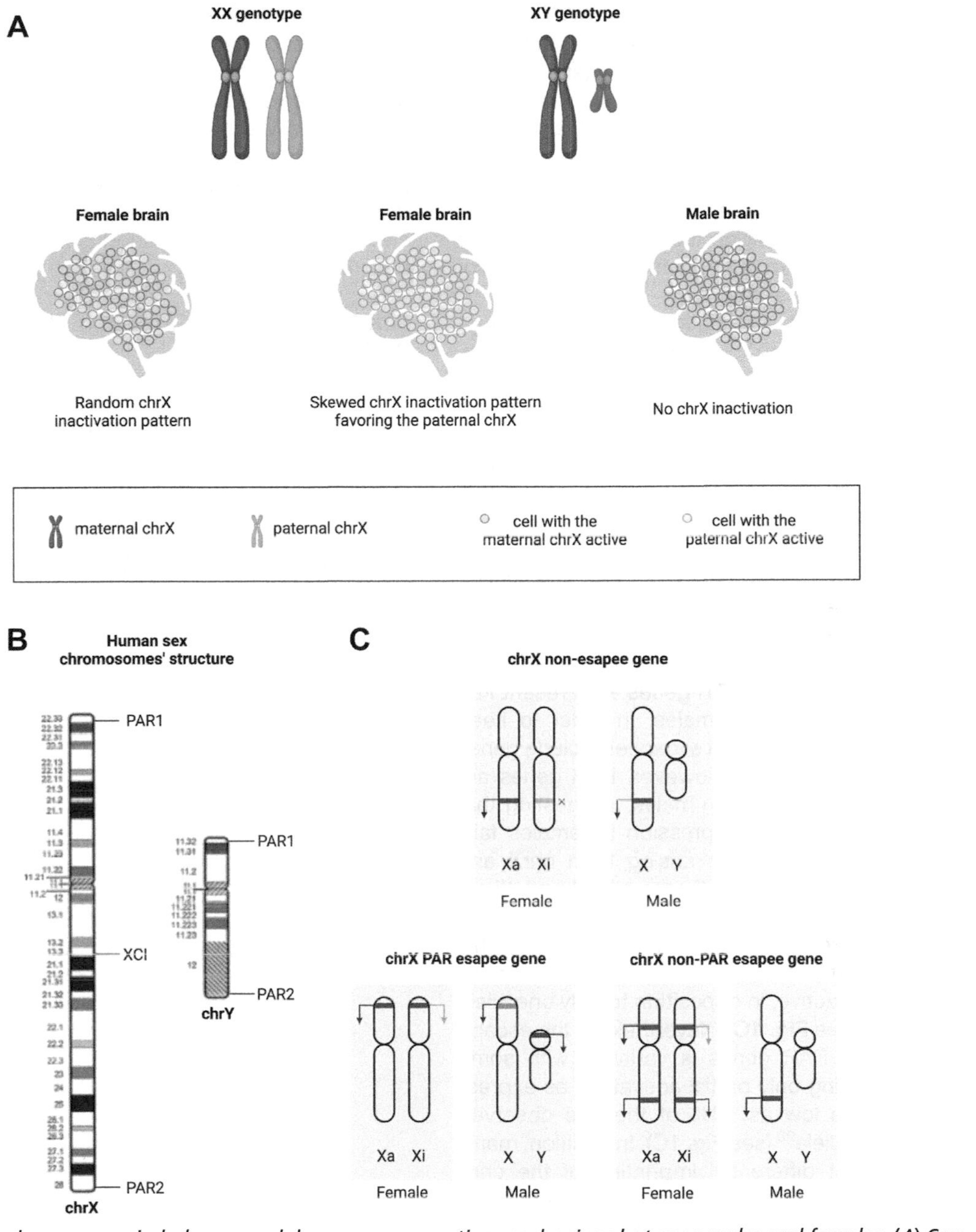

Fig. 1. *Sex-chromosome imbalances and dosage compensation mechanisms between males and females.* (*A*) Consequences of X inactivation patterns on brain cellular composition in females and the lack of X inactivation in males. (*B*) X and Y-chromosomes' ideogram showing their pseudoautosomal region (PAR) and the X inactivation center. (*C*) Functional dosage imbalances of chrX genes according to their inactivation pattern in females. Red stripes represent genes and arrows represent active transcription, with the arrow color density corresponding to the expression levels.

The choice of which X-chromosome will undergo inactivation in each cell is random, thereby the X-inactivation pattern is usually normally distributed.[19] Due to random X-inactivation, female tissues are mosaics, with about half of the cells expressing an active maternal chrX and the other half expressing an active paternal chrX (see **Fig. 1**A). The chrX inactivation mechanisms and implications make disease gene discovery on chromosome chrX a challenging task owing to its unique modes of inheritance.[20] With the possibility of presenting a skewed chrX inactivation pattern favoring the activation of one of the chrX (maternal or paternal), women have a protective mechanism against highly damaging chrX genetic variants.[21,22] For instance, in female carriers of X-linked structural rearrangements, the inactivation pattern frequently is skewed due to an apparent selection of cells with the best dosage balance. In women with large genetic deletions or duplications involving the chrX segments, the inactivation pattern is frequently skewed in favor of cells with the abnormal chrX inactive.[23,24] Consequently, chrX alterations in women can go undetected, with mild or no clinical consequences, putting men at greater risk for X-linked diseases.[25]

The chrX inactivation is, however, incomplete in humans: in female cells, a substantial portion of chrX genes is expressed from both active and inactive chrX (frequently referred to as Xa and Xi, respectively).[26] Which–and to which level–genes will be silenced in the Xi varies according to cell type, with total escape or incomplete inactivation affecting at least 23% of chrX genes in humans.[27] In this review, genes that exhibit some degree of escape from chrX inactivation are referred to as "Xi escapees." Since PAR genes are present in 2 copies in males and females, in order to keep dosage compensation, Xi escapees include genes in these chrX regions. However, PAR genes are more highly expressed in males, suggesting that combined Xa and Xi expression in females fails to reach the expression arising from chrX and chrY in males[27] (**Fig. 1**C). On the other hand, Xi escapees are not limited to PAR genes, and the non-PAR escapees are known to be more highly expressed in females, since both chrX are transcriptionally active, in opposition to only one allele in males[27] (see **Fig. 1**C). Nevertheless, the escape level of non-PAR genes is variable, with some genes reaching only partial activation, as expression level as low as 10% of the one observed from the Xa allele[28] (see **Fig. 1**C). In addition, mammals present differential imprinting of the chrX from the 2 parents. Females–and not males–inherit a paternal X chromosome (see **Fig. 1**A); therefore, any paternally imprinted X genes will be expressed in females only.[29] Thus, Xi escapees and chrX imprinting in human females contribute to sexual dimorphism not only in transcriptional profiles but also in cellular and clinical traits.[30]

The chrX comprises 829 protein-coding genes, which are significantly more frequently associated with neurological phenotypes than genes on autosomes.[25] Despite chrX being enriched in disorder-associated genes, 598 genes (71%) are not yet related to any clinical phenotype.[25] Contrasting a curated list of 1065 sleep-associated genes distributed across the entire human genome[31] to the 829 protein-coding X-linked genes, the resulting intersect contains 11 genes, including PAR and non-PAR, Xi escapees, and non-escapees (**Fig. 2**A,**Table 1**). Among those 11 sleep genes, 9 are robustly expressed in brain tissues[32] and 8 are disease-associated.[25] Many X-linked disease genes are causative of rare monogenic syndromes,[25] in which a higher prevalence of excessive daytime sleepiness and insomnia have been described.[33]

SEX-BIASED TRANSCRIPTOME IMBALANCES IN THE BRAIN

Sex-differential transcriptome has a direct impact on human evolution and human physiology in health and disease.[30] Sex influences gene expression levels and cellular composition of tissue

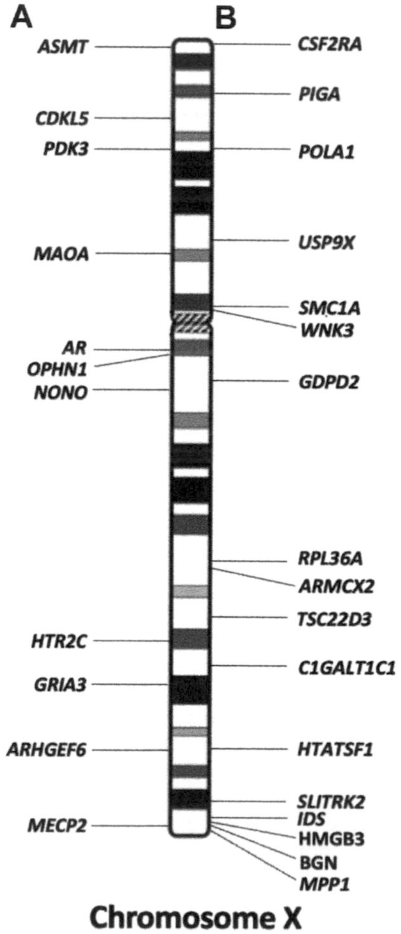

Fig. 2. *Ideogram of the chrX showing the location of genes associated with sleep disturbances and circadian rhythm.* (*A*) Sleep-associated genes located on the chrX (see genes' information in **Table 1**). (*B*) SCN rhythmic genes located on the chrX (see genes' information in **Table 2**).

Table 1
Sleep-associated genes located on chrX

Gene Symbol	PAR	chrX Inactivation	Disease Association	OMIM Disease Number	Inheritance
AR	No	Non-escapee	Yes	300068/312300//300633/313200	X-linked recessive/X-linked recessive/X-linked recessive/X-linked recessive
ARHGEF6	No	Non-escapee	No		
ASMT	Yes	Putative escapee	No		
CDKL5	No	Non-escapee	Yes	300672	X-linked dominant
GRIA3	No	Unknown	Yes	300699	X-linked recessive
HTR2C	No	Putative escapee	No		
MAOA	No	Unkown	Yes	300615	X-linked recessive
MECP2	No	Non-escapee	Yes	300673/300260/300055/312750/312750/312750	X-linked recessive/X-linked recessive/X-linked recessive/X-linked dominant/X-linked dominant/X-linked dominant
NONO	No	Non-escapee	Yes	300967	X-linked
OPHN1	No	Non-escapee	Yes	300486	X-linked recessive
PDK3	No	Non-escapee	Yes	300905	X-linked dominant

samples across the human body, and transcriptional levels of X-linked female-biased genes can accurately predict sex.[34] Genes with sex-biased expression are not primarily driven by tissue-specific gene expression and are involved in a diverse set of biological functions, such as drug and hormone response, embryonic development, sexual reproduction, fat metabolism, cancer, and immune response.[34]

Even though most transcription factors are not differentially expressed between males and females, they can exhibit sex-biased targeting patterns, demonstrating sex differences not only in the human transcriptome but also in the human epigenome.[35] Consistently, in the mouse brain, sex also affects histone marks' distribution, adding another layer to sex-biased epigenetic regulation.[36] Differentially targeted genes in humans are enriched in Xi escapees, including PAR and non-PAR Xi escapees.[35] This sex-biased gene expression regulation is associated with each tissue's function and with diseases specific to this given tissue.[35] X-linked differentially targeted genes in human brain tissues include Xi escapees previously related to sleep phenotypes, such as *ASMT* and *MAOA* genes. A polymorphism in *ASMT* has been associated with sleep and circadian rhythm in patients with bipolar disorder.[37] In *MAOA*, a regulatory polymorphism has been associated with symptoms of depression and sleep quality.[38]

Clinical consequences of the imbalances related to Xi escapees in the human brain are demonstrated by the neurologic traits observed in individuals with chrX aneuploidies, such as Turner syndrome (X0) and Klinefelter syndrome (XXY). Patients with these syndromes have only one active chrX, as males and females with normal karyotypes. However, they experience an increased risk of attention-deficit hyperactivity disorder, autism spectrum disorder, major depressive disorder, anxiety disorders,[39] poor sleep quality,[40] and elevated arousal under stressful situations.[41,42] Additionally, Xi escapees' imbalances are quantitatively associated with gene expression levels of growth hormone in the mouse hypothalamus, which was proven to contribute to sexually dimorphic metabolic traits.[43] Neurological and behavioral effects of chrX dosage have been confirmed in animal models. The number of chrX in the nuclei causes sex differences in dorsal striatal gene expression[44] and male sex behavior[45] in mice. Female mice that are haploinsufficient for Xi escapees (ie, X0 mice) have higher levels of fear reactivity compared to XX mice.[46]

SEX COMPLEMENT IN SLEEP AND CIRCADIAN PATTERNS

Despite the robust molecular evidence linking transcriptome profiles and sex-related differences in neurological functions underlying sleep, mechanistic insights connecting chrX content and sleep-relevant neurological circuits are still lacking. A mouse model now known as the "Four Core Genotypes" has been used to directly test the contributions of sex chromosome complement versus gonadal sex.[47] This model takes advantage of a spontaneous mutation that resulted in a deletion of *Sry* on the chrY, which is rescued by a transgenic insertion of *Sry* within an autosome. An animal with a chrY missing *Sry*, but with an autosomal *Sry* transgene develops normal testes and is a fertile male. Mating this male individual with a karyotypically normal (ie, XX) female produces the offspring of 4 genotypes: females with 2 chrX (XXF), females with a chrX and a *Sry*-missing chrY (XYF), males with 2 chrX and no chrY (XXM), and males with one chrX and one chrY (XYM). The Four Core Genotypes mouse model unlinks gonadal determination from the inheritance of the sex chromosomes and allows for independent analysis of those 2 factors. Using this mouse model, Kujis and colleagues[48] have demonstrated that activity duration is longer in XX individuals regardless of gonadal sex, with this circadian parameter being the most strongly modulated by sex chromosome. This finding is consistent with work demonstrating that sex differences in activity duration persist after reproductive senescence in female mice.[49] In addition, the Four Core Genotypes mice have also been used to demonstrate sex-chromosome impact on food intake.[50,51]

One of the very few studies that addressed the relationship between chrX and neuronal circuits in humans demonstrated that genetic sex impacts on GABAergic circuits in human frontal cortex.[52] Leveraging gene expression profiles from postmortem human brain samples, Seney and colleagues[52] mapped X-linked genetic polymorphisms that act as trans-expression quantitative trait loci (trans-eQTL) associated with the expression of a GABA neuron-specific marker (somatostatin, SST) and/or GABA-synthesizing enzymes (GAD67and GAD65). Trans-eQTLs correspond to single nucleotide polymorphisms which are quantitively associated with expression levels of genes located in other chromosomes, suggesting a long-range regulatory interaction. Those trans-eQTL associated with GABA key modulators were linked to 44 chrX genes,[52] including 6 Xi escapees: *COL4A6, CTPS2, DGAT2L6, PHEX, SH2D1A,* and *USP9X*.[25] Using rodent models, Seney and colleagues then confirmed that sex genotype was a driver factor underlying sex differences in GABA modulators expression and anxiety-like behaviors.

Sex-biased gene expression in the suprachiasmatic nucleus (SCN), the "master peacemaker" of circadian rhythms in mammals, might directly promote sex differences in sleep and metabolic patterns. Voltage-gated channels encoded by *Kcna4* and *Kcnd2* genes, which are A-type potassium channels, were proven to regulate the circadian period of PER2 expression in the SCN.[53] The chrX harbors voltage-gated A-type potassium channel paralogs, whose gene expression imbalances between males and females might be linked to sex-biased circadian traits.

In a recent study, Wen and colleagues[54] have used single-cell RNA sequencing to characterize the cell type composition and cell type markers in the SCN and to identify circadian gene expression patterns in those neurons. They have shown that SCN neuron subtypes exhibit quantitative differences in their light-induced gene expression changes.[54] All SCN cell types contained rhythmically expressed genes and phase differences were detected in their circadian gene expression.[54] Among those SCN "rhythmic genes," 17 are located on the chrX, 9 of them being disease-associated (**Fig. 2**B,**Table 2**). Out of those 9 rhythmic and disease-associated X-linked genes, 3 are Xi escapees (*CSF2RA*, *SMC1A*, and *USP9X*)[25] and, thus, are known to present functional imbalance between males and females in certain cell types. The PAR gene *CSF2RA* encodes a cytokine subunit related to MAP kinase cascade and interleukin signaling, which is associated with a rare lung disorder (pulmonary alveolar proteinosis)[55] and is modulated by pharmacological approaches that act on circadian rhythm.[56] *SMC1A,* a non-PAR Xi escapee, encodes a central component of the cohesion complex (i.e., a key regulator of chromatin topological organization), and is one of the main causative genes of the Cornelia de Lange syndrome, a rare genetic disorder that is associated with sleep disturbances.[57] *SMC1A* has also been reported as subjected to differential transcription factor regulation between males and females.[35] Another non-PAR Xi escapee, *USP9X*, encodes a deubiquitinase involved in the mTOR pathway and, when mutated, causes monogenic neurodevelopmental disorders.[58] In addition, *USP9X* is one of the chrX genes related to trans-eQTL associated with GABAergic regulation[52] and is also subjected to sex-biased differential transcription factor regulation,[59] being a strong candidate to promote sex-derived circadian disparities due to functional imbalances in the SCN.

Table 2
SCN rhythmic genes located on chrX

Gene Symbol	PAR	chrX Inactivation	Disease Association	OMIM Disease Number	Inheritance
ARMCX2	No	Non-escapee	No disorder		
BGN	No	Non-escapee	Confirmed monogenic disorder	300989/300106	X-linked/X-linked recessive
C1GALT1C1	No	Non-escapee	Confirmed monogenic disorder	300622	X-linked
CSF2RA	Yes	Putative escapee	Confirmed monogenic disorder	300770	X-linked
GDPD2	No	Unkown	No disorder		
HMGB3	No	Non-escapee	Putative monogenic disorder	300915	X-linked
HTATSF1	No	Non-escapee	No disorder		
IDS	No	Non-escapee	Confirmed monogenic disorder	309900	X-linked recessive
MPP1	No	Non-escapee	No disorder		
PIGA	No	Non-escapee	Confirmed monogenic disorder	300868/300818	X-linked recessive
POLA1	No	Non-escapee	Confirmed monogenic disorder	301220/301030	X-linked recessive/X-linked recessive
RPL36A	No	Non-escapee	No disorder		
SLITRK2	No	Non-escapee	No disorder		
SMC1A	No	Escapee	Confirmed monogenic disorder	300590/301044	X-linked dominant
TSC22D3	No	Non-escapee	No disorder		
USP9X	No	Escapee	Confirmed monogenic disorder	300919/300968	X-linked recessive/X-linked dominant
WNK3	No	Non-escapee	No disorder		

SEX COMPLEMENT IN MENTAL ILLNESSES RELATED TO SLEEP PATTERNS

In addition to the clinical sex disparities that directly affect sleep and circadian patterns, sex has been demonstrated to affect sleep-related diseases as well. Sleep disturbances are frequently comorbid with neuropsychiatric disorders, with a bidirectional relationship between these traits.[60] Sleep quality is strongly influenced by anxiety, depressive symptoms, and affective disorders, which are more common in women and may contribute to a higher incidence of insomnia.[61] On the other hand, two rapid-acting antidepressant strategies, low-dose ketamine, and sleep deprivation therapies dramatically reduce depressive symptoms within 24 hours in a subset of major patients with depressive disorder and cause downregulation of key clock genes in the anterior cingulate cortex.[59]

As sleep and circadian traits, neuropsychiatric phenotypes also present sex-biased prevalence and clinical manifestations, with males being at higher risk for neurodevelopmental disorders, such as autism spectrum disorder, and females being at higher risk for many later onset psychiatric diseases, such as major depression and anxiety disorders[62]. Even when considering a specific psychiatric trait, sleep phenotypes can be unequally distributed between males and females.

For instance, sleep disorders are more prevalent among female than male patients with autism spectrum disorder[63]. In accordance with those observations, chrX plays an important role in the etiology and genetic risk of psychiatric disorders[64,65].

Aiming to investigate the impact of chrX inactivation on psychiatric disorders, Ji and colleagues leveraged gene expression profiles of lymphoblastoid cell lines established from female patients with either bipolar disorder or major depression and healthy controls. They observed that *XIST*, the key regulator of chrX inactivation, and *KDM5C*, an Xi non-PAR escapee, are upregulated in patients.[66] In this same study, *XIST* was confirmed as upregulated in the disease context in female postmortem brain samples, endorsing the pathogenic significance of this putative molecular biomarker.[66] As previously discussed, chrX polymorphisms were proposed to act on the regulation of GABAergic circuits in the human brain, in a sex-biased fashion, through STT modulation.[52] Those observations are especially relevant for the biological interpretation of sex differences in major depressive disorder. It has been suggested that depression is linked to GABA/SST-related cellular phenotype,[67,68] with STT expression being reduced across multiple brain regions in patients. Importantly, SST reduction in females with depression is significantly more robust than in male patients,[52] supporting the hypothesis of sex-biased chrX functional dosage on Xi escapees.

Besides psychiatric traits, neurodegenerative disorders are also proven to be related to sleep and rhythm disorders.[69] Women experience a significantly higher tau burden and increased risk for Alzheimer's disease than men.[70] In addition to sex differences in prevalence,[71] molecular signatures in neurodegenerative disorders have also been demonstrated to differ between males and females. In brain tissues, for example, genes associated with Parkinson's disease and Alzheimer's disease are targeted by different sets of transcription factors in each sex.[35] It had been recently demonstrated that the higher risk of Alzheimer's disease is associated with a specific Xi non-PAR escapee, *USP11*, which encodes a deubiquitinase.[12] USP11 augments pathological tau aggregation via tau deubiquitination and has higher expression levels in females than in males.[12] The induction of *Usp11* loss of function in a tauopathy mouse model preferentially protects females from tau pathology and cognitive impairment, suggesting that USP11 inhibition might correspond to a putative therapeutic approach on female patients with Alzheimer's disease.[12] It is important to note that *USP11* is a paralog of gene *USP9X*, another Xi non-PAR escapee indicated in this review as a strong candidate for sex differences in circadian patterns.

SUMMARY

While much is known about the sex hormones' impact on mechanisms of sleep and circadian timing, the investigation into sex chromosome-related differences regarding the control of sleep is in its infancy. Here we sought to illustrate how chrX functional imbalances between males and females influence the neurobiological processes underlying sleep and circadian rhythms. These findings are a significant step forward in understanding how sex differences manifest in gene regulatory networks and underscore the importance of looking beyond autosomal genetic content. Most importantly, males and females often do not manifest sleep patterns in the same way or respond identically to treatment, and the exploration of the genetic causes of these differences should remain an area of active study. Here, we drafted putative research paths and indicated strong gene candidates for the further elucidation of chrX-related factors underlying circadian differences between sexes. More fully exploring sex-biased patterns of gene regulation is crucial not only for understanding how sex-specific biological processes drive health and disease but also for the development of precision therapeutics that will best treat disease in an individual, accounting for sex.

CLINICS CARE POINTS

- Sleep disturbances should be investigated on patients with X-linked syndromes associated with neurodevelopmental deficits.
- Sleep and circadian patterns on patients with X-linked neurodevelopmental syndromed might differ between sexes.
- When rare variants on X-linked genes are detected on genotyping diagnostic screenings, the X-chromosome inactivation pattern of the affected gene might indicate whereas sex biased clinical manifestations must be considered.
- Sex-related dimorphisms on brain transcriptional programs must be considered when designing health care strategies for mental and sleep illnesses with biases prevalence rates between males and females.

DISCLOSURE

Nothing to disclose.

ACKNOWLEDGMENTS

This work was supported by Associação Fundo de Incentivo à Pesquisa, Brazil and Fundação de Amparo à Pesquisa do Estado de São Paulo, Brazil (FAPESP, 2021/09089-0, recipient: MMO).

REFERENCES

1. Ober C, Loisel DA, Gilad Y. Sex-specific genetic architecture of human disease. Nat Rev Genet 2008; 9(12):911–22.
2. Morrow EH. The evolution of sex differences in disease. Biol Sex Differ 2015;6(1). https://doi.org/10.1186/S13293-015-0023-0.
3. Clocchiatti A, Cora E, Zhang Y, et al. Sexual dimorphism in cancer. Nat Rev Cancer 2016;16(5):330–9.
4. Cahill L. Why sex matters for neuroscience. Nat Rev Neurosci 2006;7(6):477–84.
5. Pengo MF, Won CH, Bourjeily G. Sleep in women across the life span. Chest 2018;154(1):196–206.
6. Mong JA, Baker FC, Mahoney MM, et al. Sleep, rhythms, and the endocrine brain: influence of sex and gonadal hormones. J Neurosci 2011;31(45): 16107–16.
7. Duffy JF, Cain SW, Chang AM, et al. Sex difference in the near-24-hour intrinsic period of the human circadian timing system. Proc Natl Acad Sci U S A 2011; 108(Suppl 3):15602–8.
8. McCarthy MM, Arnold AP. Reframing sexual differentiation of the brain. Nat Neurosci 2011;14(6): 677–83.
9. Arnold AP. Y chromosome's roles in sex differences in disease. Proc Natl Acad Sci U S A 2017;114(15): 3787–9.
10. Khramtsova EA, Davis LK, Stranger BE. The role of sex in the genomics of human complex traits. Nat Rev Genet 2019;20(3):173–90.
11. Piton A, Redin C, Mandel JL. XLID-causing mutations and associated genes challenged in light of data from large-scale human exome sequencing. Am J Hum Genet 2013;93(2):368–83.
12. Yan Y, Wang X, Chaput D, et al. X-linked ubiquitin-specific peptidase 11 increases tauopathy vulnerability in women. Cell 2022;185(21):3913–30.e19.
13. Rosenfeld CS. Brain sexual differentiation and requirement of SRY: why or why not? Front Neurosci 2017;11(NOV). https://doi.org/10.3389/FNINS.2017.00632.
14. Helena Mangs A, Morris B. The human pseudoautosomal region (PAR): origin, function and future. Curr Genomics 2007;8(2):129–36.
15. Printzlau F, Wolstencroft J, Skuse DH. Cognitive, behavioral, and neural consequences of sex chromosome aneuploidy. J Neurosci Res 2017; 95(1–2):311–9.
16. Brown SDM. XIST and the mapping of the X chromosome inactivation centre. Bioessays 1991;13(11): 607–12.
17. Lyon MF. Gene action in the X-chromosome of the mouse (Mus musculus L.). Nature 1961;190(4773): 372–3.
18. Engreitz JM, Pandya-Jones A, McDonel P, et al. The Xist lncRNA exploits three-dimensional genome architecture to spread across the X chromosome. Science 2013;341(6147). https://doi.org/10.1126/SCIENCE.1237973.
19. Amos-Landgraf JM, Cottle A, Plenge RM, et al. X chromosome-inactivation patterns of 1,005 phenotypically unaffected females. Am J Hum Genet 2006; 79(3):493–9.
20. Moysés-Oliveira M, Guilherme RDS, Dantas AG, et al. Genetic mechanisms leading to primary amenorrhea in balanced X-autosome translocations. Fertil Steril 2015;103(5). https://doi.org/10.1016/j.fertnstert.2015.01.030.
21. Moysés-Oliveira M, Di-Battista A, Zamariolli M, et al. Breakpoint mapping at nucleotide resolution in X-autosome balanced translocations associated with clinical phenotypes. Eur J Hum Genet 2019; 27(5). https://doi.org/10.1038/s41431-019-0341-5.
22. Di-Battista A, Moysés-Oliveira M, Melaragno MI. Genetics of premature ovarian insufficiency and the association with X-autosome translocations. Reproduction 2020;160(4):R55–64.
23. Di-Battista A, Meloni VA, da Silva MD, et al. Unusual X-chromosome inactivation pattern in patients with Xp11.23-p11.22 duplication: report and review. Am J Med Genet 2016;170(12). https://doi.org/10.1002/ajmg.a.37888.
24. Sisdelli L, Vidi AC, Moysés-Oliveira M, et al. Incorporation of 5-ethynyl-2′-deoxyuridine (EdU) as a novel strategy for identification of the skewed X inactivation pattern in balanced and unbalanced X-rearrangements. Hum Genet 2016;135(2). https://doi.org/10.1007/s00439-015-1622-x.
25. Leitão E, Schröder C, Parenti I, et al. Systematic analysis and prediction of genes associated with monogenic disorders on human chromosome X. Nat Commun 2022;13(1). https://doi.org/10.1038/s41467-022-34264-y.
26. Posynick BJ, Brown CJ. Escape from X-chromosome inactivation: an evolutionary perspective. Front Cell Dev Biol 2019;7. https://doi.org/10.3389/FCELL.2019.00241.
27. Tukiainen T, Villani AC, Yen A, et al. Landscape of X chromosome inactivation across human tissues. Nature 2017;550(7675):244–8.
28. Carrel L, Willard HF. X-inactivation profile reveals extensive variability in X-linked gene expression in females. Nature 2005;434(7031):400–4.

29. Cox KH, Bonthuis PJ, Rissman EF. Mouse model systems to study sex chromosome genes and behavior: relevance to humans. Front Neuroendocrinol 2014;35(4):405–19.
30. Gershoni M, Pietrokovski S. The landscape of sex-differential transcriptome and its consequent selection in human adults. BMC Biol 2017;15(1). https://doi.org/10.1186/s12915-017-0352-z.
31. Moysés-Oliveira M, Paschalidis M, Souza-Cunha LA, et al. Genetic basis of sleep phenotypes and rare neurodevelopmental syndromes reveal shared molecular pathways. J Neurosci Res 2023. https://doi.org/10.1002/jnr.25180.
32. Lonsdale J, Thomas J, Salvatore M, et al. The genotype-tissue expression (GTEx) project. Nat Genet 2013;45(6):580–5.
33. Agar G, Brown C, Sutherland D, et al. Sleep disorders in rare genetic syndromes: a meta-analysis of prevalence and profile. Mol Autism 2021;12(1):1–17.
34. Aguet F, Barbeira AN, Bonazzola R, et al. The impact of sex on gene expression across human tissues. Science (1979) 2020;369(6509). https://doi.org/10.1126/SCIENCE.ABA3066.
35. Lopes-Ramos CM, Chen CY, Kuijjer ML, et al. Sex differences in gene expression and regulatory networks across 29 human tissues. Cell Rep 2020;31(12). https://doi.org/10.1016/j.celrep.2020.107795.
36. Casciaro F, Persico G, Rusin M, et al. The histone h3 k4me3, k27me3, and k27ac genome-wide distributions are differently influenced by sex in brain cortexes and gastrocnemius of the alzheimer's disease psapp mouse model. Epigenomes 2021;5(4). https://doi.org/10.3390/EPIGENOMES5040026.
37. Geoffroy PA, Boudebesse C, Henrion A, et al. An ASMT variant associated with bipolar disorder influences sleep and circadian rhythms: a pilot study. Genes Brain Behav 2014;13(3):299–304.
38. Brummett BH, Krystal AD, Siegler IC, et al. Associations of a regulatory polymorphism of monoamine oxidase-A gene promoter (MAOA-uVNTR) with symptoms of depression and sleep quality. Psychosom Med 2007;69(5):396–401.
39. Green T, Flash S, Reiss AL. Sex differences in psychiatric disorders: what we can learn from sex chromosome aneuploidies. Neuropsychopharmacology 2019;44(1):9–21.
40. Fjermestad KW, Stokke S. Sleep problems and life satisfaction as predictors of health in men with sex chromosome aneuploidies. Behav Med 2018;44(2):116–22.
41. Keysor CS, Mazzocco MMM, McLeod DR, et al. Physiological arousal in females with fragile X or Turner syndrome. Dev Psychobiol 2002;41(2):133–46.
42. Roberts J, Mazzocco MMM, Murphy MM, et al. Arousal modulation in females with fragile X or turner syndrome. J Autism Dev Disord 2008;38(1):20.
43. Bonthuis PJ, Rissman EF. Neural growth hormone implicated in body weight sex differences. Endocrinology 2013;154(10):3826–35.
44. Chen X, Grisham W, Arnold AP. X chromosome number causes sex differences in gene expression in adult mouse striatum. Eur J Neurosci 2009;29(4):768–76.
45. Bonthuis PJ, Cox KH, Rissman EF. X-chromosome dosage affects male sexual behavior. Horm Behav 2012;61(4):565–72.
46. Isles AR, Davies W, Burrmann D, et al. Effects on fear reactivity in XO mice are due to haploinsufficiency of a non-PAR X gene: implications for emotional function in Turner's syndrome. Hum Mol Genet 2004;13(17):1849–55.
47. de Vries GJ, Rissman EF, Simerly RB, et al. A model system for study of sex chromosome effects on sexually dimorphic neural and behavioral traits. J Neurosci 2002;22(20):9005–14.
48. Kuljis DA, Loh DH, Truong D, et al. Gonadal- and sex-chromosome-dependent sex differences in the circadian system. Endocrinology 2013;154(4):1501–12.
49. Stowie AC, Glass JD. Longitudinal study of changes in daily activity rhythms over the lifespan in individual male and female C57BL/6J Mice. J Biol Rhythms 2015;30(6):563–8.
50. Seu E, Groman SM, Arnold AP, et al. Sex chromosome complement influences operant responding for a palatable food in mice. Genes Brain Behav 2014;13(6):527–34.
51. Chen X, Wang L, Loh DH, et al. Sex differences in diurnal rhythms of food intake in mice caused by gonadal hormones and complement of sex chromosomes. Horm Behav 2015;75:55–63.
52. Seney ML, Chang LC, Oh H, et al. The role of genetic sex in affect regulation and expression of GABA-related genes across species. Front Psychiatry 2013;4(SEP). https://doi.org/10.3389/fpsyt.2013.00104.
53. Granados-Fuentes D, Hermanstyne TO, Carrasquillo Y, et al. IA channels encoded by Kv1.4 and Kv4.2 regulate circadian period of Per2 expression in the suprachiasmatic nucleus. J Biol Rhythms 2015;30(5):396–407.
54. Wen S, Ma D, Zhao M, et al. Spatiotemporal single-cell analysis of gene expression in the mouse suprachiasmatic nucleus. Nat Neurosci 2020;23(3):456–67.
55. Suzuki T, Sakagami T, Rubin BK, et al. Familial pulmonary alveolar proteinosis caused by mutations in CSF2RA. J Exp Med 2008;205(12):2703–10.
56. Kwon EY, Shin SK, Choi MS. Ursolic acid attenuates hepatic steatosis, fibrosis, and insulin resistance by modulating the circadian rhythm pathway in diet-induced obese mice. Nutrients 2018;10(11). https://doi.org/10.3390/NU10111719.

57. Zambrelli E, Fossati C, Turner K, et al. Sleep disorders in Cornelia de Lange syndrome. Am J Med Genet C Semin Med Genet 2016;172(2):214–21.
58. Wrobel L, Siddiqi FH, Hill SM, et al. mTORC2 assembly is regulated by USP9X-mediated deubiquitination of RICTOR. Cell Rep 2020;33(13). https://doi.org/10.1016/J.CELREP.2020.108564.
59. Orozco-Solis R, Montellier E, Aguilar-Arnal L, et al. A circadian genomic signature common to ketamine and sleep deprivation in the anterior cingulate cortex. Biol Psychiatry 2017;82(5):351–60.
60. van Someren EJW. Brain mechanisms of insomnia: new perspectives on causes and consequences. Physiol Rev 2021;101(3):995–1046.
61. Zhang B, Wing YK. Sex differences in insomnia: a meta-analysis. Sleep 2006;29(1):85–93.
62. Wigdor EM, Weiner DJ, Grove J, et al. The female protective effect against autism spectrum disorder. Cell Genomics 2022;2(6):100134.
63. Martini MI, Kuja-Halkola R, Butwicka A, et al. Sex differences in mental health problems and psychiatric hospitalization in autistic young adults. JAMA Psychiatr 2022. https://doi.org/10.1001/JAMAPSYCHIATRY.2022.3475.
64. Zhao C, Gong G. Mapping the effect of the X chromosome on the human brain: neuroimaging evidence from turner syndrome. Neurosci Biobehav Rev 2017;80:263–75.
65. Chang D, Gao F, Slavney A, et al. Accounting for eX-entricities: analysis of the X chromosome in GWAS reveals X-linked genes implicated in autoimmune diseases. PLoS One 2014;9(12):e113684.
66. Ji B, Higa KK, Kelsoe JR, et al. Over-expression of XIST, the Master Gene for X chromosome inactivation, in females with major affective disorders. EBioMedicine 2015;2(8):909–18.
67. Seney ML, Sibille E. Sex differences in mood disorders: perspectives from humans and rodent models. Biol Sex Differ 2014;5(1). https://doi.org/10.1186/s13293-014-0017-3.
68. Seney ML, Ekong KI, Ding Y, et al. Sex chromosome complement regulates expression of mood-related genes. Biol Sex Differ 2013;4(1). https://doi.org/10.1186/2042-6410-4-20.
69. Borges CR, Poyares D, Piovezan R, et al. Alzheimer's disease and sleep disturbances: a review. Arq Neuropsiquiatr 2019;77(11):815–24.
70. Palta P, Rippon B, Tahmi M, et al. Sex differences in in vivo tau neuropathology in a multiethnic sample of late middle-aged adults. Neurobiol Aging 2021;103:109–16.
71. Rajan KB, Weuve J, Barnes LL, et al. Population estimate of people with clinical Alzheimer's disease and mild cognitive impairment in the United States (2020–2060). Alzheimer's Dementia 2021;17(12):1966–75.

Night Shift Work and Sleep Disturbances in Women

A Scoping Review

Suleima P. Vasconcelos, PhD[a], Lucia C. Lemos, PhD[b], Claudia R.C. Moreno, PhD[b,*]

KEYWORDS

• Sleep • Shifwork • Female • Disturbed sleep

KEY POINTS

- Most women who work in shifts are in the health area.
- Diversity in shift schedules make it difficult to compare the results of the studies.
- Rotating shifts seem to be the worst in relation to the other types of shifts, with regard to sleep duration and sleepiness of female shift workers.
- Sex differences related to sleep disturbances need to be on the research agenda.

INTRODUCTION

Shift work is a type of work that allows essential services to be available to the population uninterruptedly. The number of shift or night workers in the world is not precise, as there are no statistical data on this work organization in many countries, in addition to differences in relation to the criteria adopted to define shift work. However, it is said that there is a trend in increasing the proportion of these workers in most western countries,[1] which has been observed since the 1990s when Moore-Ede used the expression "the 24 h society".[2] Especially when shift work includes night work (night shift work), it can cause circadian misalignment[3,4] and is associated with several health problems such as inflammatory and cardiovascular diseases, obesity, type 2 diabetes, and cancer.[5,6] In addition, it is an important modifier of social and family relationships.[7] One of the main consequences of night work is the reduction in sleep duration,[8] caused by the temporal changes in the homeostatic pressure of sleep and in the circadian pressure for wakefulness. As a result, there is a sleep debt leading to excessive sleepiness during wakefulness and reduced performance during the night work.[9,10]

Night shift work can have even more significant impact on women, considering that in most societies, even in developed countries, women are still responsible for activities beyond work, such as childcare and housework. Therefore, the combination of work and household is a stressor for women, which make difficult recovering after working nights.[7] In addition, the distinct types of shift work can affect the mental health of professionals differently, with a greater impact on the mental health of female workers.[11]

A study carried out with female workers showed that shift work, poor sleep quality, and high stress at work were significantly associated with depression and suicidal.[12] Another consequence of sleep disturbances in women who work in shifts is related to aspects of reproductive health and fertility.[13] It is recommended, for example, that pregnant workers do not perform night work more than one night a week.[14] In addition, it is possible to verify the importance of the gender focus in studies on night work, as the impacts on physical and mental health can

[a] Public Health Graduate Program, Federal University of Acre, Campus da Universidade Federal Do Acre, Rio Branco - AC, Rio Branco 69917-400, Brazil; [b] Department of Health, Life Cycles and Society, School of Public Health, University of São Paulo, Av. Dr. Arnaldo, 715, São Paulo, Brazil
* Corresponding author. Department of Health, Life Cycles and Society, School of Public Health, University of São Paulo, Av. Dr. Arnaldo, 715, 1246-904, São Paulo, Brazil.
E-mail address: crmoreno@usp.br

Sleep Med Clin 18 (2023) 533–543
https://doi.org/10.1016/j.jsmc.2023.06.016

be different considering not only biological, but social issues. Thus, this study aims to identify the evidence on sleep disturbances in female night shift work.

METHODS

Type of Study

This study is a scoping review. This type of study is developed with the aim of exploring the literature broadly and deeply, mapping and synthesizing the scientific evidence on a topic, as well as identifying knowledge gaps in a given field.[15] The present scoping review was conducted in accordance with the Joanna Briggs Institute guidelines in the article "Updated methodological guidance for conducting scoping reviews".[16] The Preferred Reporting Items for Systematic Reviews and Meta-Analyses extension for Scoping Reviews (PRISMA-ScR) update was used to write this review.

Search Strategy

The PCC format (population, concept, and context) was adopted as search strategy as described below.

1. Population—women;
2. Concept—sleep disturbances;
3. Context—shift work/night work.

The search for articles was carried out from November 16 to 22, 2022, in the Medline databases via Pubmed, Embase, Cochrane, and Lilacs. The search strategy was formulated using the controlled vocabulary of the Medical Subject Headings (Mesh), Embase Subject Headins (Entree), and Health Sciences Descriptors (DeCs) databases. The references identified in the databases were exported to the Rayyan application of the Qatar Computing Research Institute (QCRI). **Table 1** presents the terms used in the search.

Inclusion and Exclusion Criteria

The aim of the study and the mnemonic PCC (population, concept, and context) were used as a guide for defining the inclusion criteria. Primary observational (cross-sectional, case–control cohort) and experimental studies (randomized clinical trials) and systematic reviews were included in the review. Articles not published in English, gray literature, opinion articles, editorials, and those published more than 10 years ago were excluded from the review.

Selection of Studies

After removing duplicates, according to the study eligibility criteria, the selection process (screening of titles and abstracts and complete reading of articles) was carried out independently by 2 reviewers and in cases of disagreement, a third reviewer issued the opinion about the inclusion of the article in the review. The independence of the reviewers was ensured by blinding the reviewers using the Blind ON tool of the Rayyan application of the Qatar Computing Research Institute, QCRI.

Data Extraction

After careful analysis of the selected articles, data were extracted using a previously prepared Microsoft Excel spreadsheet with the following information: author, year of publication, study location, research objective, design, population, outcome, and results.

RESULTS

Search Procedure

The search comprised 1859 records in the Pubmed, Embase, Lilacs and Cochrane databases (**Fig. 1**). The selection process followed the procedure of PRISMA–ScR (Preferred Reporting Items for Systematic reviews and Meta-analyses for Scoping Reviews). After removing the duplicates, 1677 remained for evaluation of titles and abstracts. Around 96 (5.7%) articles were selected for full reading and of these 12 studies were selected for synthesis.

Study Characteristics

Table 2 presents the main characteristics of the studies included in the synthesis (author, country, year of publication, objective, number of participants, result, and conclusion). The average number of participants in the studies was 638.66 (SD = 824.18) ranging from 16 to 2.818. All participants were women, age ranging from 20 to 65 year old. We observed a variation in relation to the types of shifts, with 41.6% of participants working day and night shifts,[17,20,22,24,28] 33.3% in rotating shifts,[18,21,25,26] and 16.6% only in night work. Among the activities carried out, the role of nurse, nursing assistant, midwife and caregiver covered most of the studies, except for the study by Kim and colleagues,[21] which has investigated industry workers. It was found that most of the selected studies were carried out in countries on the Asian continent (75%), namely China,[20,24] Taiwan,[18] Republic of Korea,[21,28] Japan,[25] Israel,[23] India,[22] and United Arab Emirates.[26] The other studies were developed in the United States of America[17,19] and Finland.[27] Most studies had a cross-sectional design (75%),[17–22,24–26] whereas

Table 1
Search strategy in database according to the population, concept, context framework for scoping review

Population	("Female") OR ("Woman") OR ("Women") OR ("Woman, Working" OR "Working Woman" OR "Working Women")
CONTEXT	("schedule shift work" OR "schedules shift work" OR "work schedule shift" OR "night shift work" OR "shift work night" OR "rotating shift work" OR "shift work rotating")
CONCEPT	("Sleeping Habits" OR "Sleep Habits" OR "Habit, Sleep" OR "Habits, Sleep" OR "Sleep Habit" OR "Habit, Sleeping" OR "Habits, Sleeping") OR ("Sleep-Wake Schedule Disorder" OR "Sleep Wake Schedule Disorders" OR "Sleep-Wake Schedule Disorder" OR "Sleep Wake Schedule Disorder" OR "Circadian Rhythm Sleep Disorders" OR "Sleep-Wake Cycle Disorder" OR "Sleep Wake Cycle Disorder" OR "Circadian Rhythm Sleep Disorder" OR "Sleep-Wake Cycle Disorders" OR "Sleep Wake Cycle Disorders" OR "Shift-Work Sleep Disorder" OR "Shift Work Sleep Disorder" OR "Sleep Disorder, Shift-Work" OR "Shift-Work Sleep Disorders" OR "Sleep Disorder, Shift Work" OR "Sleep Disorders, Shift-Work" OR "Advanced Sleep Phase Syndrome" OR "Delayed Sleep Phase Syndrome" OR "Delayed Sleep-Phase Syndrome"

Source: DECS, MESH, ENTREE (2022).

16.7% were longitudinal prospective,[27,28] and 8.3% were experimental.[23]

Sleep Variables

Actigraphy was carried out in 4 studies[17,20,23,27] and the most commonly analyzed variables were sleep duration, sleep efficiency, sleep latency; wake after sleep onset. In general, actigraphy is used in the assessment of activity-rest data, with recordings for 24 hours a day, for days or weeks, allowing the assessment of sleep in a real condition.

Subjective sleep quality was assessed in 7 studies using the Pittsburgh Sleep Quality Index (PSQI).[18,20–23,25,26,29] In the study carried out by Lin and colleagues,[18] workers in rotating shifts had poor sleep quality when compared with day workers. Kim and colleagues[21] identified that subjective reports of poor sleep quality were more frequent among workers in rotation shifts with short intervals between night shifts (12 days) when compared with shifts with intervals of 4 and 6 weeks, respectively. In addition, Uekata and colleagues[25] identified that 60.4% of workers in rotating night shifts had low sleep quality (PSQI > 6). Vijaykumar and colleagues[22] found that night workers had poor sleep quality when compared with day workers and those who had never worked shifts. In the experimental study conducted by Zion and Shochat[23] to evaluate the effectiveness of naps on the quality of sleep of night workers (night shift with and without 30 min scheduled nap at 4:00 h), no statistically significant difference was observed between the experimental and control groups. In the study by Kang and colleagues[20] there was no statistical significant difference in sleep quality scores between shifts (day shift, evening shift, and night shift). Zhang and colleagues[24] assessed subjective sleep quality using a General Sleep Disturbance Scale-Chinese version–GSDS.[30,31] They found out that workers who worked shifts reported poor sleep quality (69.4%).[24]

Sleepiness was assessed in three studies. Ruggiero and colleagues[17] used the Stanford Sleepiness Scale[32] to compare day and night shift workers, but found no differences in sleepiness scores between subjects on each shift. Zion and Shochat[23] using the Karolinska Sleepiness Scale–KSS[33] identified an increase in sleepiness throughout all shifts. In addition, the authors observed less sleepiness in the mornings after nights with naps compared with nights without naps at 5:00 h, 6:00 h, and 7:00 h. Zhang and colleagues[24] assessed daytime sleepiness using a subitem of the GSDS.[30,31] According to GSDS subscale, the mean of daytime sleepiness in all participants (n = 647) was 3.60 (SD = 1.33); however, in those who experienced sleep disturbances (n-454) the mean of subscale (daytime sleepiness) was 4.22 (SD = 1.00).

Chronotype was analyzed in 5 studies[19,23,25–27] and the instruments used to access this variable were Biological Clocks Questionnaire[19]; Munich Chronotype Questionnaire[23,25,34]; Morningness–eveningness (rMEQ-5)[26,35]; and Diurnal Type Scale.[27,36] Lastly, the concentration of melatonin was evaluated by a single study. Bani and colleagues[26] evaluated salivary melatonin levels,

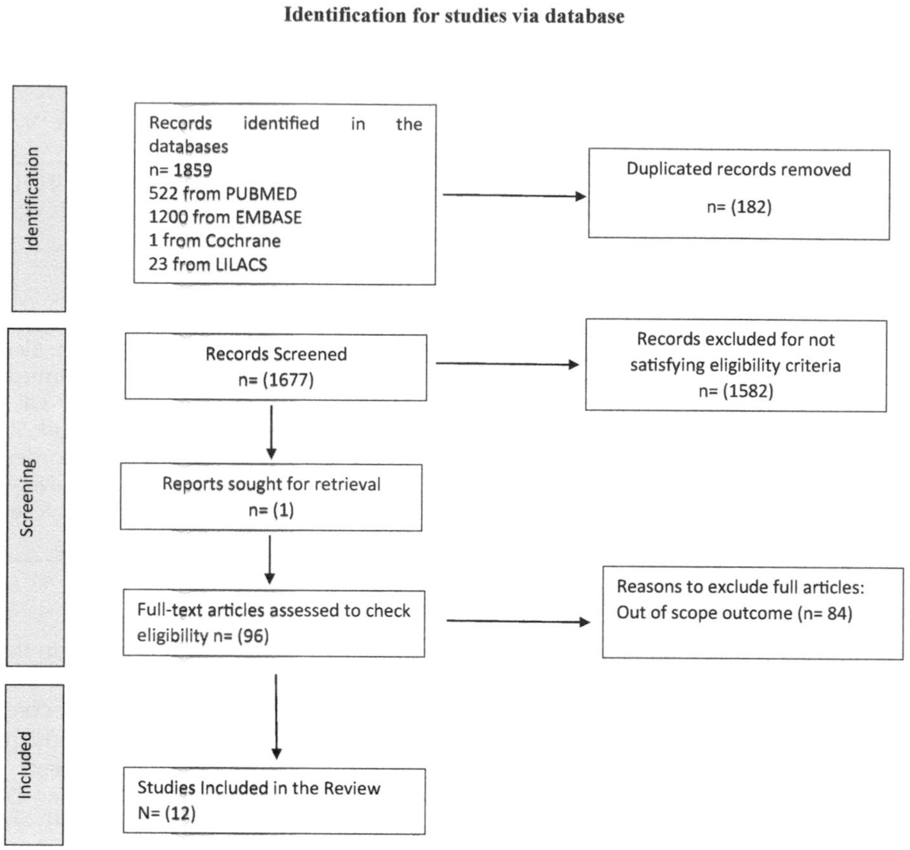

Fig. 1. PRISMA-ScR flow diagram.

showing a reduction in its nocturnal concentration in nurses in rotating night shifts. Salivary samples were collected during the first hour of the day shift (between 07:00 h and 08:00 h) and at night of the same day (between 21:00 h and 22:00 h). When working at night, the data collection took place between 21:00 h and 22:00 h and between 7:00 h and 8:00 h the next day. Rotating night shift nurses had lower evening melatonin compared with the day shift, and night melatonin levels were significantly higher in the day shift. There was no difference in perceived sleep quality between the two groups. Nurses on the rotating night shift had better scores for subjective sleep quality, sleep duration, and sleep disturbances compared with nurses on the day shift. Nurses on the rotating night shift had worse sleep efficiency compared with nurses on the day shift.

DISCUSSION

In this scoping review, most of the participants were health care providers working at night. Although injuries related to shift work have been studied in different populations of workers,[37] many studies were conducted with health professionals, mainly nurses. This professional category has been evaluated in relation to psychomotor attention, decision-making, and several disorders associated with unusual working hours.[38,39]

The retrieved studies in this review have shown evidence of worsening sleep quality and changes in circadian rhythm responses in women who worked in shift work schedules. In one of the studies accessed, for example, nurses who worked at night napped more often and had more changes in the length of their main sleep episodes than those who worked during the day. In addition, night workers were sleepier after work.[17] According to the authors, nurses who worked at night did not get enough sleep with a tendency to have few episodes of awakenings during sleep. The authors suggest that planned napping during the night shift may be effective in reducing the sleep restriction, fatigue, and sleepiness. Sleep restriction and an irregular sleep pattern are important problems for nurses who work in shifts.[17]

Moreover, it called our attention the differences in the shift types in the retrieved studies, what makes difficult any comparison among them. However,

Table 2
Descriptive summary of the included studies (n = 12)

Author, Year	Design	N	Shift Schedule	Occupation	Method for Assessing Outcomes	Main Results
Ruggiero et al,[17] 2012	Cross-sectional	16	Day and night shifts	Nurse	Actigraph; Sleep diary; Stanford Sleepiness Scale	Night nurses napped more frequently and had more changes in the length of their main sleep periods than day nurses. Night nurses were sleepier after work than day nurses.
Lin et al,[18] 2012	Cross-sectional (survey)	1360	Rotation shift	Nurses	Pittsburgh Sleep Quality Index (PSQI); Chinese Health Questionnaire 12-item (CHQ-12)	Nurses on rotation shift had the poor sleep quality and mental health compared with nurses on day shift.
Petrov et al,[19] 2014	Cross-sectional (survey)	213	Night shift	Nurses	Biological Clocks Questionnaire (BCQ); Standard Shiftwork Index (SSI)	Nap proxy and no sleep types were associated with poorer adaptation to night shift work; switch sleeper and incomplete switcher types were identified as more adaptive strategies.
Kang et al,[20] 2014	Cross-sectional (aurvey)	35	Day and night shifts	Nurses	Actigraph; Sleep Diary; PSQI	Night-shift nurses exhibited the lowest values of circadian rhythm amplitude, acrophase, autocorrelation, and mean of the circadian relative power (CRP), whereas evening-shift workers exhibited the greatest standard deviation of the CRP among the three shift groups.
Kim et al,[21] 2015	Cross-sectional (survey)	2.818	Rotation shift	Manufacturing	PSQI	The group with the shortest night shift rotation interval (group C) had the lowest sleep quality.

(*continued on next page*)

Table 2
(*continued*)

Author, Year	Design	N	Shift Schedule	Occupation	Method for Assessing Outcomes	Main Results
Vijaykumar et al,[22] 2018	Cross-sectional study	150	Day and night shifts	Nurses	PSQI; Reaction time test	Global score of PSQI, subjective sleep quality, sleep duration, and sleep medication was statistically high among night shift nurses suggesting poor sleep quality compared to day shift and controls.
Zion & Shochat,[23] 2019	Experimental study	119	Night shift	Nurses	Munich Chronotype Questionnaire for Shiftwork; Pittsburgh Sleep Quality Index; Pre-Sleep Arousal Scale at study onset; Actigraph; Pre-Sleep Arousal Scale (PSAS); Karolinska Sleepiness Scale (KSS), Digit Symbol Substitution Task (DSST); a subtest of the Wechsler Adult Intelligence Scale	Differences in sleepiness appeared following the nap period, with higher sleepiness levels in the no-nap compared with the nap condition.
Zhang et al,[24] 2019	Cross-sectional study	647	Day and night shifts	Nurses	General Sleep Disturbance Scale-Chinese version (GSDS), Fatigue Scale-Short Form (C-LFS-SF)	More than two-thirds of the participants (70.3%) scored at least three on the GSDS, indicating that the RNs in the current study experienced clinically significant sleep disturbance.
Uekata et al,[25] 2019	Cross-sectional (survey)	1253	Rotation shift	Nurses and midwives	PSQI; Munich Chronotype Questionnaire; Cambridge-Hopkins questionnaire-restless legs syndrome 13	Participants with later mid-sleep time's exhibited delayed sleep phases, which was more significant for work-free days than working day.

Bani-Issa et al,[26] 2020	Cross-sectional	510	Fixed; rotation shift	Nurses	Pittsburgh Sleep Quality Index; Morningness–eveningness (rMEQ-5); salivary melatonin	Rotating night shift nurses had significantly lower evening melatonin compared with the fixed day shift group. No significant difference was found in sleep quality between the groups.
Honkalampi et al,[27] 2022	Longitudinal	52	Morning and evening shifts	Home care Workers	Diurnal Type Scale; Actigraph	On night N3, E-types had a significantly shorter total sleep time and spent less time in bed compared to M- and N-types. There were no statistically significant differences in actigraphy-based sleep quality parameters between M-, N-, and E-types on nights N1, N2, and N4.
Ki & Choi-Kwon,[28] 2022	Longitudinal prospective cohort study	491	Day shit; rotating shift work	Nurses	Insomnia Severity Index (ISI), Fatigue Severity Scale (FSS), Center for Epidemiologic Studies Depression Scale (CES-D)	Sleep disturbance was present in 62.5 of studied population. There was association between sleep disturbance and turnover intention.

the studies showed some evidence that the women working in rotating shifts presented a worse condition compared with those working during the day. In the study by Lin and colleagues,[18] for instance, sleep quality and mental health were significantly worse in rotation shift compared with other work schedules. The number of consecutive shifts seems to reduce cognition and increase sleepiness, as shown by James and colleagues[40] in a quasi-experimental study with 94 nurses (men and women) in 3 consecutive shifts. Honkalampi and colleagues[27] found similar results in a study with women only. Petrovic and colleagues[19] evaluated the strategies used on days off, namely (a) night stay, (b) nap proxy, (c) switch sleeper, (d) no sleep, and (e) incomplete switcher. The author found that most participants (96.7%) preferred to switch to sleeping at night on their day off, and only 23.9% of the sample reported high adaptation levels to their shift schedule. However, the small sample size for night stay types may prevent strong conclusions. In addition, the adaptive strategies for reducing sleep disturbances may not be suitable for everyone as each individual can respond differently to the work schedule. Circadian hygiene strategies that include the knowledge of an individual's internal timing is crucial to define sleep/awake times.[41]

The studies selected for this review did not discuss sex differences regarding the outcome of interest. Yet, it is important to highlight that there is no consensus in the literature on sex differences in terms of sleep characteristics and patterns. Polysomnography sleep studies with healthy subjects showed that findings of sex differences in sleep are mixed, probably due to differences in study design, variability in the populations and sample size.[42] However, some studies suggest better sleep quality among women compared with men.[43,44] A recent study conducted with healthy adults who did not work in shifts found lower sleep fragmentation in women compared with men.[45] According to the authors, differences in lifestyle and age may contribute to the observation of differences between the sexes in relation to sleep. For example, sleep efficiency in the group of younger women was higher not only compared with elderly women but also when compared with younger men. On the other hand, there was a tendency to low sleep efficiency in the group of elderly women compared with elderly men[45] whereas another study with the elderly showed that among the 44.9% who reported sleep disturbances, 51.5% were female.[46]

Aiming to discuss factors associated with sleep disorders, Zhang and colleagues[24] estimated a prediction model for sleep disorders including the work environment, biological characteristics, and lifestyle. The results showed that the most important predictors are morning fatigue (100%), body mass index (30.5%), gastrointestinal symptoms (17.6%), and intake of caffeinated beverages at work (17.3%). The authors discuss the importance of detecting these factors to identify nurses working shifts with a higher risk of sleep disorders. It is important to note that some workers may develop circadian rhythm disorders as well as other sleep disorders. Circadian rhythm disorders are associated with changes of the circadian timing system, with shift work being a variable that contributes to circadian misalignment.[47] Vijaykumar and colleagues[22] suggested that circadian rhythm alterations could explain the observed differences in sleep quality in day shift nurses, night shift nurses, and those who never exposed to shift work. The authors' findings showed that subjective sleep quality and sleep duration were statistically worse among night shift nurses suggesting poor sleep quality compared with day shift and controls, corroborating other studies.[17,18,20] These findings are not surprising as night work invades the biological night, while sleep occurs during the biological day. This internal circadian misalignment and modified times for rest and work may lead to shorter sleep duration and bad sleep quality.[48]

As circadian misalignment shows individual responses, it is interesting to compare whether there were sleep disturbances according to chronotype. Honkalampi and colleagues[27] suggested that morning and intermediate types may have better sleep quality than evening types, which was also reflected in heart rate variability parameters. The evening types had a significantly shorter total sleep duration and spent less time in bed compared with morning and intermediate types on the third night shift. Uekata and colleagues[25] also evaluated the chronotype in nurses and midwives, in addition to the impact of rotating shift work on sleep quality and Willis-Ekbom syndrome. Difficulty initiating sleep represented 40% of workers on three-shift rotation, while those who worked rotating 16 h night shifts reported good sleep quality. Morning types were more frequent among diurnal workers, who also presented a lower social jet lag than the other studied groups. Insomnia was observed both on workdays and days off, and subjective sleep quality was more affected by the three-shift rotation. According to the authors,[25] a short interval between working days during rotation shifts alters the circadian rhythm, generating biological misalignment and insomnia, an hypothesis corroborated by 2 studies in this review.[18,21] Evening type was an independent risk factor for decreased subjective sleep quality. In addition, total sleep duration was shorter on working days among the evening types compared with other chronotypes, however, during the days off occurred the opposite.[25]

Only one study in this review analyzed melatonin concentration in connection with sleep quality and chronotype.[26] The authors found that rotating night shift nurses had significantly lower evening melatonin compared with the day shift group. No significant difference was found in sleep quality between the groups. Rotating night shift workers were more likely to have evening or intermediate types as well as to report alignment of work hours to their chronotype compared with day shift workers. Hittle and colleagues[49] also suggested that when chronotype and work hours are incongruent, the probability of health problems and differences in sleep quality are noted.

Of the 12 studies in this review, 4 used actigraphy, 2 with sleep diaries, while 7 studies used the PSQI.[19,21–24,26,27] The daily sleep–wake behavior assessed by the actigraphs and the completion of sleep diaries provide information about the sleep–wake cycle and the daily routine of the workers during the study protocol. Although polysomnography has considered the "gold standard" for sleep tracking, several studies use actigraphy with satisfactory results.[50]

This scoping review is the first, as far as we know, to present specific studies with adult women and night shift workers, exclusively evaluating sleep disturbances and the influence of this on health repercussion. Therefore, we presented consistent evidence and highlighted the gaps in the knowledge of the subject. However, the reduced number of articles that met the inclusion criteria, reducing the ability to measure robust conclusion, is a limitation of this review. It is important to highlight that only one study did not refer to nursing workers. It is also noteworthy that the selection criteria of the studies excluded pregnant and puerperal women, and not a single study had controlled the menstrual phase.

The studies presented in the review suggest that night shift work reduces the free time and sleep duration as well as affects workers' alertness, attention, and health. However, it is important to emphasize that more research is needed to investigate specific issues of female shift workers, as well as the social context in which they are inserted and its impact on health.

CLINICS CARE POINTS

In the case of the development of sleep or other health problems, relevant clinical points must be taken into account, such as:

- careful anamnesis and physical examination.
- information from family members of patients, doctors and previous records about working hours and the time when symptoms appeared.

DISCLOSURE

The authors have nothing to disclose.

FUNDING

Claudia RC Moreno is a recipient of a fellowship from CNPq (ID 307875/2022-9).

REFERENCES

1. ILO. International Labour Conference, 107th Session. Ensuring decent working time for the future. General survey concerning working-time instruments. Report No.:ILC.107/III(B). Geneva, Switzerland: International Labour Organization; 2018.
2. Moore-Ede M. The twenty-four-hour society: understanding human limits in a world that never stops. Boston, MA: Addison-Wesley; 1993. p. 600.
3. Moreno CRC, Marqueze EC, Sargent C, et al. Working Timing Society consensus statements: evidence-based effects of shift work on physical and mental health. Ind Health 2019;57:139–57.
4. Vetter C. Circadian disruption: what do we actually mean? Eur J Neurosci 2020;51:531–50.
5. Kecklund G, Axelsson J. Health consequences of shift work and insufficient sleep. BMJ 2016;1:355.
6. Iarc. Night shift work. IARC Monogr Identif Carcinog Hazards Hum 2020;124:1–371.
7. Arlinghaus A, Bohle P, Iskra-Golec I, et al. Working Time Society consensus statements: evidence-based effects of shift work and non-standard working hours on workers, family and community. Ind Health 2019;57:184–200.
8. Åkerstedt T. Shift work and disturbed sleep/wakefulness. Occup Med 2003;53:89–94.
9. Van Dongen HPA. Shift work and inter-individual differences in sleep and sleepiness. Chronobiol Int 2006;23:11391147.
10. Folkard S, Lombardi DA, Tucker PT. Shiftwork: safety, sleepiness and sleep. Ind Health 2005;43:20–3.
11. Kalmbach DA, Pillai V, Cheng P, et al. Shift work disorder, depression, and anxiety in the transition to rotating shifts: the role of sleep reactivity. Sleep Med 2015;16:1532–8.
12. Junseok S, Lee Sangyoon. Effects of work stress, sleep, and shift work on suicidal ideation among female workers in an electronics company. Am J Ind Med 2021;64:519–27.

13. Kloss JD, Perlis M, Zamzowa J, et al. Sleep, sleep disturbance and fertility in women. Sleep Med Rev 2015;22:78–87.
14. Garde AH, Begtrup L, Bjorvatn B, et al. How to schedule night shift work in order to reduce health and safety risks. Scand J Work Environ Health 2020;46:557–69.
15. Tricco AC, Lillie E, Zarin W, et al. A scoping review on the conduct and reporting of scoping reviews. BMC Med Res Methodol 2016;16:15.
16. Peters MDJ, Marnie C, Tricco AC, et al. Updated methodological guidance for the conduct of scoping reviews. JBI Evid Synth 2020;18:2119–26.
17. Ruggiero JS, Redeker NS, Fiedler N, et al. Sleep and psychomotor vigilance in female shiftworkers. Biol Res Nurs 2012;14:225–35.
18. Lin PC, Chen CH, Pan SM, et al. Atypical work schedules are associated with poor sleep quality and mental health in Taiwan female nurses. Int Arch Occup Environ Health 2012;85:877–84.
19. Petrov ME, Clark CB, Molzof HE, et al. Sleep strategies of night-shift nurses on days off: which ones are most adaptive? Front Neurol 2014;5:1–8.
20. Kang JH, Miao NF, Tseng IJ, et al. Circadian activity rhythms and sleep in nurses working fixed 8-hr shifts. Biol Res Nurs 2014;3:1–8.
21. Kim JY, Chae CH, Kim YO, et al. The relationship between quality of sleep and night shift rotation interval. Ann Occup Environ Med 2015;27:31.
22. Vijaykumar N, Kiran S, Karne SL. Influence of altered circadian rhythm on quality of sleep and its association with cognition in shift nurses. Natl J Physiol Pharm Pharmacol 2018;8:643–9.
23. Zion N, Shochat T. Let them sleep: the effects of a scheduled nap during the night shift on sleepiness and cognition in hospital nurses. J Adv Nurs 2019;00:1–13.
24. Zhang X, Lee SY, Luo H, et al. A prediction model of sleep disturbances among female nurses by using the BP-ANN. J Nurs Manag 2019;27:1123–30.
25. Uekata S, Kato C, Nagaura Y, et al. The impact of rotating work schedules, chronotype, and restless legs syndrome/Willis-Ekbom disease on sleep quality among female hospital nurses and midwives: a cross-sectional survey. Int J Nurs Stud 2019;95:103–12.
26. Bani-Issa W, Rahman HA, Albluwi N, et al. Morning and evening salivary melatonin, sleepiness and chronotype: a comparative study of nurses on fixed day and rotating night shifts. J Adv Nurs 2020;00:1–13.
27. Honkalampi K, Kupari S, Järvelin-Pasanen S, et al. The association between chronotype and sleep quality among female home care Workers performing shift work. Chronobiology Int 2022;39:747–56.
28. Ki J, Choi-Kwon S. Health problems, turnover intention, and actual turnover among shift work female nurses: analyzing data from a prospective longitudinal study. PLoS One 2022;17:e0270958.
29. Buysse DJ, Reynolds III CF, Monk TH, et al. The Pittsburgh sleep quality index: a new instrument for psychiatric practice and research. Psychiatr Res 1988;28:193–213.
30. Lee KA, Hicks G, Nino-Murcia G. Validity and reliability of a scale to assess fatigue. Psychiatr Res 1991;36(3):291–8.
31. Lee SY. Validating the general sleep disturbance scale among Chinese American parents with hospitalized infants. J Transcult Nurs 2007;18(2):111–7.
32. Hoddes E, Dement W, Zarcone V. The development and use of the Stanford sleepiness scale. Psychophysiology 1972;9:150.
33. Åkerstedt T, Gillberg M. Subjective and objective sleepiness in the active individual. Int J Neurosci 1991;52:29–37.
34. Roenneberg T, Wirs-Justice A, Merrow M. Life between clocks: daily temporal patterns of human chronotypes. J. Biol. Rhythms 2003;18:80–90.
35. Horne JA, Östberg O. A self-assessment questionnaire to determine morningness-eveningness in human circadian rhythms. Int J Chronobiol 1976;4:97–110.
36. Torsvall L, Akerstedt T. A diurnal type scale. Construction, consistency and validation in shift work. Scand J Work Environ Health 1980;6:283–90.
37. Schneider D, Harknett K. Consequências da instabilidade do horário de trabalho rotineiro para a saúde e o bem-estar do trabalhador. Am Socio Rev 2019;84(1):82–114.
38. Kaliyaperumal D, Elango Y, Alagesan M, et al. Effects of sleep deprivation on the cognitive performance of nurses working in shift. J Clin Diagn Res 2017;11(8):CC01–3.
39. Vasconcelos SP, Fischer FM, Reis AO, Moreno CR. Factors associated with work ability and perception of fatigue among nursing personnel from Amazonia. Rev Bras Epidemiol 2011;14(4):688–97.
40. James L, Elkins-Brown N, Wilson M, et al. The effects of three consecutive 12-hour shifts on cognition, sleepiness, and domains of nursing performance in day and night shift nurses: a quasi-experimental study. Int J Nurs Stud 2021;123:104041.
41. Moreno CRC, Raad R, Gusmão WDP, et al. Are we ready to implement circadian hygiene interventions and programs? Int J Environ Res Public Health 2022;19(24):16772.
42. Mong JA, Cusmano DM. Sex differences in sleep: impact of biological sex and sex steroids. Philos Trans R Soc Lond B Biol Sci 2016;19:20150110.

43. Bixler EO, Papaliaga MN, Vgontzas AN, et al. Women sleep objectively better than men and the sleep of young women is more resilient to external stressors: effects of age and menopause. J Sleep Res 2009;18:221–8.
44. Ohayon MM, Carskadon MA, Guilleminault C, et al. Meta-analysis of quantitative sleep parameters from childhood to old age in healthy individuals: developing normative sleep values across the human lifespan. Sleep 2004;27:1255–73.
45. Kováčová K, Stebelová K. Sleep characteristics according to gender and age measured by wrist actigraphy. Int J Environ Res Public Health 2021 15;18:13213.
46. Moreno CRC, Santos JLF, Lebrão ML, et al. Sleep disturbances in older adults are associated to female sex, pain and urinary incontinence. Rev Bras Epidemiol 2019;4(21Suppl):e180018.
47. Duffy JD, Abbott SM, Burgess HJ, et al. Workshop report. Circadian rhythm sleep–wake disorders: gaps and opportunities. SLEEPJ 2021;44(5):zsaa281.
48. Lim YC, Hoe VCW, Darus A, et al. Association between night-shift work, sleep quality and metabolic syndrome. Occup Environ Med 2018;75:716–23.
49. Hittle BM, Caruso CC, Jones HJ, et al. Nurse health: the influence of chronotype and shift timing. West J Nurs Res 2020;42:1031–41.
50. Chinoy ED, Cuellar JA, Huwa KE, et al. Performance of seven consumer sleep-tracking devices compared with polysomnography. Sleep 2021;44:zsaa291.

Sleep Disorders and Aging in Women

Ritika Gadodia, MD[a], Deepika Nandamuru, MD[b], Wahida Akberzie, MD[c], Lynn Kataria, MD[d,*]

KEYWORDS

• Sleep • Aging in women • Insomnia • Sleep-disordered breathing

KEY POINTS

- Sleep disorders can increase in aging women such as insomnia and sleep-disordered breathing.
- Disruptions in sleep leading up to menopause and thereafter can have a significant impact on females and focused history is paramount to tailor treatment.
- If a patient is a limited historian, reliance on family and caregivers may be necessary along with diagnostic testing, such as, actigraphy and PSG.

INTRODUCTION

Projections of the US Census Bureau show the nation's 65-and-older population is expected to double from 49 million in 2016 to 95 million in 2060 that is, nearly a quarter of the US population.[1] This is of particular significance because sleep disturbances are more common in older adults.[2] Patients over the age of 65 report increased sleep latency, increased arousals during sleep and decreased sleep maintenance.[3] The Cardiovascular Health Study surveyed 4467 participants of advancing age, and found the incidence of trouble falling asleep was 2.8%, frequent awakenings were 12.3% and excessive daytime sleepiness was 4.4%.[4] Moreover, women were specifically more likely to have trouble falling asleep.[4] In addition to evidence of subjective sleep disturbances in this population, studies using polysomnography (PSG) have objectively confirmed that age-related changes in sleep predispose older individuals to increased sleep-fragmentation and wakefulness at night.[5] Numerous studies have consistently shown that the female gender is an independent risk factor for poor sleep quality, as measured by scales such as the Pittsburgh Sleep Quality Index and the Epworth Sleepiness Scale.[6–8] This is of particular importance because poor quality of sleep has been showed to correlate to limitations in activities of daily living in women.[9,10] An interesting study showed that women with shorter sleep times had double the odds of decline in their hand grip strength as compared to those with longer sleep times.[11] More recent studies have also looked at pathologic sleep related conditions such as restless leg syndrome and obstructive sleep apnea and found them to be more prevalent in advancing age. These disorders further elderly females at risk for cardiovascular diseases, headaches, memory loss and depression.[12] Sleep disorders such as insomnia have been linked to increased caregiver burden, and have been identified as factor in caregivers' decision regarding nursing home placement.[13,14] When looking at healthcare burden and cost-effectiveness, undiagnosed obstructive sleep apnea has been projected to cost the healthcare system nearly 149.7 billion dollars annually.[15]

[a] Department of Medicine, Medstar Washington Hospital Center, 110 Irving Street Northwest, Washington, DC 20010, USA; [b] Department of Neurology, George Washington University School of Medicine, GW Medical Faculty Associates, 2150 Pennsylvania Avenue Northwest, Washington, DC 20037, USA; [c] Department of Primary Care Medicine, Primary Care Service, Martinsburg VA Medical Center, 510 Butler Avenue, Martinsburg, WV 25405, USA; [d] Sleep Laboratory, Washington DC VA Medical Center, George Washington University School of Medicine, 3rd Floor, 50 Irving Street Northwest, Washington, DC 20422, USA
* Corresponding author. Sleep Laboratory, Washington DC VA Medical Center, George Washington University School of Medicine, 3rd Floor, 50 Irving Street Northwest, Washington, DC 20422.
E-mail address: Lynn.kataria@va.gov

Sleep Med Clin 18 (2023) 545–557
https://doi.org/10.1016/j.jsmc.2023.06.017
1556-407X/23/Published by Elsevier Inc.

The sleep physiology in women of advancing age is unique for many reasons, one of the most notable being hormonal changes. Estrogen and progesterone affect sleep patterns from puberty to menopause and during specific periods such as pregnancy and the menstrual cycle.[16] The incidence of numerous conditions is altered by menopause, exampled by a significantly higher apnea index in postmenopausal as compared to premenopausal females.[16]

This article will review sleep requirements and hormonal changes, and discuss the evaluation of disorders including insomnia, circadian disorders, restless leg syndrome, hypersomnia, and sleep-disordered breathing with a focus on women of advancing age including prevalence and recommended treatment options.

SLEEP ACROSS THE LIFESPAN

Changes in sleep architecture

Sleep is composed of two main states: rapid eye movement (REM) and non-rapid eye movement sleep (NREM). NREM sleep involves a synchronous cortical electroencephalogram, including sleep spindles, K-complexes, and slow waves.[17] It is associated with low muscle tone and minimal psychological activity. REM sleep has a desynchronized electroencephalogram, muscles are atonic, and dreaming occurs during this stage.[18] In adults the natural progression of sleep involves sleep beginning in NREM sleep and progressing into deeper NREM stages and then eventually REM sleep. As people age, the composition of sleep changes. Starting in preteenager years slow wave sleep (SWS; stage N3) starts declining by 40% and continues a slower decline into old age.[17] In advanced age populations, PSG studies of sleep architecture display decreases in total sleep time, sleep efficiency, and SWS with age.[19–23]

In women 65 years of age and older there is a greater association between declining total sleep time and aging.[5] Age-related changes in Stage 1 sleep are more apparent in women including less percentage of stage 2 sleep and a greater percentage of SWS than age-matched men.[5] The SIESTA study found that men had a 1.7% decrease in SWS per decade of age compared to women who had no change in SWS with age.[24] This same study found that women had a smaller rate of increase in Stage 1 sleep, a greater rate of increase in stage 2 sleep, and a greater rate of decline in REM, in comparison with men.[24] Changes in sleep architecture may be one reason why women are more likely to report sleep problems. Another important component that may be playing a role in sleep quality and contributing to changes in sleep architecture are the hormonal changes that occur throughout a woman's lifespan.

Hormonal changes and sleep in women

Women report more sleep disturbances and poor sleep quality around the time of menses.[25] Despite subjective sleep complaints, polysomnographic variables have shown that sleep continuity and sleep efficiency remain stable at different phases of the ovulatory menstrual cycle in young healthy women.[25] Percentages of SWS and slow wave activity in NREM sleep are unchanged across the menstrual cycle.[25] As women transition into menopause, lower estradiol levels were associated with poorer sleep over time.[26] The decline of endogenous estrogen that occurs in menopause, poses a great factor in sleep quality with consequences of sleep fragmentation in this population.[27]

In a community-based survey of women's health and menopausal symptoms, it was found that perimenopausal and postmenopausal women are more likely to report difficulty sleeping compared with premenopausal women.[28] During this time period, there is an increase in follicle-stimulating hormone (FSH) and luteinizing hormone, with a decline in estradiol levels.[29] Kravitz and colleagues investigated the effects of estradiol and FSH on sleep disturbances and noticed that a reduction of estradiol levels correlated with trouble falling asleep and staying asleep.[30] An increase in FSH levels was associated with reports of difficulty staying asleep.[30] Although the specific effects of estrogen, FSH, and luteinizing hormone on sleep as women go through menopause is controversial their contribution to sleep disruption cannot be ignored and may have lasting effects as women age.

Sleep requirements

According to the National Sleep Foundation, sleep time duration recommended is 7 to 8 hours for healthy aging adults.[31] As individuals age, the ability to sleep becomes more difficult with an increase in disturbed sleep.[32] Some research suggests that the quantity of sleep differs by age not because of changes in the necessity, but more that the ability to obtain needed sleep decreases with age.[33] The ability to sleep declines and may be related to medical and/or psychiatric illness and circadian changes.[33]

Ohayon and Vecchierini looked at 1000 older French adults who reported approximately 7 hours of sleep with men sleeping slightly more than women.[32] On average, total sleep time declines by 10 minutes per decade; however, this decline was more prominent in women than in men.[32] Empana and colleagues (39) included 9294 subjects aged greater than or equal to 65 years (60% of them being women) and found that 18.7% of the participants had regular or frequent excessive daytime sleepiness. A decline in the quantity and quality of sleep in women with advanced age are contributors to sleep disorders in this population.

Patient evaluation

Women of advancing age can suffer from an array of sleep disorders. They may present with sleep disturbance resulting in hypersomnolence, delirium, and impaired cognition, which can contribute to low a lower functional activity level and increased risk of accidents and injury. Obtaining a thorough history is imperative and may often involve family members, caregivers, and/or bed partners. Secondary collateral information can provide useful information regarding any unusual nocturnal events such as acting out of dreams, limb movements, snoring and witnessed apneic events. When obtaining a sleep-focused history of presenting illness (**Box 1**), it is important to ask about sleep/wake schedules, weekend routines, the sleep environment, and typical sleep habits. It is also important to ask about substance use including caffeine, alcohol, illicit drug use, and herbals, with particular focus on the timing of consumption with relation to sleep timings.

Sleep-disordered breathing is common in women 65 years and older.[34,35] There are several sleep questionnaires that can be used to screen for sleep-disordered breathing. A helpful tool for screening patients for sleep-disordered breathing is the STOP-BANG questionnaire, which is based on eight yes/no questions related to clinical features of sleep apnea (snoring, tiredness, observed apnea, hypertension, BMI>35 kg/m2, age>50, neck size>40 cm, male gender).[36] The questionnaire has shown to have a high sensitivity when using a cutoff score of 3 or more, with a sensitivity of 84% in detecting sleep apnea, 93% in detecting moderate sleep apnea and 100% for severe sleep apnea.[37] Another commonly used questionnaire in the sleep clinic is the Insomnia Severity Index (ISI). It consists of seven items used to assess the subjective symptoms and consequences of insomnia, as well as the severity of concerns.[38] A score of 15 or greater suggests moderate to severe insomnia, with a sensitivity of 47.7% to 78.1% and a specificity of 98.3% to 100%.[39]

Excessive daytime sleepiness is a common clinical consequence of pathologic sleep conditions including OSA, narcolepsy, and idiopathic hypersomnia. A commonly used validated questionnaire is the Epworth Sleepiness Scale (ESS). This is a self-administered questionnaire whereby patients score their chances of falling asleep in eight unique situations commonly encountered in their daily lives. Patients rate their chances of falling asleep from 0 (never) to 3 (high) and a score of 10 or higher suggests pathologic daytime sleepiness.[40] However, it is important to note that many studies have demonstrated clinically relevant variability in ESS scores, likely secondary to situational sleepiness influencing the subjective scoring system. Changes in ESS should therefore be interpreted with caution.[41,42] An interesting cross-sectional study reported that taking patient-completed and partner-completed ESS

Box 1
Sleep questionnaire for women in advancing age and caretakers

Focused Sleep Questionnaire for Women of Advancing Age and Caretakers

When do you wake up in the morning?

When do you fall asleep at night?

How long does it take you to fall asleep?

How many hours do you sleep per night?

How many times do you wake up during a typical night?

Do you feel that you are excessively sleepy during the daytime and take naps?

Do you have difficulties falling asleep or staying asleep?

Do you take medications or use alcohol to help you sleep?

Does pain bother you doing sleep?

Do you snore, gasp or stop breathing at night? Did this get worse during menopause?

Do you have uncomfortable sensations in your legs at night or unusual movements at night?

Do you have symptoms of sleep paralysis, hallucinations at sleep onset or waking, or cataplexy?

Are there any environmental noises or disturbances such as TV, bright lights, pets, or noises that disturb your sleep?

When did you reach menopause?

What was your sleep like during, before and after menopause?

Do you have medical, neurologic or psychiatric conditions that interfere with sleep?

scores into consideration together can improve the diagnostic utility of the ESS.[43]

A simplistic approach can be adopted when considering the sleep complaints in women of advancing age (**Figs. 1** and **2**). Clinical providers can evaluate whether sleep complaints are focused on excessive daytime sleepiness versus difficulty falling asleep or maintaining sleep throughout the night. There is certainly overlap between the two; however, this approach can help determine possible etiologies and appropriate next steps with respect to screening and testing.

Sleep disorders in women aged 65 and above

Women have high rates of insomnia.[44,45] Several epidemiologic studies have found that prevalence of insomnia symptoms reaches close to 40% in individuals 65 years of age and older.[46–48] Also, women above the age of 45 are 1.7 times more likely to have insomnia than men.[46] Patients may present with symptoms of difficulty initiating or maintaining sleep. According to the International Classification of Sleep Disorders 3, insomnia is defined as "a persistent difficulty with sleep initiation, duration, consolidation, or quality that occurs despite adequate opportunity and circumstances for sleep, and results in some form of daytime impairment."[49] Chronic insomnia consists of symptoms for at least 3 months at least three times per week, and short-term as being less than 3 months.[49] Performing a thorough sleep history and past medical history is needed, paying attention to medical, neurologic and psychiatric co-morbidities. Substances and medications that may disturb sleep are over-the-counter decongestants, beta agonists, corticosteroids, selective serotonin reuptake inhibitors (SSRIs), antipsychotics, diuretics, anticholinergics, alcohol, caffeine, and stimulants.[50] Obtaining information regarding sleep hygiene, including sleep time, wake time, and use of electronics before bed is necessary. A sleep diary can be used to further assess sleep patterns and actigraphy may also provide more information regarding the regular sleep-wake schedule and disturbances.

Regardless of medical history, the treatment of insomnia in adults ages 65 and above includes maintaining a regular sleep-wake schedule.[51] Cognitive behavioral therapy-Insomnia (CBT-I) is first-line treatment for insomnia in older adults with a multi-behavioral approach.[52,53] Several prospective studies have compared the efficacy of CBT-I, medications, and combination of CBT-I with medication.[54–56] Extending CBT-I may also prove to be beneficial in this patient population to maintain short term gains.[54–57] CBT-I consists of cognitive and behavioral techniques like stimulus control therapy, sleep restriction therapy, cognitive restructuring, relaxation techniques, and sleep hygiene education.[58] There are several risks with pharmacotherapy due to changing pharmacodynamics and pharmacokinetics in advanced age adults. Therefore, the discussion of risks should occur with patients and caregivers, which include falls, over sedation, confusion, and

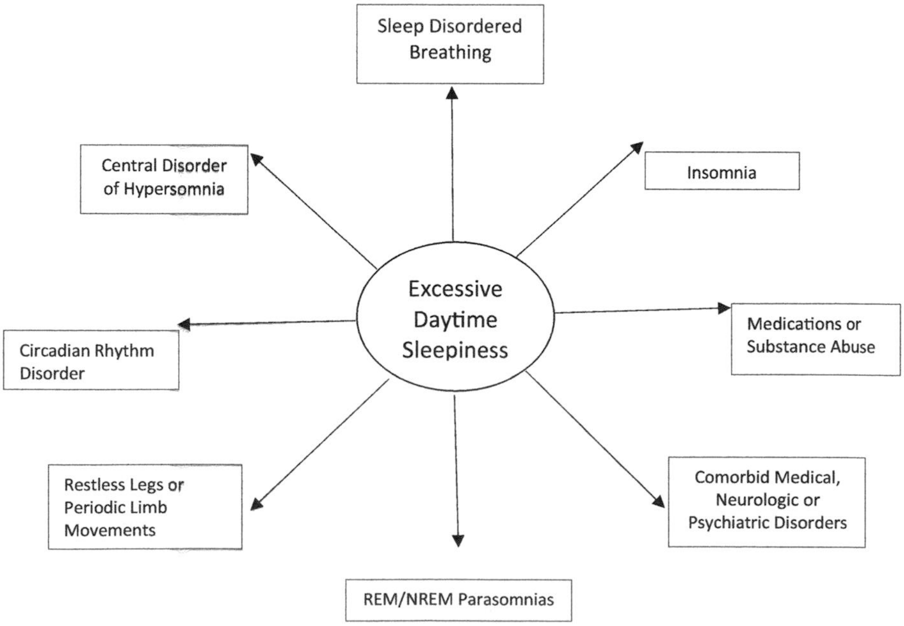

Fig. 1. Etiologies for complaints of excessive daytime sleepiness in women of advancing age.

cognitive impairment. Long-acting benzodiazepines should be avoided due to these risks mentioned. Nonbenzodiazepines such as zolpidem and eszopiclone are considered shorter acting, although they are not completely devoid of significant side effects either.[13] Ramelteon and other melatonin receptor agonists are Food and Drug Administration approved for insomnia and have been shown to effective with sleep initiation insomnia.[59] Other medications that are often used for the treatment of insomnia include trazodone, mirtazapine, tricyclic antidepressants, gabapentin, and first-generation antihistamines, however several of these medications may cause significant side effects including orthostatic hypotension and increase risk of falls and caution should be exercised in older individuals. Antidepressants should only be considered for insomnia when there is underlying depression.[53]

There is evolving data regarding alternative nonpharmacologic therapies in women and randomized controlled trials are warranted. Small studies have found that yoga may produce a reduction in insomnia severity in perimenopausal and postmenopausal women.[60,61] There is limited data regarding therapeutic massage, however one small study looking at 44 postmenopausal volunteers that were randomly distributed into three groups of therapeutic massage, passive movements, and control.[62] Habitual physical activity has also showed benefit in menopausal women.[53] The individuals in the therapeutic massage group demonstrated improvement in Insomnia Severity Index and the menopause quality of life questionnaire.[62]

Obstructive sleep apnea

Sleep-disordered breathing (SDB) is an umbrella term which includes OSA, central sleep apnea (CSA) disorders, sleep related hypoventilation disorders and sleep related hypoxemia disorders.[63] OSA is characterized by repeated episodes of partial or complete obstruction of the respiratory passages during sleep, with continued respiratory effort.[63] OSA increases with advanced age one study showed that the prevalence of SDB was 18.1% in the 61 to 100-year age group, as compared to 11.3% in the 45 to 64-year age group.[64] Other studies have also shown that the prevalence of OSA increases with age and may be up to 90% in men and 78% in women aged 60 to 85 year old.[34,65] Notably, the gender differences are less evident after menopause,[65] which may be secondary to the respiratory stimulant effect of progesterone in premenopausal women.[66] A recent study showed that the doubling of serum concentrations of estrogen and progesterone were associated with 19% and 9% decreased odds of snoring respectively.[67] Interestingly, the prevalence of OSA was also relatively low in postmenopausal women with hormone replacement therapy (HRT), further suggestive a protective effect.[68] Given the higher association in postmenopausal women, a diagnosis of OSA should be appropriately considered as part of the evaluation of women of advancing age presenting with sleep disruption.

SDB is associated with a lower physical health-related quality of life and cognitive function in older age, and the presence of these may guide further management and be used as treatment target measures in this age group.[69] Another significant finding was in advanced age edentulous patients, where it was found that early prosthetic rehabilitation with denture wear and mandibular advancement improves the morbidity associated with OSA.[70] Symptoms of SDB include excessive daytime sleepiness (EDS), snoring, witnessed apneic events, choking, or gasping in sleep, and morning

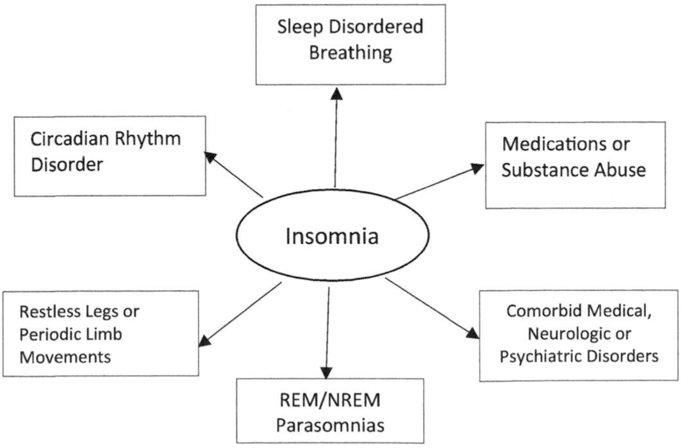

Fig. 2. Etiologies for complaints of insomnia in women of advancing age.

headaches. Fatigue and insomnia, rather than snoring and sleepiness may be the predominant symptoms in women, and the STOP-BANG scoring favors males.[71] In fact, the Berlin Questionnaire has been shown to have the highest sensitivity in both genders.[71]

A sleep study is indicated for the confirmation of diagnosis of OSA. Home sleep apnea testing that is technically adequate may also be used in patients with no significant cardiopulmonary disease, neuromuscular disease, history of stroke, chronic opiate use, or concerns of hypoventilation.[72] OSA is diagnosed in patients with at least 5 obstructive respiratory events on PSG or out-of-center sleep study, and treatment is guided by the presence of symptoms or co-morbid conditions. First-line therapy is Continuous Positive Airway Pressure (CPAP), but may be limited by patient adherence ranging anywhere between 20% and 80%.[73] Auto titrating, self-adjusting devices (APAP) have shown improved adherence as compared to CPAP, but its impact on EDS was similar to patients on CPAP.[74] When changes designed specifically for women such as increased sensitivity to airflow limitation and lower pressure rise were used, women showed better control of OSA.[71] Several alternate therapeutic options are available for mild OSA, including mandibular assist devices and positional devices.[75] A novel alternative is daytime neuromuscular electrical therapy of the tongue muscles, which has demonstrated efficacy in reducing snoring as well as improvement in EDS. It is therefore promising for women in advanced age due to its minimal transient side effect profile.[76] Recently, Hypoglossal Nerve Stimulation (HNS) has been developed for use in individuals with moderate to severe OSA who are unable to use CPAP therapy.[77] HSN is an implantable device that acts as a pacemaker and delivers electrical stimuli to the hypoglossal nerve. This treatment option necessitates a drug-induced sleep endoscopy followed by surgery, and it is imperative that risks and benefits be discussed with the patient when evaluating for candidacy in females of advancing age. Other invasive surgical options may not normalize the AHI and are associated with pain and long healing times, therefore potentially limiting their use in older patients.[78] Given the recent surge in treatment modalities for OSA, it is important to promote shared decision-making with the consideration of factors such as degree of OSA, patient preference, surgical candidacy, and likelihood of adherence to PAP.

Central sleep apnea

CSA syndromes are defined as a reduction or cessation in airflow due to reduced or absent respiratory effort.[63] Data from the Sleep Heart Health Study showed the prevalence of CSA and Cheyne Strokes Respiration to be 0.9% and 0.4% respectively, and predominant OSA with a component of CSA was found in 2.7% of adults aged 40 and older.[79] In a different cohort including men aged 65 years and older, the prevalence was found to be as high as 7.5%.[80] CSAs due to Cheyne-Stokes respiration (CSR) is characterized by absence of air flow and respiratory effort followed by hyperventilation in a crescendo-decrescendo pattern and can occur in 30% to 50% of patients with congestive heart failure.[81] While evaluating a patient, it is important to keep in mind that a patient may have both central and obstructive sleep apnea, especially since the prevalence of both increases with age.

Patients may present with EDS, insomnia, or nocturnal dyspnea. It is important to remember that due to the association of CSA with CHF, a patient's symptoms of frequent night-time awakening or disturbed sleep may be falsely assumed to be a consequence of their heart failure.[63] CSA is also associated with atrial fibrillation, renal failure, and chronic opiate use.[82–84] These are all conditions that are increasingly common with advancing age, and older females with these co-morbidities and sleep complaints should undergo thorough evaluation for CSA. Diagnosis of CSA in the presence of these comorbidities may also guide therapy, and there is some evidence that sleep apnea in patients with chronic renal failure may be corrected with the use of nocturnal hemodialysis instead of conventional hemodialysis.[85]

CSA is diagnosed in individuals with at least 5 central respiratory events on PSG, and most respiratory events should be central in nature. Treatment is guided by the severity of CSA, symptoms, and the presence of co-morbid conditions. The different options include CPAP, Bi-level PAP in a spontaneous timed (ST) mode, and Adaptive-Serve-Ventilation (ASV). Although ASV was previously used as a second-line therapy for patients with CSA who did not tolerate CPAP, the results of the SERVE-HF trial showed that the ASV device increased mortality without improving quality of life in heart failure with reduced ejection fraction patients with CSA.[86] Based on current evidence, it may still be considered as an option in patients with EF>45%.[87] There is also low-level evidence supporting the use of acetazolamide and theophylline in the treatment of CSA if PAP therapy is not tolerated, but its use is limited by its side effect provide which includes electrolyte imbalances, tinnitus, and gastrointestinal side effects.[81] Currently, the overall quality of evidence regarding therapeutic options in CSA is moderate at best, particularly in women of advancing age, and more data is needed to optimize patient care strategies in this cohort.

Restless leg syndrome evaluation

Restless leg syndrome (RLS) is a sensorimotor disorder characterized by uncomfortable sensations in the lower limb, followed by a strong urge to move them to alleviate discomfort.[63] The REST study showed that the prevalence of RLS was 2.7% per a self-filled patient questionnaire, but that only 6.1% had received a formal diagnosis.[88] Prevalence and severity of RLS increases with age, and is twice as high in women.[89] In the MEMO study with women aged 65 to 73 years, women had a higher prevalence of 13.9%, as compared to the overall prevalence of 9.8%.[90] Pregnant and post-menopausal states increase the risk of RLS. It is hypothesized that changes in hormonal levels, rather than absolute values may result in symptoms of RLS. Iron and fluctuating estrogen levels influence dopamine and glutamate transmission, which may explain the higher prevalence in these demographic subgroups.[91] RLS symptoms typically worsen with rest and are improved with movement. Therefore, they can cause sleep disruption and be a source of distress. Amongst women 65 years and older, those with RLS have a significantly higher cardiovascular disease related mortality, even after adjustment for all potential confounders.[92]

RLS is diagnosed through focused questions rather than diagnostic testing.[93] Per the International Restless Leg Syndrome Study Group, 5 clinical criteria must be met to establish the diagnosis.[94] During patient evaluation, it is essential to review medications as some may cause sleep-related leg cramps and mimic RLS. Some of the medications are commonly used in older individuals including diuretics, raloxifene, and statins. On the other hand, some medications are known to precipitate or exacerbate RLS, including hydroxyzine, diphenhydramine, metoclopramide, and anti-depressants including sertraline and fluoxetine.[95]

RLS is associated with iron deficiency anemia, and initial work-up includes a ferritin level. Iron supplementation is recommended if levels are $\leq$75 mcg/L, or if the transferrin saturation is $<$20%.[96] Non-pharmacologic therapies include regular exercise, reducing intake of caffeine and other stimulants, proper sleep hygiene, cold-water massages or leg baths, vibratory stimulation devices, yoga or acupuncture.[89] If symptoms persist, medications used for initial treatment include dopaminergic agonists (pramipexole, ropinirole) and alpha-2 ligands (gabapentin, pregabalin). Common side effects of dopamine agonists include nausea, headache, sleepiness, and impulse control disorders.[89] Impulse control disorders have been reported in 6% to 17% of patients when treated for RLS with dopamine agonists.[97] Therefore, patients should be evaluated regarding a history of impulse control, and patients on treatment with dopamine agonists should be monitored for the development of symptoms such as compulsive shopping, pathologic gambling, or compulsive eating. Alpha-2 ligands also have a significant side effect profile including somnolence, dizziness, fatigue, weight gain and headaches.[89] Given the sedative effects of both classes of medications, it is particularly important to use these medications with caution in women of advancing age. They are not only at an increased risk of falls, but also at risk for the development of subsequent osteoporotic fractures. Therefore, when considering various therapeutic options for RLS, it is important to have thorough discussion regarding risks and benefits of each option.

Parasomnia evaluation

Parasomnias are undesirable physical events or experiences that occur during the initiation of sleep, within sleep, or during arousal from sleep.[63] Parasomnias can be divided as NREM-related, REM-related, or other parasomnias. NREM parasomnias are more prevalent in the pediatric population. However, REM parasomnias, particularly REM sleep behavior disorder (RBD), occurs more commonly in men and patients over the age of 50 years.[98] In a cohort of elderly Korean patients, the estimated prevalence of RBD was approximately 2%, of which 22.1% were females.[61] It is speculated that women have less aggressive RBD behaviors, which may result in underdiagnosis.[99]

Patients with RBD experience lack of muscle atonia in REM sleep, resulting in vivid dreams and dream enactment. While RBD is more common in men, it can have significant effects on bed partners including injuries, sleep disruption, and adverse health effects. Spouses of RBD patients have exhibited a higher prevalence of insomnia and mood problems, and RBD negatively affects the spouses' quality of life.[100] Up to 32% of patients with RBD had injured themselves at initial presentation, and 64% had assaulted their spouses.[101] Therefore, the optimization of RBD treatment, and evaluation of sleep and mental health aspects in bed partners is an important component of the patient evaluation.[100] There is a similar prevalence of RBD amongst men and women of advanced age with neurologic disorders such as narcolepsy and Parkinson's disease, and evaluation in the clinic setting should include history and physical exam focused on these conditions as well[99]

Individuals often present after bed partners notice dramatic and intense motor activity during sleep as the individual acts out dreams. RBD has been shown to have an association with alpha-synucleinopathy neurodegenerative diseases including Parkinson's disease, Multiple System Atrophy (MSA) and Lewy Body Dementia. There are also numerous medications that can precipitate and exacerbate symptoms of RBD such as SSRIs, TCAs, and MAOIs. Medication-associated RBD may occur in 6% of patients using them.[101,102] Obtaining a PSG with 4-limb EMG is helpful in identification or REM without atonia and dream enactment and can help rule out RBD mimics such as OSA causing pseudo-RBD. The first steps of treatment include ensuring a safe bedroom environment via the removal of firearms, other weapons, or sharp objects and even lamps or alarm clocks. Due to the high risk of falls, the height of the bed should be lowered, and bed partners should be advised to sleep in a separate room.[103] Pharmacotherapy includes melatonin or clonazepam. Both can decrease both dream enactment and sleep-related injuries. Common side effects of melatonin include abdominal discomfort and sleep fragmentation. Clonazepam can cause sedation and cognitive disturbances, and hence it should be used with caution, and after adequate counseling in women of advancing age.[103]

Circadian rhythm sleep-wake disorder evaluation

A circadian rhythm sleep-wake disorder (CRSWD) is defined by the alterations of the circadian time-keeping system, its entrainment mechanisms, or a misalignment of the endogenous circadian rhythm and the external environment.[63] It is estimated that the prevalence is <3% in the general population, but there is limited data amongst women of advancing age. Since CRSWDs are often confused with insomnia, there may be a component of underdiagnosis.[104]Some forms of CRSWDs such as jet lag may be self-limiting, but others can have severe adverse medical, psychological and social consequences.[104]

There are different types of CRSWD, but one commonly seen disorder in advanced age individuals is advanced sleep-wake phase disorder. These patients will have features of early or advanced timing of the major sleep episode in relation to the desired sleep and wakeup time. A 2014 population survey evaluating advanced sleep-wake phase disorder demonstrated a prevalence of 0.25% to 7%.[105] Advanced sleep-wake phase disorder is found more commonly in advancing age adults, however it is a diagnostic challenge since many of these patients have depression, pain, physical limitations and respiratory symptoms that may contribute to or cause similar symptoms such as early morning awakenings.[104] During patient evaluation, it is important to use tools such as a sleep log and actigraphy to help assess sleep-wake patterns and to obtain at least 7 days of data though preferably 14 days.[63] The primary recommendation for the treatment of advanced sleep-wake phase disorder is the implementation of evening bright light to delay circadian rhythms.[106]

Other CRSWD seen more commonly in older adults include irregular sleep-wake rhythm disorder(ISWRD), whereby patients may have multiple irregular bouts of sleep within a day, and non-24-h-sleep wake disorder, which is characterized by sleep timing that moves progressively later every night, and is particularly common amongst patients with vision loss.[104] Irregular sleep-wake rhythm disorder is more common in individuals with neurodegenerative disorders. Therapy focuses on using a multimodal strategy of structured activities with time cues and bright-light to regularize sleep-wake schedule. Melatonin, which is commonly used in adolescents, may cause depression or worsen cognitive impairment in elderly patients with dementia.[106] Adults of advancing age may also be prone to shift-work disorder.[104] In the evaluation and management of CRSWD in patients of advancing age, physicians must understand that they are more severely affected than the younger patient cohort, because of their decreased ability to sleep at adverse circadian times. Further research is needed to understand the implications of CRSWDs and the benefits of treatment on quality of life, morbidity, and mortality in women of advancing age.

Central disorders of hypersomnia evaluation

A patient may present with hypersomnia that is not due to disturbed nocturnal sleep, or misaligned circadian rhythm. Some examples of central disorders of hypersomnia include narcolepsy type 1 or 2, idiopathic hypersomnia, kleine-levin Syndrome, hypersomnia due to a medical disorder/medication, and insufficient sleep syndrome. In an Australian study, the prevalence of patient reported hypersomnia amongst women aged 70 to 79 tears was 13.2%, and amongst women aged ≥80 year old was 17%. However, there is a lack of data of prevalence data of PSG-confirmed hypersomnia in this population.[107]

Central disorders of hypersomnia disorders are not generally diagnosed in patients aged 65 and above as they tend to present with symptoms at a younger age. However, if a patient has persisting hypersomnolence, it is important to consider these disorders. This is particularly significant when patients are obtaining the recommended hours of sleep, have appropriate sleep hygiene, and do not have a contributing comorbid condition or take a medication that could explain the hypersomnolence. To evaluate for a disorder of hypersomnolence, overnight PSG is recommended with next day Multiple Sleep Latency Test (MSLT). Actigraphy prior to the PSG/MLT is recommended to evaluate for sleep-wake cycle disturbance or insufficient sleep. A study showed progressive decrease in the number of SOREMP and an increase in the meal sleep latency in MSLT as a function of age, which suggests that the current diagnostic criteria may be too stringent in the diagnosis of narcolepsy in patients with advancing age.[108] OSA and periodic limb movements are more common in patients with narcolepsy, and should be suspected when previously well controlled older narcolepsy patients exhibit a new worsening of symptoms.[109]

Non-pharmacological treatment consists of frequent scheduled naps. Medications that are used to treat narcolepsy or idiopathic hypersomnolence include modafinil and armodafinil, traditional stimulations, sodium oxybate, solriamfetol, and pitolisant.[110] However, there are several serious side effects of these medications such as psychosis, suicidal ideation, cardiac arrhythmias, hypertension, QT -prolongation or sedation. Therefore, when discussing pharmacologic therapy, it is important to consider comorbid conditions, interactions with other medications, and overall risks of therapy.

SUMMARY

Evaluation of sleep disorders in women of advancing age requires understanding changes in sleep architecture with aging and the impact of hormonal changes on sleep to determine appropriate differential diagnoses and focused clinical evaluations. Obtaining a thorough history and detailed medical reconciliation can provide useful clues to the underlying diagnosis. A focused history in this cohort should include reviewing the temporal relation of symptoms to menopause, as well as comorbid conditions. Caregiver and family involvement are crucial where individuals may have dementia or mild cognitive impairment. It is important for clinicians to understand sleep physiology and architectural changes in women with advancing age and consider how treatment strategies may be tailored to improve sleep and quality of life.

DISCLOSURE

The authors have nothing to disclose.

CLINICS CARE POINTS

- As individuals age the ability to sleep becomes more difficult and older individuals tend to show an increase in disturbed sleep.
- Obtaining a thorough history is imperative and may often involve family members, caregivers and/or bed partners.
- Clinical providers can evaluate whether sleep complaints are focused on excessive day time sleepiness versus difficulty falling asleep or maintaining sleep throughout the night.

REFERENCES

1. Vespa J, Medina L, Armstrong DM. Population Estimates and Projections. :15.
2. Huntley J, Ostfeld AM, Taylor JO, et al. Established populations for epidemiologic studies of the elderly: study design and methodology. Aging Clin Exp Res 1993;5(1):27–37.
3. Martin J, Shochat T, Ancoli-Israel S. Assessment and treatment of sleep disturbances in older adults. Clin Psychol Rev 2000;20(6):783–805.
4. Quan SF, Enright PL, Katz R, et al. Factors associated with incidence and persistence of symptoms of disturbed sleep in an elderly cohort: the cardiovascular health study. Am J Med Sci 2005;329(4): 163–72.
5. Ohayon MM, Carskadon MA, Guilleminault C, et al. Meta-analysis of quantitative sleep parameters from childhood to old age in healthy individuals: developing normative sleep values across the human lifespan. Sleep 2004;27(7):1255–73.
6. Malakouti SK, Foroughan M, Nojomi M, et al. Sleep patterns, sleep disturbances and sleepiness in retired Iranian elders. Int J Geriatr Psychiatry 2009;24(11):1201–8.
7. Blazer DG, Hays JC, Foley DJ. Sleep complaints in older adults: a Racial comparison. J Gerontol Ser A 1995;50A(5):M280–4.

8. Chiu HF, Leung T, Lam LC, et al. Sleep problems in Chinese elderly in Hong Kong. Sleep 1999;22(6):717–26.
9. Newman AB, Enright PL, Manolio TA, et al. Sleep disturbance, psychosocial correlates, and cardiovascular disease in 5201 older adults: the Cardiovascular Health Study. J Am Geriatr Soc 1997;45(1):1–7.
10. Goldman SE, Stone KL, Ancoli-Israel S, et al. Poor sleep is associated with poorer physical performance and greater functional limitations in older women. Sleep 2007;30(10):1317–26.
11. Poor Sleep Quality and Functional Decline in Older Women - PMC. Accessed December 7, 2022. https://www.ncbi.nlm.nih.gov/pmc/articles/PMC3375617/.
12. Gulia KK, Kumar VM. Sleep disorders in the elderly: a growing challenge. Psychogeriatr 2018;18(3):155–65.
13. McCall WV. Sleep in the elderly: burden, diagnosis, and treatment. Prim Care Companion J Clin Psychiatry 2004;6(1):9–20.
14. Spira AP, Covinsky K, Rebok GW, et al. Objectively measured sleep quality and nursing home placement in older women. J Am Geriatr Soc 2012;60(7):1237–43.
15. Seegert L. Study: Older adults with obstructive sleep apnea have higher health costs. Association of Health Care Journalists. Published March 19, 2020. Accessed December 7, 2022. https://healthjournalism.org/blog/2020/03/study-older-adults-with-obstructive-sleep-apnea-have-higher-health-costs/.
16. Terán-Pérez G, Arana-Lechuga Y, Esqueda-León E, et al. Steroid hormones and sleep regulation. Mini Rev Med Chem 2012;12(11):1040–8.
17. Carskadon MA, Dement WC. Chapter 2 – Normal Human Sleep : An Overview. :21.
18. Fuller PM, Gooley JJ, Saper CB. Neurobiology of the sleep-wake cycle: sleep architecture, circadian regulation, and regulatory feedback. J Biol Rhythms 2006;21(6):482–93.
19. Landolt HP, Dijk DJ, Achermann P, et al. Effect of age on the sleep EEG: slow-wave activity and spindle frequency activity in young and middle-aged men. Brain Res 1996;738(2):205–12.
20. Carrier J, Land S, Buysse DJ, et al. The effects of age and gender on sleep EEG power spectral density in the middle years of life (ages 20-60 years old). Psychophysiology 2001;38(2):232–42.
21. Gaudreau H, Carrier J, Montplaisir J. Age-related modifications of NREM sleep EEG: from childhood to middle age. J Sleep Res 2001;10(3):165–72.
22. Crowley K, Trinder J, Kim Y, et al. The effects of normal aging on sleep spindle and K-complex production. Clin Neurophysiol 2002;113(10):1615–22.
23. Parrino L, Boselli M, Spaggiari MC, et al. Cyclic alternating pattern (CAP) in normal sleep: polysomnographic parameters in different age groups. Electroencephalogr Clin Neurophysiol 1998;107(6):439–50.
24. Dorffner G, Vitr M, Anderer P. The effects of aging on sleep architecture in healthy subjects. Adv Exp Med Biol 2015;821:93–100.
25. Baker FC, Driver HS. Circadian rhythms, sleep, and the menstrual cycle. Sleep Med 2007;8(6):613–22.
26. Hollander LE, Freeman EW, Sammel MD, et al. Sleep quality, estradiol levels, and behavioral factors in late reproductive age women. Obstet Gynecol 2001;98(3):391–7.
27. Sleep in Women Across the Life Span - ScienceDirect. Accessed January 5, 2023. https://www.sciencedirect.com/science/article/abs/pii/S0012369218305701.
28. Kravitz HM, Ganz PA, Bromberger J, et al. Sleep difficulty in women at midlife: a community survey of sleep and the menopausal transition. Menopause N Y N 2003;10(1):19–28.
29. Moline ML, Broch L, Zak R. Sleep in women across the life cycle from adulthood through menopause. Med Clin North Am 2004;88(3):705–36.
30. Kravitz HM, Joffe H. Sleep during the perimenopause: a SWAN story. Obstet Gynecol Clin North Am 2011;38(3):567–86.
31. Hirshkowitz M, Whiton K, Albert SM, et al. National Sleep Foundation's sleep time duration recommendations: methodology and results summary. Sleep Health 2015;1(1):40–3.
32. Ohayon MM, Vecchierini MF. Normative sleep data, cognitive function and daily living activities in older adults in the community. Sleep 2005;28(8):981–9.
33. Ancoli-Israel S, Alessi C. Sleep and aging. Am J Geriatr Psychiatry 2005;13(5):341–3.
34. Senaratna CV, Perret JL, Lodge CJ, et al. Prevalence of obstructive sleep apnea in the general population: a systematic review. Sleep Med Rev 2017;34:70–81.
35. Heinzer R, Vat S, Marques-Vidal P, et al. Prevalence of sleep-disordered breathing in the general population: the HypnoLaus study. Lancet Respir Med 2015;3(4):310–8.
36. STOP-Bang Questionnaire: A Practical Approach to Screen for Obstructive Sleep Apnea - PubMed. Accessed December 8, 2022. https://pubmed.ncbi.nlm.nih.gov/26378880/.
37. Chung F, Yegneswaran B, Liao P, et al. STOP questionnaire: a tool to screen patients for obstructive sleep apnea. Anesthesiology 2008;108(5):812–21.
38. Bastien CH, Vallières A, Morin CM. Validation of the Insomnia Severity Index as an outcome measure for insomnia research. Sleep Med 2001;2(4):297–307.
39. Morin CM, Belleville G, Bélanger L, et al. The Insomnia Severity Index: psychometric indicators

to detect insomnia cases and evaluate treatment response. Sleep 2011;34(5):601–8.
40. Johns MW. A new method for measuring daytime sleepiness: the Epworth sleepiness scale. Sleep 1991;14(6):540–5.
41. Grewe FA, Roeder M, Bradicich M, et al. Low repeatability of Epworth Sleepiness Scale after short intervals in a sleep clinic population. J Clin Sleep Med JCSM 2020;16(5):757–64.
42. Lee JL, Chung Y, Waters E, et al. The Epworth sleepiness scale: Reliably unreliable in a sleep clinic population. J Sleep Res 2020;29(5):e13019.
43. The utility of patient-completed and partner-completed Epworth Sleepiness Scale scores in the evaluation of obstructive sleep apnea - PubMed. https://pubmed.ncbi.nlm.nih.gov/27301400/. Accessed December 8, 2022.
44. Hall MH, Kline CE, Nowakowski S. Insomnia and sleep apnea in midlife women: prevalence and consequences to health and functioning. F1000Prime Rep 2015;7. https://doi.org/10.12703/P7-63.
45. Martin JL, Schweizer CA, Hughes JM, et al. Estimated prevalence of insomnia among women veterans: results of a postal survey. Wom Health Issues 2017;27(3):366–73.
46. Ohayon MM. Epidemiology of insomnia: what we know and what we still need to learn. Sleep Med Rev 2002;6(2):97–111.
47. Crowley K. Sleep and sleep disorders in older adults. Neuropsychol Rev 2011;21(1):41–53.
48. Foley D, Ancoli-Israel S, Britz P, et al. Sleep disturbances and chronic disease in older adults: results of the 2003 national sleep foundation sleep in America survey. J Psychosom Res 2004;56(5):497–502.
49. American Academy of Sleep Medicine. International classification of sleep disorders. 3rd edition. Darien, IL: American Academy of Sleep Medicine; 2014.
50. Misra S, Malow BA. Evaluation of sleep disturbances in older adults. Clin Geriatr Med 2008;24(1):15–26.
51. Tatineny P, Shafi F, Gohar A, et al. Sleep in the elderly. Mo Med 2020;117(5):490–5.
52. Morgenthaler T, Kramer M, Alessi C, et al. Practice parameters for the psychological and behavioral treatment of insomnia: an update. An american academy of sleep medicine report. Sleep 2006;29(11):1415–9.
53. Khan SS, Khawaja IS. Disorders of sleep in women: insomnia. Psychiatr Ann 2019;49(12):518–23.
54. Morin CM, Colecchi C, Stone J, et al. Behavioral and pharmacological therapies for late-life insomnia: a randomized controlled trial. JAMA 1999;281(11):991.
55. Jacobs GD, Pace-Schott EF, Stickgold R, et al. Cognitive behavior therapy and pharmacotherapy for insomnia: a randomized controlled trial and direct comparison. Arch Intern Med 2004;164(17):1888.
56. Morin CM, Vallières A, Guay B, et al. Cognitive-behavior therapy, singly and combined with medication, for persistent insomnia: acute and maintenance therapeutic effects. JAMA, J Am Med Assoc 2009;301(19):2005–15.
57. Beaulieu-Bonneau S, Ivers H, Guay B, et al. Long-term maintenance of therapeutic gains associated with cognitive-behavioral therapy for insomnia delivered alone or combined with zolpidem. Sleep 2017;40(3). https://doi.org/10.1093/sleep/zsx002.
58. Morin CM, Bootzin RR, Buysse DJ, et al. Psychological and behavioral treatment of insomnia:update of the recent evidence (1998-2004). Sleep 2006;29(11):1398–414.
59. Roth T, Seiden D, Sainati S, et al. Effects of ramelteon on patient-reported sleep latency in older adults with chronic insomnia. Sleep Med 2006;7(4):312–8.
60. Afonso RF, Hachul H, Kozasa EH, et al. Yoga decreases insomnia in postmenopausal women: a randomized clinical trial. Menopause N Y N 2012;19(2):186–93.
61. Guthrie KA, Larson JC, Ensrud KE, et al. Effects of pharmacologic and nonpharmacologic interventions on insomnia symptoms and self-reported sleep quality in women with hot flashes: a pooled analysis of individual participant data from four MsFLASH trials. Sleep 2018;41(1). https://doi.org/10.1093/sleep/zsx190.
62. Oliveira DS, Hachul H, Goto V, et al. Effect of therapeutic massage on insomnia and climacteric symptoms in postmenopausal women. Climacteric J Int Menopause Soc 2012;15(1):21–9.
63. Sateia MJ. International classification of sleep disorders-third edition: highlights and modifications. Chest 2014;146(5):1387–94.
64. Bixler EO, Vgontzas AN, Ten Have T, et al. Effects of age on sleep apnea in men: I. Prevalence and severity. Am J Respir Crit Care Med 1998;157(1):144–8.
65. McMillan A, Morrell MJ. Sleep disordered breathing at the extremes of age: the elderly. Breathe Sheff Engl 2016;12(1):50–60.
66. Block AJ, Wynne JW, Boysen PG. Sleep-disordered breathing and nocturnal oxygen desaturation in postmenopausal women. Am J Med 1980;69(1):75–9.
67. Sigurðardóttir ES, Gislason T, Benediktsdottir B, et al. Female sex hormones and symptoms of obstructive sleep apnea in European women of a population-based cohort. PLoS One 2022;17(6):e0269569.
68. Bixler EO, Vgontzas AN, Lin HM, et al. Prevalence of sleep-disordered breathing in women: effects of

gender. Am J Respir Crit Care Med 2001;163(3 Pt 1):608–13.
69. Ward SA, Storey E, Gasevic D, et al. Sleep-disordered breathing was associated with lower health-related quality of life and cognitive function in a cross-sectional study of older adults. Respirol Carlton Vic 2022;27(9):767–75.
70. Tripathi A, Gupta A, Rai P, et al. Correlation between duration of edentulism and severity of obstructive sleep apnea in elderly edentulous patients. Sleep Sci Sao Paulo Braz 2022;15(Spec 2):300–5.
71. Sex and Gender in Lung Disease and Sleep Disorders: A State-of-the-Art Review - PubMed. Accessed December 11, 2022. https://pubmed.ncbi.nlm.nih.gov/35300976/.
72. Clinical Practice Guideline for Diagnostic Testing for Adult Obstructive Sleep Apnea: An American Academy of Sleep Medicine Clinical Practice Guideline - PubMed. Accessed December 9, 2022. https://pubmed.ncbi.nlm.nih.gov/28162150/.
73. Patil SP, Ayappa IA, Caples SM, et al. Treatment of adult obstructive sleep apnea with positive airway pressure: an American academy of sleep medicine clinical practice guideline. J Clin Sleep Med JCSM 2019;15(2):335–43.
74. Hudgel DW, Fung C. A long-term randomized, cross-over comparison of auto-titrating and standard nasal continuous airway pressure. Sleep 2000;23(5):645–8.
75. Mashaqi S, Patel SI, Combs D, et al. The hypoglossal nerve stimulation as a novel therapy for treating obstructive sleep apnea-A literature review. Int J Environ Res Public Health 2021;18(4):1642.
76. Baptista PM, Martínez Ruiz de Apodaca P, Carrasco M, et al. Daytime neuromuscular electrical therapy of tongue muscles in improving snoring in individuals with primary snoring and mild obstructive sleep apnea. J Clin Med 2021;10(9):1883.
77. Costantino A, Rinaldi V, Moffa A, et al. Hypoglossal nerve stimulation long-term clinical outcomes: a systematic review and meta-analysis. Sleep Breath Schlaf Atm 2020;24(2):399–411.
78. Aurora RN, Casey KR, Kristo D, et al. Practice parameters for the surgical modifications of the upper airway for obstructive sleep apnea in adults. Sleep 2010;33(10):1408–13.
79. Prevalence and Characteristics of Central Compared to Obstructive Sleep Apnea: Analyses from the Sleep Heart Health Study Cohort - PMC. Accessed December 10, 2022. https://www.ncbi.nlm.nih.gov/pmc/articles/PMC4909617/.
80. Prevalence and correlates of sleep-disordered breathing in older men: osteoporotic fractures in men sleep study - PubMed. Accessed December 10, 2022. https://pubmed.ncbi.nlm.nih.gov/17767677/.
81. Aurora RN, Chowdhuri S, Ramar K, et al. The treatment of central sleep apnea syndromes in adults: practice parameters with an evidence-based literature review and meta-analyses. Sleep 2012;35(1):17–40.
82. Javaheri S, Parker TJ, Liming JD, et al. Sleep apnea in 81 ambulatory male patients with stable heart failure. Types and their prevalences, consequences, and presentations. Circulation 1998;97(21):2154–9.
83. Leung RST, Huber MA, Rogge T, et al. Association between atrial fibrillation and central sleep apnea. Sleep 2005;28(12):1543–6.
84. Wang D, Teichtahl H, Drummer O, et al. Central sleep apnea in stable methadone maintenance treatment patients. Chest 2005;128(3):1348–56.
85. Hanly PJ, Pierratos A. Improvement of sleep apnea in patients with chronic renal failure who undergo nocturnal hemodialysis. N Engl J Med 2001;344(2):102–7.
86. Douglas Bradley T, Floras JS. The SERVE-HF trial. Can Respir J J Can Thorac Soc 2015;22(6):313.
87. Aurora RN, Bista SR, Casey KR, et al. Updated adaptive servo-ventilation recommendations for the 2012 AASM guideline: "the treatment of central sleep apnea syndromes in adults: practice parameters with an evidence-based literature review and meta-analyses.". J Clin Sleep Med JCSM 2016;12(5):757–61.
88. Restless legs syndrome prevalence and impact: REST general population study - PubMed. Accessed December 11, 2022. https://pubmed.ncbi.nlm.nih.gov/15956009/.
89. Garcia-Malo C, Peralta SR, Garcia-Borreguero D. Restless legs syndrome and other common sleep-related movement disorders. Contin Minneap Minn 2020;26(4):963–87.
90. Rothdach AJ, Trenkwalder C, Haberstock J, et al. Prevalence and risk factors of RLS in an elderly population: the MEMO study. Memory and Morbidity in Augsburg Elderly. Neurology 2000;54(5):1064–8.
91. Seeman MV. Why are women prone to restless legs syndrome? Int J Environ Res Public Health 2020;17(1):368.
92. Li Y, Li Y, Winkelman JW, et al. Prospective study of restless legs syndrome and total and cardiovascular mortality among women. Neurology 2018;90(2):e135–41.
93. Diagnosis of Restless Leg Syndrome (Willis-Ekbom Disease) - PubMed. Accessed December 11, 2022. https://pubmed.ncbi.nlm.nih.gov/26329433/.
94. Restless legs syndrome/Willis-Ekbom disease diagnostic criteria: updated International Restless Legs Syndrome Study Group (IRLSSG) consensus criteria–history, rationale, description, and significance - PubMed. Accessed December 11, 2022. https://pubmed.ncbi.nlm.nih.gov/25023924/.
95. Kolla BP, Mansukhani MP, Bostwick JM. The influence of antidepressants on restless legs syndrome

and periodic limb movements: a systematic review. Sleep Med Rev 2018;38:131–40.

96. Restless Legs Syndrome: clinical features, diagnosis and a practical approach to management - PubMed. Accessed December 11, 2022. https://pubmed.ncbi.nlm.nih.gov/29097554/.
97. Cornelius JR, Tippmann-Peikert M, Slocumb NL, et al. Impulse control disorders with the use of dopaminergic agents in restless legs syndrome: a case-control study. Sleep 2010;33(1):81–7.
98. Singh S, Kaur H, Singh S, et al. Parasomnias: a comprehensive review. Cureus 2018;10(12):e3807.
99. Bodkin CL, Schenck CH. Rapid eye movement sleep behavior disorder in women: relevance to general and specialty medical practice. J Womens Health 2009;18(12):1955–63.
100. Lam SP, Wong CCY, Li SX, et al. Caring burden of REM sleep behavior disorder - spouses' health and marital relationship. Sleep Med 2016;24:40–3.
101. Olson EJ, Boeve BF, Silber MH. Rapid eye movement sleep behaviour disorder: demographic, clinical and laboratory findings in 93 cases. Brain J Neurol 2000;123(Pt 2):331–9.
102. Bf B. REM sleep behavior disorder: updated review of the core features, the REM sleep behavior disorder-neurodegenerative disease association, evolving concepts, controversies, and future directions. Ann N Y Acad Sci 2010;1184. https://doi.org/10.1111/j.1749-6632.2009.05115.x.
103. Rapid Eye Movement Sleep Behavior Disorder and Other Rapid Eye Movement Parasomnias - PubMed. Available at: https://pubmed.ncbi.nlm.nih.gov/32756229/. Accessed December 13, 2022.
104. Kim JH, Duffy JF. Circadian rhythm sleep-wake disorders in older adults. Sleep Med Clin 2018;13(1): 39–50.
105. Identifying advanced and delayed sleep phase disorders in the general population: a national survey of New Zealand adults - PubMed. Available at: https://pubmed.ncbi.nlm.nih.gov/24548144/. Accessed December 13, 2022.
106. Auger RR, Burgess HJ, Emens JS, et al. Clinical practice guideline for the treatment of intrinsic circadian rhythm sleep-wake disorders: advanced sleep-wake phase disorder (ASWPD), delayed sleep-wake phase disorder (DSWPD), non-24-hour sleep-wake rhythm disorder (N24SWD), and irregular sleep-wake rhythm disorder (ISWRD). An update for 2015. J Clin Sleep Med 2015;11(10): 1199–236.
107. Prevalence of excessive daytime sleepiness in a sample of the Australian adult population - PubMed. Available at:https://pubmed.ncbi.nlm.nih.gov/24513435/. Accessed December 13, 2022.
108. Dauvilliers Y, Gosselin A, Paquet J, et al. Effect of age on MSLT results in patients with narcolepsy-cataplexy. Neurology 2004;62(1):46–50.
109. Chakravorty SS, Rye DB. Narcolepsy in the older adult: epidemiology, diagnosis and management. Drugs Aging 2003;20(5):361–76.
110. Central Disorders of Hypersomnolence: Focus on the Narcolepsies and Idiopathic Hypersomnia - PubMed. Available at: https://pubmed.ncbi.nlm.nih.gov/26149554/. Accessed December 13, 2022.

Sleep Deficiency in Pregnancy

Arlin Delgado, MD, Judette M. Louis, MD, MPH*

KEYWORDS

• Pregnancy • Sleep deficiency • Maternal outcomes • Labor outcomes • Sleep health equity

KEY POINTS

- Sleep is critical and necessary for a person to maintain a healthy lifestyle, requiring 7 to 8 hours nightly during adulthood.
- During pregnancy, sleep deficiency may be caused by many physiologic, emotional, and mental health changes.
- Sleep deficiency is associated with an increased risk of adverse maternal outcomes (gestational diabetes, hypertensive disorders, and depression) as well as preterm labor and delivery.
- Socioeconomic factors and social determinants of health are critical factors that must be evaluated further to best address sleep health disparities in these at-risk populations.
- Future research needs to evaluate if sleep deficiency is a causal factor in adverse maternal and neonatal outcomes.

INTRODUCTION

Sleep is considered a critical and necessary aspect of one's daily life for overall health. The National Sleep Foundation recommends that a person sleep approximately 7 to 9 hours per 24 hour during adulthood, ages 26 to 64 years of age.[1] However, in 2014, up to 35% of adults reported short sleep duration, and up to 34% (CI 34.4%–35.2%) of women were affected.[2] Abnormalities in sleep duration, poor sleep quality, and abnormal timing of sleep all contribute to morbidity in the affected individual. Although studies in pregnancy are limited, in the general populations, existing data indicate that these sleep disturbances are associated with mortality risk, impaired metabolism, impaired learning and cognitive functioning, and overall poorer quality of life.[3,4] In the 2018 "Sleep in America Poll," women reported a lower effectiveness, defined as ability to complete daily tasks and responsibilities, when analyzing their sleep health compared with men.[5] This finding is further supported by several studies in which women were found to report higher levels of self-reported sleep deprivation and sleep problems.[6,7]

Despite these concerning statistics, this literature fails to comprehensively address the challenges specific to women. Sleep in women is affected by a multitude of factors—including socioeconomic factors, natural physiologic changes, and demographic characteristics.

One impactful socioeconomic factor is the entrance of women into the work force. As women enter careers, they are now juggling family-related responsibilities and the demands of a workforce that are negatively affecting their sleep hygiene. This was found in a secondary analysis of data from The Sister Study, a prospective cohort study of women aged 35 to 74 years. Cross-sectional and longitudinal sleep data was available for more than 20,000 women. Patient perceived sex-specific and sexual orientation-specific job discrimination was significantly and independently associated with shorter sleep duration and higher odds of having short sleep duration (less than 7 hours/night) at the start of the study. Among

This article originally appeared in *Clinics in Chest Medicine*, Volume 43 Issue 2, June 2022.
Department of Obstetrics and Gynecology, Morsani College of Medicine, University of South Florida Morsani College of Medicine, 2 Tampa General Circle, Tampa, FL 33606, USA
* Corresponding author.
E-mail address: Jlouis1@usf.edu

Sleep Med Clin 18 (2023) 559–571
https://doi.org/10.1016/j.jsmc.2023.06.011
1556-407X/23/

those who did not have abnormal sleep, age-specific job discrimination was associated with the new onset of short sleep at time 2 (OR = 1.21, 95% CI: 1.03, 1.43).[8] Considering these competing responsibilities and tasks, women reported they ran out of time to sleep more frequently than men.[9]

Physiologically, natural hormone fluctuations across varying time points in life (from puberty to menstruation and through postmenopausal states) affect sleep differently. This effect is due to established associations between the fluctuations in estrogen and progesterone that are associated with changes in sleep–wake cycles, affecting the quality and quantity of sleep.[10,11]

Sleep Pattern Changes in Pregnancy

During pregnancy, there are different hormonal and physiologic changes that adversely affect a woman's ability to sleep (**Table 1**).[11] Mindell, Cook, and Nikolovski (2015)[12] distributed a survey to more than 2400 pregnant women and found that 76% reported insufficient nighttime sleep, 49% reported significant daytime sleepiness, and 78% required daytime naps. Meanwhile, Hedman and colleagues (2002)[13] surveyed women before, during, and after pregnancy and found self-reported sleep duration increased during the first trimester of pregnancy but subsequently decreased after delivery. The mean sleep duration was 7.8 hours before pregnancy, 8.2 hours in the first trimester ($P < .001$), and 7 hours after delivery ($P < .001$). Objectively, women who were followed using activity tracking devices during pregnancy were found to have a significant inverse association between gestational age and sleep duration (-B = 0.2; $P < .001$).[14] The nuMoM2b Sleep Duration and Continuity Substudy is a prospective study of a subset of the women enrolled in the nuMoM2b parent study. The primary objective of this substudy was to examine the relationship of objectively assessed sleep duration, continuity, and timing, with cardiovascular and metabolic morbidity related to pregnancy. A total of 782 nulliparous women wore a wrist actigraphic monitor and completed a sleep log for 7 consecutive days before 23 weeks of gestation. Approximately one-third (27.9%) of these women had a sleep duration less than 7 hours.[15] A meta-analysis of 5 studies using polysomnography to quantify and define sleep patterns in pregnancy supports the findings. There was an overall significantly reduced total sleep time from the first to the third trimester of pregnancy by 26.8 minutes (pooled WMD, 95% CI = 12.14–41.56).[16] Increases in a woman's wake after sleep onset, and transition from N3 sleep stage and rapid eye movement sleep to more superficial nonrapid eye movement sleep are hypothesized to cause the observed sleep structure changes. These changes then lead to a subjectively perceived less restorative sleep pattern.

These sleep stage transitions, in part, are due to an increase in estrogen production, which also leads to increasing hyperemia and collapsibility of the upper airways, possibly worsening underlying sleep-related disorders.[17] Furthermore, changes in the metabolism of supplements, such as iron and folate, are associated with increasing restless leg syndrome. An increase in water retention increases renal blood flow that leads to urinary frequency, often requiring multiple awakenings per night, especially in the third trimester.[17] Melatonin, a hormone well established in regulation of the circadian rhythm, is also impacted during pregnancy–with an initial increase in the first trimester, a decrease in the middle of pregnancy, and then a final increase in the third trimester associated with the onset of labor. Although no data in humans is established, rat studies suggest the placenta is a source of melatonin and can cross the maternal–fetal interface increasing serum levels.[18] All of these changes can interact to contribute negatively to a woman's ability to sleep.[11]

SLEEP HEALTH DISPARITIES IN PREGNANCY

Sleep health disparities defined as differences in one or more dimensions of sleep health (duration, efficiency, timing, regularity, alertness, and quality) that adversely affect designated disadvantaged populations are prevalent yet understudied. In a

Table 1
Factors contributing to sleep deficiency in pregnancy

	First Trimester	Second Trimester	Third Trimester
Factors decreasing sleep	Nausea/vomiting Urinary frequency Backache	Fetal movement Heartburn Cramps Tingling in extremities Shortness of breath Night awakening	

multisite survey and chart review of 267 pregnant women by Kalmbach and colleagues (2019),[19] the researchers found a high prevalence of self-reported sleep disturbance. Short sleep duration was reported in 24% of women who were on average 28 weeks of gestation women (±1.20, range 25–37). Women living in poverty (defined as less than $20K annual household income) were 72% more likely to have an increased score (>8) on the Pittsburgh sleep quality index (PSQI), with higher scores indicating worsening sleep. Moreover, although not statistically significant, it was noted that women in poverty reported less sleep compared with women not in poverty (6.31 hours vs 6.66 hours, respectively). Additionally, women living in poverty were more likely to identify as Black race (67.5% vs 23.9%, $P < .001$). Similarly, in a study of 133 women surveyed during each trimester and between 4 and 11 weeks postpartum, using the PSQI, it was found that African American women subjectively had poor sleep.[20] Most recently, Feinstein, and colleagues (2020),[21] published findings on the evaluation of 14 years of cross-sectional National Health Interview Survey showing that compared with pregnant White women, pregnant Black women had a higher short sleep prevalence (prevalence ratio for pregnant Black women = 1.35; 95% CI, 1.08–1.6). Article published by Okun and colleagues[22] further supported this in which 170 pregnant women were assessed between 10 and 20 weeks gestation in which it was found women with household income less than $50K per year was associated with poorer sleep quality on the PSQI ($P < .05$) and greater sleep fragmentation ($P < .05$), using PSQI as well as actigraphy, respectively. These findings are supported by the Nulliparous Pregnancy Outcomes Study: monitoring mothers-to-be sleep activity substudy. The Sleep Duration and Continuity substudy included pregnant women (16–21 weeks of gestation) who underwent 7 days of actigraphy. Among the 782 participants, 27.9% had short sleep duration (<7 hours). Increasing age, race-ethnicity (specifically non-Hispanic Black, and Asian), increasing BMI, insurance (specifically commercial), and recent smoking history were significantly associated with shorter sleep duration.[15] Further, in that sample, there were differences in sleep efficiency and fragmentation. Social inequalities do exist, and their presence predisposes these populations to sleep-related adverse health outcomes.

Sleep Deficiency and Risk for Depression, Antepartum, and Postpartum

Depression is considered one of the most common complications of pregnancy. Research shows that quality and quantity of sleep in pregnancy are predictors of depression in the postpartum period.[23–25] Peripartum and postpartum depression affects approximately 10% to 20% of women.[26] The prevalence has been increasing with as evidenced by a doubling in the rate of antidepressant use during pregnancy since 1999.[27,28] Peripartum depression is defined as the onset of a major depressive disorder during pregnancy. Postpartum depression is defined as the onset of a major depressive episode within 4 weeks from delivery; however, some will argue for inclusions of onset up to 12 weeks from delivery (**Table 2**).[29] Episodes of depression are, in turn, linked with many adverse maternal and neonatal outcomes. Maternal outcomes include risk of preterm delivery, lack of infant bonding, increased risk of suicidality, and use of substances and other risky behaviors.[30] Adverse neonatal outcomes including increased risk of small for gestational age, and potentially low birth weight infants,[31] failure to thrive, and difficulties with development in cognitive, behavioral, and emotional domains.[30]

Field (2007) studied sleep quality, defined as the number of nightly sleep disturbances, and found was linked to an increased risk of depression symptoms in the second and third trimesters.[32] In a prospective study, 63 women were followed through the latter stage of pregnancy (defined between 36 weeks gestation and term), and results indicated a history of sleep disruption during this time was associated with the onset of postnatal blues, a transient mood disturbance within the weeks after delivery.[33] Skouteris and colleagues (2008)[23] established sleep quality early in pregnancy would predict levels of depressive symptoms later in pregnancy, after following women starting at 15 to 23 weeks gestation for 3 times at 8-week intervals. This association held even after controlling for already present depressive symptoms. Similarly, in a cross-sectional study of 360 women who completed a PSQI questionnaire and the Edinburgh Postnatal Depression Scale (EPDS), women with poor sleep quality were 3.34 more times higher than women who reported good sleep quality to have high depression scores (odds ratio = 3.34, CI 2.04–5.48, $P < .001$).[34]

However, these studies do not evaluate the impact of sleep duration on a woman and her pregnancy. In a study by Jomeen and Martin (2007),[35] women with depression in pregnancy were more likely to report short sleep duration on the PSQI (PSQI subscale mean scores of 0.32 vs 0.79, $P = .002$) at 14 weeks gestation. In a prospective study by Okun and colleagues (2013)[36]

Table 2
Definitions of maternal and pregnancy-related health outcomes

Health Outcomes	Timing of Onset	Diagnostic Criteria
Maternal-Related Health Disorders and Outcomes		
Peripartum depression	Any gestational age	Depressive episode meeting criteria per the DSMV criteria
Postpartum depression	After delivery until 12 wk from delivery	Depressive episode meeting criteria per the DSMV criteria
GDM	Any gestational age	Two or more elevated glucose values during a 3-h 100g glucose tolerance test[a]
Chronic hypertension	<20 wk gestation	Two or more blood pressures with: • SBP[a] > 140 and/or DBP [b] > 90
Gestational hypertension	>20 wk gestation	2 or more blood pressures with: • SBP[b] > 140 and/or DBP[c] >90
Preeclampsia	–	Chronic or gestational hypertension diagnosis and: 24 h protein >300g or Urine protein/creatinine > 0.3
Preeclampsia with severe features	–	Preeclampsia and (at least one of the following): • Thrombocytopenia (platelets <100K) • Elevated liver enzymes twice upper limit of normal • Severe persistent right upper quadrant or epigastric pain • Abnormal renal clearance (creatinine > 1.1 or twice patient baseline) • New onset headache unresponsive to medical management or visual disturbances • Pulmonary edema
Shoulder dystocia	At time of delivery	Vaginal delivery requiring additional maneuvers to deliver a fetus after gentle traction and pulling have failed to deliver the infant shoulder
Neonate and Infant-Related Health Disorders and Outcomes		
Preterm birth	20 wk 0 d–36 wk 6 d gestation	Periviable and viable delivery (via vaginal delivery or cesarean section)
Stillbirth	–	Delivery of dead infant, previously viable
Macrosomia	–	Infant weighing >4000 g at time of delivery

[a] Based off Carpenter and Coustan.
[b] SBP: systolic blood pressure.
[c] DBP: diastolic blood pressure.

of 160 pregnant women, up to 38% of women met criteria for sleep deficiency. This was defined as deficiency in duration (with 7 hours as threshold), insufficiency (determined by 5 question measure), or insomnia symptoms (positive case based on Insomnia Sleep Quality scoring criteria) in at least 1 time point during their early gestation (either between 10 and 12, 14 and 16, or 18 and 20 weeks gestation). At 10 to 12 weeks gestation, 14 to 16 weeks gestation, and 18 to 20 weeks gestation, the prevalence of reported short sleep duration decreased from approximately 10% to 5%. Women who were sleep deficient across all 3 study time points reported more perceived stress when comparing the Perceived Stress Scale (PSS) scores between the sleep-deficient and nonsleep-deficient groups ($F_{2,157} = 5.53$; $P < .01$), as well as an increase in depressive symptoms calculated from the Inventory of Depressive Symptomatology scale (IDS; $F_{2,157} = 3.85$; $P = .02$). Wrist actigraphs with a sleep deficiency defined as less than 6 hours supported these qualitative findings—regardless of which gestational age time point (either between

10 and 12, 14 and 16, or 18 and 20 weeks gestation), a woman's score for depressive symptomology and pregnancy-related distress (using PSS and IDS, respectively) did not differ among those sleep deficient or not ($F_{2,157}$ = 1.71; P = .18 and $F_{2,157}$ = 2.86; P = .06, respectively). A woman's perceived stress level was significantly related to sleep deficiency ($F_{2,157}$ = 5.31, $P < .01$; **Table 3**).

The association between sleep deficiency and depression is challenging to delineate as it is uncertain which factors impact or leads to the other first. The studies suggesting an association between sleep quality and quantity with depression are often based on self-reported data with minimal objective data and are often cross-sectional, precluding the establishment of causation. In addition, the association between sleep quality, quantity, and depression is confounded and impacted by socioeconomics, age, education, occupation, and familial responsibilities and expectations among women.[27,37,38] Future literature should seek to establish causation between sleep deficiency and depression as the adverse neonatal and maternal outcomes associated with depression are economically and emotionally costly.

Sleep Deficiency and Risk for Gestational Diabetes

Gestational diabetes (GDM) in pregnancy is defined as carbohydrate intolerance that develops during pregnancy. It is one of the most common medical complications faced during pregnancy, and it is the cause of up to 86% of all reported diabetes during pregnancy.[39–41] Physiologically, a woman's increase in hormones (estrogen, progesterone, leptin, cortisol, placental lactogen, and growth hormone) promotes a state of insulin resistance and gluconeogenesis. This state can lead to hyperglycemia, and therefore promotes an imbalance of oxidants leading to oxidative stress and increasing inflammatory state in tissues (muscle and/or adipose). Insulin resistance additionally creates neurohormonal imbalances that upregulate satiety and hunger signals, leading to increased caloric intake, which further exacerbates the situation.[42]

Women diagnosed with GDM are at increased risk for adverse maternal and neonatal outcomes. Maternal outcomes include an increased risk for preeclampsia,[43] and development of diabetes long term.[44] The affected neonates are at increased risk for macrosomia, neonatal hypoglycemia, shoulder dystocia, and stillbirth[45,46] (see **Table 2**).

Several studies within the last 12 years have sought to study the association between sleep and the development of GDM. Early work found self-reported sleep less than 7 hours per night was associated with an increased risk for GDM.[47] In another study of more than 1200 women, self-reported sleep duration of less than 4 hours per night was associated with a significantly increased relative risk of GDM compared with those reporting 9 hours per night even after adjusting for age and ethnicity (RR = 5.56, 95% CI 1.31–23.69.[48] However, this study's definition of sleep duration (<4 hours per night) was considered extreme as it only represented 1.6% of the cohort and is not an accepted definition. Recently, several studies[49–51] sought to study these associations among Asian women and once again found associations between sleep deficiency and GDM. Zhou and colleagues (2016)[49] and Cai and colleagues (2017)[51] both found an increased risk of GDM with short sleep duration (less than 7 hours and less than 6 hours nightly, respectively). Conversely, a study by Reutrakul and colleagues (2011)[52] did not find the same association. In a group of 169 women with 26 cases of GDM, the association between GDM and short sleep duration defined as less than 7 hours was not statistically significant (unadjusted OR = 2.4, 95% CI 1.0–5.9, P = .06). Additionally, Wang and colleagues (2017)[50] found self-reported sleep duration less than 7 hours was not associated with GDM (aOR = 1.36, 95% CI 0.87–2.14).

These studies were limited by their sample size and limited power to detect an association between sleep duration and GDM. The cohorts were also not generalizable as they tended to be homogenous in race/ethnicity among the patient population and from single-site centers. These concerns were subsequently addressed between two studies recently published within the last 5 years. In a study across 12 clinical sites with more than 2581 women when exposed to short or long sleep durations were compared with GDM regardless of obesity, no association was found, but when compared among nonobese women, sleep duration in the second trimester only was associated with GDM after adjustment for multiple confounding factors (prepregnancy BMI, family history, age, ethnicity, gestational age, parity, and marital status).[53] Finally, a study by Facco and colleagues (2017)[54] objectively assessed sleep parameters and found exposure to less than 7 hours of sleep per night during pregnancy was associated with an increased odds of GDM compared with longer sleep, adjusting for other confounding factors (like BMI) with a 2-fold increased risk.

Overall, the literature suggests a clear association between sleep deficiency and GDM. However,

Table 3
Sleep deficiency and depression, antepartum, and postpartum

Study	Study Type	Study Population	Evaluation	Conclusions
Field et al (2007)	Prospective cohort	83 depressed; 170 depressed (divided by formal interview) in second and third trimester	Self-reported scales: CES-D, STAI, STAXI, VITAS, and sleep scale[a]; Urine assays—cortisol and norepinephrine	Depressed women had high depression ($P < .05$), anxiety ($P < .01$), and sleep disturbance scores ($P < .01$) in both trimesters
Wilkie, et al (1992)	Prospective cohort	63 women in third trimester and postnatal period	Self-reported scale: Stein questionnaire; Kendell score	90% reported worse sleep at end of third trimester Poorer sleep quality recorded the increasing emotional distress recorded
Skouteris, et al (2008)	Prospective cohort	273 women followed at 15–23 wk with q8week intervals for 3 follow-ups	Self-reported scale: PSQI[b] and Beck depression inventory	Sleep quality in early pregnancy predicted levels of depressive symptoms later in pregnancy
Iranpour, et al (2016)	Cross-sectional	360 pregnant women	Self-reported scale: PSQI and EPDS[c]	Women with poor sleep quality were more likely to have higher depression score
Jomeen and Martin, 2007	Cross-sectional	148 pregnant women	Self-reported scale: PSQI and EPDS[c]	Women with higher depression scores had shorter sleep duration ($P = .002$)
Okun, et al (2013)	Prospective cohort	160 pregnant at 10–12, 14–16, and 18–20 wk gestation	Self-reported sleep diary Actigraphy	Women who were sleep deficiency across all time points perceived higher stress ($P < .01$) and depressive levels ($P = .02$)

[a] CES-D = Clinical Epidemiologic Studies Depression Scale; STAI = State/trait anxiety index; STAXI = State/trait anger inventory; VITAS = VITAS healthcare corporation.
[b] PSQI = Pittsburgh sleep questionnaire index.
[c] EPDS = Edinburgh postnatal depression scale.

Table 4
Sleep deficiency and preterm birth

Study	Study Type	N (Preterm/Full Term)	Comparison Made	Relative Risk (95% CI)	Adjusted Odds Ratio (95% CI)
Michell, et al 2011	Prospective cohort	131/960	<5 h vs	1.7 (1.1–2.8)[a]	
			6–7 h vs	0.9 (0.6–1.4)	
			>8 h	1.0	
Kajeepeta, 2014	Case-control	479/480	<6 h vs		**1.53 (1.08–2.17)**[b]
			7–8 h vs		1 (referent)
			>9 h		1.5 (1.04–2.16)
Okun, et al (2012)	Prospective cohort	26/186	<7 h vs		0.86 (0.29–0.2.59)
			>9 h		1.19 (0.38–3.75)

Bold indicates ratio was significant, at $P < .05$.
[a] Adjusted for maternal age, education, prepregnancy BMI, and smoking status.
[b] Adjusted for maternal age, prepregnancy weight, unplanned pregnancy, no vitamin use and sleep duration, as well as vital exhaustion.

it is unclear whether that association is limited to populations that would otherwise be at low risk for GDM. Future work should establish if there is causation and the implementation of protective factors to reduce the risk of GDM.

Sleep Deficiency and Risk for Hypertensive Disorders

Hypertensive disorders in pregnancy include chronic hypertension, gestational hypertension, and preeclampsia. Chronic hypertension and gestational hypertension, as well as preeclampsia, are disorders defined based on elevated blood pressure values and laboratory abnormalities[55] (see **Table 2**). These disorders have been previously associated with adverse maternal outcomes,[56] including myocardial infarct, acute respiratory distress, renal failure, coagulopathy, and adverse fetal outcomes,[57] including oligohydramnios, intrauterine growth restriction, and preterm delivery. One earlier study by Edwards and colleagues (2000)[58] found women with these disorders may have underlying altered sleep patterns. The authors studied sleep architecture using a polysomnogram in 25 preeclamptic patients and compared them to 17 primigravida women to find that preeclamptic patients had an increased percentage of time spent in slow-wave sleep ($P < .001$), as well as a decrease in rapid eye movement; however, these patients were simultaneously on clonidine—an antihypertensive medication known to alter sleep architecture.

Very few studies have examined the association between sleep quantity or quality and hypertension. Williams and colleagues (2010)[59] completed a prospective cohort study of 1272 healthy pregnant women. Medical records were extracted to find blood pressure values and sleep deficiency assessed using self-reported sleep duration. Women with short sleep (defined as less than 5 hours) had an increased likelihood of pregnancy-induced hypertension and development of preeclampsia (OR 9.52, 95% CI 1.82–49.4). In a case series of 9 women with preeclampsia and 8 women with normal term pregnancy, sleep quality was evaluated using recorded nocturnal body movement activity with a static charge-sensitive bed and found women with preeclampsia had a significantly increased total frequency of body movements.[60] However, both groups self-reported similar subjective sleep complaints, and this study did not define sleep duration as a complaint. Furthermore, although essential demographic characteristics were collected in these studies, no further analysis was performed to risk stratify women (**Table 5**).

Sleep Deficiency and Risk of Preterm Birth

Preterm birth is defined as birth between 20 weeks 0 days and 36 weeks 6 days gestation and is a leading cause of perinatal morbidity and mortality in the United States (see **Table 2**).[61] It affects approximately 10% of all pregnancies[62] and accounts for up to 50% of long-term disability (neurodevelopmental or physical) among children.[63] Analysis of health-care costs shows these disabilities cost billions annually within the first 6 months alone.[64]

The pathophysiological link between sleep deficiency and preterm birth has been a topic of interest for researchers worldwide. It has been long thought inflammatory cytokines play a role in the initiation of labor. Okun and colleagues (2007)[65] subsequently studied 19 women in late pregnancy (defined at 36 weeks gestation) and found that those who self-reported poorer sleep quality as measured by the PSQI had higher serum interleukin 6, a known proinflammatory cytokine.

In a study by Micheli and colleagues (2011),[66] sleep patterns of Greek women were analyzed. It was found that women who self-reported less than 5 hours of sleep nightly during the third trimester were at high risk for preterm birth (relative risk 1.7, CI 1.1–2.8) even after controlling for maternal age, education, smoking exposure, and prepregnancy BMI. However, when the types of preterm birth were evaluated, medically indicated preterm birth, defined as maternal or fetal complications necessitating earlier delivery (RR 2.4, CI 1.0–6.4), was associated with sleep deprivation but not spontaneous preterm birth (RR 1.6, CI 0.8–2.9). This association was supported by a case-control study of 479 Peruvian women who had a preterm birth compared with 480 women with a full-term delivery at the same hospital.[67] In this study, it was found that short sleep duration (defined as $\leq$6 hours) when compared with women who slept 7 to 8 hours was significantly associated with preterm birth. This association persisted after accounting for potential confounders such as maternal age, weight, use of vitamins, and planned pregnancy status (adjusted odds ratio [aOR] = 1.56; 95% CI 1.11–2.19). In 2021, Okun, Obetz, and Feliciano[68] used sleep diaries, as well as actigraphy (an objective measure), to assess sleep for three 2-week periods in early gestation (between 10 and 20 weeks) in addition to laboratory testing for fasting levels of interleukin 6 (ILK-6), interferon gamma (IFN y), and tumor necrosis factor alpha (TNF-α). During weeks 10, 14, and 18, it was found that ILK-6, IFN y, and TNF-α did not vary significantly (IL-6: 0.27 vs 0.25 vs 0.37; $F_{2170} = 1.85$; IFN y: 1. 6 vs 1. 66 vs 1.66, $F_{2168} = 0.17$; IFN-y: 6.98 vs 10.22 vs 5.37, $F_{2164} = 0.75$) and were not predictive of neonatal birth weight or gestational age. However,

Table 5
Sleep deficiency and hypertensive disorders

Study	Study Type	Population	Evaluation Methods	Conclusions
Ekholm, et al (1992)	Cross-sectional	9 preeclamptic, 8 nonpreeclamptic	Nocturnal body movement activity	Preeclamptic women had increased body movement frequency
Edwards, et al (2000)	Cross-sectional	25 preeclamptic, 17 nonpreeclamptic	Polysomnogram	Preeclamptic patients with increased time spent in slow-wave sleep, and less rapid eye movement sleep
Williams, et al (2010)	Prospective cohort	1272 pregnant followed through pregnancy	Self-reported sleep duration Chart extraction	Sleep duration <5 h associated with increased likelihood of pregnancy-induced hypertension and preeclampsia development

analysis showed diary assessed total sleep time and actigraphy assessed sleep latency were negatively associated with gestational age ($\beta = -0.21$, $t = -2.11$, $P < .05$) and $\beta = -0.26$, $t = -1.95$, $P = .05$, respectively).

Conversely, Okun et.al (2012)[69] found no significant difference in preterm birth among a cohort of 217 women who self-reported less than 7 hours of sleep in unadjusted and adjusted models ($P = 0.77$ and $P = .88$, respectively). Preterm birth was found among women that reported an increased amount of time in bed; however, when adjusted for the presence of major depressive disorder, selective serotonin receptor use, employment, age, and history of preterm birth, this no longer was significant ($P = .15$). This study was limited by its small sample size. It was not powered to answer the question regarding whether sleep deficiency is an independent risk factor in addition to knowing the used self-reported sleep analysis is subject to recall bias (see **Table 4**). More sleep studies gathering objective clinical data are required to further address and delineate the relationship between sleep deficiency and preterm birth.

Sleep Deficiency and Labor Outcomes

Not only does sleep deficiency affect maternal health and pregnancy outcomes, but limited data also indicates a link to a patient's perception and experience during labor and delivery. Studies have shown a link between sleep deficiency and a patient's labor course and duration of labor. In a cohort of 131 healthy primiparous women, 48-hour actigraphy and subjective sleep questionnaires were used to assess the association among fatigue, sleep disturbance, and duration, as well as the mode of delivery.[70] Women were categorized into 3 categories: average of 6 hours or less per night (<6 hours), average of 6 to 6.9 hours per night (6–6.9 hours), or greater than average of 7 hours per night (7+ hours). It was found women who reported an average of 6 hours of sleep or less during the last month of pregnancy had a statistically longer duration of labor (<6 hours: average 29 hours vs 6–6.9 hours: average 20 hours vs 7+ hours: average 17.7 hours, $P < .05$). These women also had a higher rate of cesarean birth (<6 hours: 37% vs 7+ hours:11%, $P < .05$). Similarly, in a study of 88 women who completed the PSQI three times per week during their last 3 weeks of prenatal care as well as at the initial postpartum visit, it was found that women who described poor sleep quality defined by higher PSQI scores were found to have shorter sleep duration (average 6.45 ± 2.07 hours) and were 20% more likely to have a cesarean section and longer duration of labor.[71] A study by Beebe and Lee (2007)[72] assessed a woman's sleep patterns in the 5 days before labor and noted in 35 nulliparous women that those with worst reported sleep, especially the evening before hospitalization, had increased perception of pain with spontaneous labor onset. These women were enrolled at greater than 38 weeks gestation (to avoid preterm delivery in the sample) and recruited in childbirth classes. Sleep was recorded via wrist actigraphy monitors. The total amount of sleep decreased in the last 5 nights of pregnancy progressively from on average 452 minutes ± 58 (approximately 7.5 hours) to an average of 274 minutes ± 145 (approximately 4.5 hours); this change was significant between 2 nights before delivery and the night of delivery ($t = -4.94$, $P < .001$). The women's scores on fatigue in early labor had a moderate correlation with a woman's total sleep time the night before birth (r's = −0.39), yet not statistically significant given the small sample size. Although these studies suggest an association, they do not establish causation of whether the sleep duration was the cause of longer labor or if other emotional and physical stressors (not examined) are the cause of these perceptions.

SUMMARY

In conclusion, sleep deficiency is a common problem faced among our population, especially among pregnant women. Sleep deprivation during pregnancy may be due to multiple physiologic, emotional, and physical factors. The existing literature supports an association between sleep deficiency and an increased risk for pregnancy-related complications, including GDM and hypertensive disorders in pregnancy. Moreover, a woman's mental health may be placed at risk secondary to peripartum depression. However, major gaps in knowledge remain. Future clinical research should focus on establishing causation as well as exploring effective interventions to mitigate and reduce the occurrence of adverse maternal and neonatal outcomes with sleep deficiency.

CLINICS CARE POINTS

- Sleep Deficiency affects up to one third of women throughout their life, and pregnancy related changes may lead to onset of sleep deficiency.
- Women should be screened and evaluated early in pregnancy for predisposing risk factors, such as low socioeconomic status, and provided resources when possible.

- Causation of pregnancy related complications (gestational diabetes, depression, hypertensive disorders) in patients with sleep deficiency has not been evaluated in research.

DISCLOSURE

The authors have no conflicting interests to report.

REFERENCES

1. Nation Sleep Foundation. National sleep foundation recommends new sleep times. National Sleep Foundation; 2019. Available at: https://www.sleepfoundation.org/press-release/national-sleep-foundation-recommends-new-sleep-times. Accessed February 1, 2021.
2. Center for Disease Control and Prevention. Cdc - data and statistics - sleep and sleep disorders. Sleep 2017;1. Available at: https://www.cdc.gov/sleep/data_statistics.html. Accessed February 1, 2021.
3. Rod NH, Vahtera J, Westerlund H, et al. Sleep disturbances and cause-specific mortality. results from the GAZEL cohort study. Am J Epidemiol 2011; 173(3):300–9.
4. Choi JW, Song JS, Lee YJ, et al. Increased mortality in relation to insomnia and obstructive sleep apnea in Korean patients studied with nocturnal polysomnography. J Clin Sleep Med 2017;13(1):49–56.
5. National Sleep Foundation. Sleep & effectiveness are linked, but few plan their sleep 2018. Available at: https://sleepfoundation.org/sites/default/files/Sleep in America 2018_prioritizing sleep.pdf. Accessed February 14, 2021.
6. Lindberg E, Janson C, Gislason T, et al. Sleep disturbances in a young adult population: can gender differences be explained by differences in psychological status? Sleep 1997;20(6):381–7.
7. Arber S, Bote M, Meadows R. Gender and socio-economic patterning of self-reported sleep problems in Britain. Soc Sci Med 2009;68(2):281–9.
8. Lee S, Chang AM, Buxton OM, et al. Various types of perceived job discrimination and sleep health among working women: findings from the sister study. Am J Epidemiol 2020;189(10):1143–53.
9. National sleep foundation. Summary of findings 2005. (March 2005). Retrieved from: https://www.sleepfoundation.org/wp-content/uploads/2018/10/2005_summary_of_findings.pdf.
10. Pengo MF, Won CH, Bourjeily G. Sleep in women across the life span. Chest 2018;154(1):196–206.
11. Reichner CA. Insomnia and sleep deficiency in pregnancy. Obstet Med 2015;8(4):168–71.
12. Mindell JA, Cook RA, Nikolovski J. Sleep patterns and sleep disturbances across pregnancy. Sleep Med 2015;16(4):483–8.
13. Hedman C, Pohjasvaara T, Tolonen U, et al. Effects of pregnancy on mothers' sleep. Sleep Med 2002; 3(1):37–42.
14. Kominiarek MA, Yeh C, Balmert LC, et al. Sleep duration during pregnancy using an activity tracking device. AJP Rep 2020;10(3):E309–14.
15. Reid KJ, Facco FL, Grobman WA, et al. Sleep during pregnancy: the nuMoM2b pregnancy and sleep duration and continuity study. Sleep 2017;40(5):zsx045.
16. Garbazza C, Hackethal S, Riccardi S, et al. Polysomnographic features of pregnancy: a systematic review. Sleep Med Rev 2020;50.
17. Santiago JR, Nolledo MS, Kinzler W, et al. Sleep and sleep disorders in pregnancy. Ann Intern Med 2001; 134(5):396–408.
18. McCarthy R, Jungheim ES, Fay JC, et al. Riding the rhythm of melatonin through pregnancy to deliver on time. Front Endocrinol (Lausanne) 2019;10:616.
19. Kalmbach DA, Cheng P, Sangha R, et al. Insomnia, short sleep, and snoring in mid-to-late pregnancy: disparities related to poverty, race, and obesity. Nat Sci Sleep 2019;11:301–15.
20. Christian LM, Carroll JE, Porter K, et al. Sleep quality across pregnancy and postpartum: effects of parity and race. Sleep Heal 2019;5(4):327–34.
21. Feinstein L, McWhorter KL, Gaston SA, et al. Racial/ethnic disparities in sleep duration and sleep disturbances among pregnant and non-pregnant women in the United States. J Sleep Res 2020;29(5):e13000.
22. Okun ML, Tolge M, Hall M. Low socioeconomic status negatively affects sleep in pregnant women. J Obstet Gynecol Neonatal Nurs 2014;43(2):160–7.
23. Skouteris H, Germano C, Wertheim EH, et al. Sleep quality and depression during pregnancy: a prospective study. J Sleep Res 2008;17(2):217–20.
24. Bei B, Milgrom J, Ericksen J, et al. Subjective perception of sleep, but not its objective quality, is associated with immediate postpartum mood disturbances in healthy women. Sleep 2010;33(4):531–8.
25. Dørheim SK, Bjorvatn B, Eberhard-Gran M. Can insomnia in pregnancy predict postpartum depression? A longitudinal, population-based study. PLoS One 2014;9(4):e94674.
26. Kettunen P, Koistinen E, Hintikka J. Is postpartum depression a homogenous disorder: time of onset, severity, symptoms and hopelessness in relation to the course of depression. BMC Pregnancy Childbirth 2014;14(1):402.
27. Gale S, Harlow BL. Postpartum mood disorders: a review of clinical and epidemiological factors. J Psychosom Obstet Gynecol 2003;24(4):257–66.
28. Yonkers K, Wisner KL, Stewart DE, et al. Management of depression during pregnancy. Obstet Gynecol 2014;114(3). https://doi.org/10.1002/pnp.113.

29. Langan RC, Goodbred AJ. Identification and management of peripartum depression. Vol 93. 2016. Available at: http://www.wpspublish.com/. Accessed May 18, 2021.
30. Bonari L, Pinto N, Ahn E, Einarson A, Steiner M, Koren G. Perinatal risks of untreated depression during pregnancy. Canadian journal of psychiatry 2004; 49(11):726–35.
31. Szegda K, Markenson G, Bertone-Johnson ER, et al. Depression during pregnancy: a risk factor for adverse neonatal outcomes? A critical review of the literature. J Matern Fetal Neonatal Med 2014; 27(9):960–7.
32. Field T, Diego M, Hernandez-Reif M, et al. Sleep disturbances in depressed pregnant women and their newborns. Infant Behav Dev 2007;30(1):127–33.
33. Wilkie G, Shapiro CM. Sleep deprivation and the postnatal blues. J Psychosom Res 1992;36(4): 309–16.
34. Iranpour S, Kheirabadi GR, Esmaillzadeh A, et al. Association between sleep quality and postpartum depression. J Res Med Sci 2016;21(8):110.
35. Jomeen J, Martin C. Assessment and relationship of sleep quality to depression in early pregnancy. J Reprod Infant Psychol 2007;25(1):87–99.
36. Okun ML, Kline CE, Roberts JM, et al. Prevalence of sleep deficiency in early gestation and its associations with stress and depressive symptoms. J Women's Health (Larchmt) 2013;22(12):1028–37.
37. Lusskin SI, Pundiak TM, Habib SM. Perinatal depression: hiding in plain sight. Can J Psychiatry 2007;52(8):479–88.
38. Beck CT. Predictors of postpartum depression: an update. Nurs Res 2001;50(5):275–85.
39. Correa A, Bardenheier B, Elixhauser A, et al. Trends in prevalence of diabetes among delivery hospitalizations, United States, 1993–2009. Matern Child Health J 2015;19(3):635–42.
40. Coustan DR. Gestational diabetes mellitus. Clin Chem 2013;59(9):1310–21.
41. American Diabetes Association. American diabetes standards of medical care in diabetes. Diabetes Care 2016;39(Supplement 1):S1–106.
42. Plows JF, Stanley JL, Baker PN, et al. Molecular sciences the pathophysiology of gestational diabetes mellitus. doi:10.3390/ijms19113342.
43. Yogev Y, Xenakis EMJ, Langer O. The association between preeclampsia and the severity of gestational diabetes: the impact of glycemic control. Am J Obstet Gynecol 2004;191(5):1655–60.
44. England LJ, Dietz PM, Njoroge T, et al. Preventing type 2 diabetes: public health implications for women with a history of gestational diabetes mellitus. Am J Obstet Gynecol 2009;200(4):365.e1–8.
45. Rosenstein MG, Cheng YW, Snowden JM, et al. The risk of stillbirth and infant death stratified by gestational age in women with gestational diabetes. American journal of obstetrics and gynecology, 206. Mosby Inc.; 2012. p. 309.e1–7.
46. O'sullivan JB. Body weight and subsequent diabetes mellitus. JAMA 1982;248(8):949–52.
47. Facco FL, Grobman WA, Kramer J, et al. Self-reported short sleep duration and frequent snoring in pregnancy: impact on glucose metabolism. Am J Obstet Gynecol 2010;203(2):142.e1–5.
48. Qiu C, Enquobahrie D, Frederick IO, et al. Glucose intolerance and gestational diabetes risk in relation to sleep duration and snoring during pregnancy: a pilot study. BMC Womens Health 2010;10:17.
49. Zhou FM, Yang LQ, Zhao RP, et al. Effect of sleep in early pregnancy on gestational diabetes; a prospective study. J Sichuan Univ (Medical Sci Ed 2016;47(6):964–8. Available at: https://pubmed.ncbi.nlm.nih.gov/28598132/. Accessed January 20, 2021.
50. Wang H, Leng J, Li W, et al. Sleep duration and quality, and risk of gestational diabetes mellitus in pregnant Chinese women. Diabet Med 2017;34(1): 44–50.
51. Cai S, Tan S, Gluckman PD, et al. Sleep quality and nocturnal sleep duration in pregnancy and risk of gestational diabetes mellitus. Sleep 2017;40(2). https://doi.org/10.1093/sleep/zsw058.
52. Reutrakul S, Zaidi N, Wroblewski K, et al. Sleep disturbances and their relationship to glucose tolerance in pregnancy. Diabetes Care 2011;34(11): 2454–7.
53. Rawal S, Hinkle SN, Zhu Y, et al. A longitudinal study of sleep duration in pregnancy and subsequent risk of gestational diabetes: findings from a prospective, multiracial cohort. American journal of obstetrics and gynecology, 216. Mosby Inc.; 2017. p. 399. e1–8.
54. Facco FL, Grobman WA, Reid KJ, et al. Objectively measured short sleep duration and later sleep midpoint in pregnancy are associated with a higher risk of gestational diabetes. Am J Obstet Gynecol 2017;217(4):447.e1–13.
55. Roccella EJ. Report of the national high blood pressure education program working group on high blood pressure in pregnancy. Am J Obstet Gynecol 2000;183(1):s1–22.
56. Steegers EAP, Von Dadelszen P, Duvekot JJ, et al. Pre-eclampsia. In: The lancet, 376. Elsevier B.V.; 2010. p. 631–44.
57. Bokslag A, Van Weissenbruch M, Mol BW, et al. Preeclampsia; short and long-term consequences for mother and neonate. 2016. doi:10.1016/j.earlhumdev.2016.09.007.
58. Edwards N, Blyton DM, Kesby GJ, et al. Preeclampsia is associated with marked alterations in sleep architecture. Sleep 2000;23(5):619–25.
59. Williams MA, Miller RS, Qiu C, et al. Associations of early pregnancy sleep duration with trimester-

specific blood pressures and hypertensive disorders in pregnancy. Sleep 2010;33(10):1363–71.
60. Ekholm EMK, Polo O, Rauhala ER, et al. Sleep quality in preeclampsia. Am J Obstet Gynecol 1992; 167(5):1262–6.
61. Byrne B, Morrison JJ. Preterm birth. Clin Evid (Online) 2003;10:1700–15. Available at: https://www.who.int/news-room/fact-sheets/detail/preterm-birth. Accessed June 1, 2021.
62. Martin JA, Brady MPH, Hamilton E, et al. National vital statistics reports, Volume 66, Number 1, January 5, 2017. Vol 66. 2015. Available at: http://www.cdc.gov/nchs/data_access/Vitalstatsonline.htm. Accessed February 27, 2021.
63. Wood NS, Marlow N, Costeloe K, et al. Neurologic and developmental disability after extremely preterm birth. N Engl J Med 2000;343(6):378–84.
64. Beam AL, Fried I, Palmer N, et al. Estimates of healthcare spending for preterm and low-birthweight infants in a commercially insured population: 2008â€"2016. J Perinatol 2020;40:1091–9.
65. Okun ML, Hall M, Coussons-Read ME. Sleep disturbances increase interleukin-6 production during pregnancy: implications for pregnancy complications. Reprod Sci 2007;14(6):560–7.
66. Micheli K, Komninos I, Bagkeris E, et al. Sleep patterns in late pregnancy and risk of preterm birth and fetal growth restriction. Epidemiology 2011; 22(5):738–44.
67. Kajeepeta S, Sanchez SE, Gelaye B, et al. Sleep duration, vital exhaustion, and odds of spontaneous preterm birth: a case-control study. BMC Pregnancy Childbirth 2014;14(1):337.
68. Okun ML, Obetz V, Feliciano L. Sleep disturbance in early pregnancy, but not inflammatory cytokines, may increase risk for adverse pregnancy outcomes. Int J Behav Med 2021;28(1):48–63.
69. Okun ML, Luther JF, Wisniewski SR, et al. Disturbed sleep, a novel risk factor for preterm birth? J Women's Heal 2012;21(1):54–60.
70. Lee KA, Gay CL. Sleep in late pregnancy predicts length of labor and type of delivery. Am J Obstet Gynecol 2004;191(6):2041–6.
71. Naghi I, Keypour F, Ahari SB, et al. Sleep disturbance in late pregnancy and type and duration of labour. J Obstet Gynaecol 2011; 31(6):489–91.
72. Beebe KR, Lee KA. Sleep disturbance in late pregnancy and early labor. J Perinat Neonatal Nurs 2007;21(2):103–8.

UNITED STATES POSTAL SERVICE®

Statement of Ownership, Management, and Circulation (All Periodicals Publications Except Requester Publications)

1. Publication Title	2. Publication Number	3. Filing Date
SLEEP MEDICINE CLINICS	025 – 053	9/18/2023
4. Issue Frequency	5. Number of Issues Published Annually	6. Annual Subscription Price
MAR, JUN, SEP, DEC	4	$243.00

7. Complete Mailing Address of Known Office of Publication (*Not printer*) (*Street, city, county, state, and ZIP+4®*)
ELSEVIER INC.
230 Park Avenue, Suite 800
New York, NY 10169

Contact Person: Malathi Samayan
Telephone (*Include area code*): 91-44-4299-4507

8. Complete Mailing Address of Headquarters or General Business Office of Publisher (*Not printer*)
ELSEVIER INC.
230 Park Avenue, Suite 800
New York, NY 10169

9. Full Names and Complete Mailing Addresses of Publisher, Editor, and Managing Editor (*Do not leave blank*)

Publisher (*Name and complete mailing address*)
DOLORES MELONI, ELSEVIER INC.
1600 JOHN F KENNEDY BLVD. SUITE 1600
PHILADELPHIA, PA 19103-2899

Editor (*Name and complete mailing address*)
JOANNA COLLETT, ELSEVIER INC.
1600 JOHN F KENNEDY BLVD. SUITE 1600
PHILADELPHIA, PA 19103-2899

Managing Editor (*Name and complete mailing address*)
PATRICK MANLEY, ELSEVIER INC.
1600 JOHN F KENNEDY BLVD. SUITE 1600
PHILADELPHIA, PA 19103-2899

10. Owner (*Do not leave blank. If the publication is owned by a corporation, give the name and address of the corporation immediately followed by the names and addresses of all stockholders owning or holding 1 percent or more of the total amount of stock. If not owned by a corporation, give the names and addresses of the individual owners. If owned by a partnership or other unincorporated firm, give its name and address as well as those of each individual owner. If the publication is published by a nonprofit organization, give its name and address.*)

Full Name	Complete Mailing Address
WHOLLY OWNED SUBSIDIARY OF REED/ELSEVIER, US HOLDINGS	1600 JOHN F KENNEDY BLVD SUITE 1600 PHILADELPHIA, PA 19103-2899

11. Known Bondholders, Mortgagees, and Other Security Holders Owning or Holding 1 Percent or More of Total Amount of Bonds, Mortgages, or Other Securities. If none, check box → ☐ None

Full Name	Complete Mailing Address
N/A	

12. Tax Status (*For completion by nonprofit organizations authorized to mail at nonprofit rates*) (*Check one*)
The purpose, function, and nonprofit status of this organization and the exempt status for federal income tax purposes:
☒ Has Not Changed During Preceding 12 Months
☐ Has Changed During Preceding 12 Months (*Publisher must submit explanation of change with this statement*)

PS Form **3526**, July 2014 [*Page 1 of 4 (see instructions page 4)*] PSN: 7530-01-000-9931 **PRIVACY NOTICE:** See our privacy policy on *www.usps.com*.

13. Publication Title	14. Issue Date for Circulation Data Below
SLEEP MEDICINE CLINICS	JUNE 2023

15. Extent and Nature of Circulation		Average No. Copies Each Issue During Preceding 12 Months	No. Copies of Single Issue Published Nearest to Filing Date
a. Total Number of Copies (*Net press run*)		143	129
b. Paid Circulation (*By Mail and Outside the Mail*)	(1) Mailed Outside-County Paid Subscriptions Stated on PS Form 3541 (Include paid distribution above nominal rate, advertiser's proof copies, and exchange copies)	96	93
	(2) Mailed In-County Paid Subscriptions Stated on PS Form 3541 (*Include paid distribution above nominal rate, advertiser's proof copies, and exchange copies*)	0	0
	(3) Paid Distribution Outside the Mails Including Sales Through Dealers and Carriers, Street Vendors, Counter Sales, and Other Paid Distribution Outside USPS®	33	24
	(4) Paid Distribution by Other Classes of Mail Through the USPS (e.g., First-Class Mail®)	7	6
c. Total Paid Distribution [*Sum of 15b (1), (2), (3), and (4)*] ▶		136	123
d. Free or Nominal Rate Distribution (*By Mail and Outside the Mail*)	(1) Free or Nominal Rate Outside-County Copies included on PS Form 3541	6	5
	(2) Free or Nominal Rate In-County Copies Included on PS Form 3541	0	0
	(3) Free or Nominal Rate Copies Mailed at Other Classes Through the USPS (e.g., First-Class Mail)	0	0
	(4) Free or Nominal Rate Distribution Outside the Mail (*Carriers or other means*)	1	1
e. Total Free or Nominal Rate Distribution (*Sum of 15d (1), (2), (3) and (4)*)		7	6
f. Total Distribution (*Sum of 15c and 15e*) ▶		143	129
g. Copies not Distributed (*See Instructions to Publishers #4 (page #3)*) ▶		0	0
h. Total (*Sum of 15f and g*)		143	129
i. Percent Paid (*15c divided by 15f times 100*) ▶		95.1%	95.35%

* If you are claiming electronic copies, go to line 16 on page 3. If you are not claiming electronic copies, skip to line 17 on page 3.

PS Form **3526**, July 2014 (*Page 2 of 4*)

16. Electronic Copy Circulation	Average No. Copies Each Issue During Preceding 12 Months	No. Copies of Single Issue Published Nearest to Filing Date
a. Paid Electronic Copies ▶		
b. Total Paid Print Copies (Line 15c) + Paid Electronic Copies (Line 16a) ▶		
c. Total Print Distribution (Line 15f) + Paid Electronic Copies (Line 16a) ▶		
d. Percent Paid (Both Print & Electronic Copies) (16b divided by 16c × 100) ▶		

☒ **I certify that 50% of all my distributed copies (electronic and print) are paid above a nominal price.**

17. Publication of Statement of Ownership
☒ If the publication is a general publication, publication of this statement is required. Will be printed in the DECEMBER 2023 issue of this publication.
☐ Publication not required.

18. Signature and Title of Editor, Publisher, Business Manager, or Owner
Malathi Samayan - Distribution Controller — *Malathi Samayan* — Date: 9/18/2023

I certify that all information furnished on this form is true and complete. I understand that anyone who furnishes false or misleading information on this form or who omits material or information requested on the form may be subject to criminal sanctions (including fines and imprisonment) and/or civil sanctions (including civil penalties).

PS Form **3526**, July 2014 (*Page 3 of 4*) **PRIVACY NOTICE:** See our privacy policy on *www.usps.com*.

9780443182426